Workplace Wellness: From Resiliency to Suicide Prevention and Grief Management

Judy E. Davidson · Marcus Richardson
Editors

Workplace Wellness: From Resiliency to Suicide Prevention and Grief Management

A Practical Guide to Supporting Healthcare Professionals

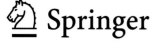 Springer

Editors
Judy E. Davidson
Division of Nursing
Department of Psychiatry
University of California, San Diego
La Jolla, CA, USA

Marcus Richardson
Division of Nursing
University of California, San Diego
La Jolla, CA, USA

ISBN 978-3-031-16982-3   ISBN 978-3-031-16983-0   (eBook)
https://doi.org/10.1007/978-3-031-16983-0

This Springer imprint is published by the registered company Springer Nature Switzerland AG
The registered company address is: Gewerbestrasse 11, 6330 Cham, Switzerland

Preface

The Wellness Continuum: From Resiliency to Managing Grief Following Suicide

Wellness initiatives cover a broad, even seemingly endless spectrum of concepts, with individual efforts at building resiliency at one end, to dealing with the worst-case scenario of death of a colleague at the other. We have crafted this text to provide strategies and practices to enhance wellness for healthcare professionals: physicians, nurses, pharmacists, therapists, chaplains, and others. Strategies to be adopted by healthcare leaders and wellness directors are offered with a wide variety of opportunities to build a holistic meaningful wellness practice at the individual, academic, and system level.

Though healthcare professionals desire information to inform their personal practice it would be remiss to focus only on individual wellness. Therefore, each chapter includes implications for academics, training the next generation of health professionals, and leaders who have fiduciary power to provide needed services and strategies at an institutional level. As a value-added service to readers, many chapters are accompanied by a short 3–5 min video that can be used to stimulate discussion at a team meeting, book club, or academic exercise. Discussion questions conclude each chapter to be used by professors or facilitators of book clubs.

The chapters have been intentionally organized to start with resiliency building practices such as mindfulness, cognitive-based therapy skill building, and developing effective empathic communication. The chapters progress to more controversial, complex, and challenging issues concerning helping staff heal after medical errors, coping with substance use disorders, and dealing with workplace violence and incivility. In early chapters, unique techniques to build resilience through physical and metaphysical activities have been explored, such as the use of improvisation exercises, diet, fitness, and animal and art therapy. Later chapters delve into heavier topics on wellness and explore techniques to develop skills to recognize and overcome challenges associated with working in healthcare. One topic focuses on tackling burnout among healthcare, which has become a national initiative [1]. However, focusing on burnout without assessing for comorbid depression could lead to suicide. Therefore, an entire chapter is devoted to the topic of the difference between burnout and depression and why it is important.

We now know that healthcare professionals are at a high risk of suicide [2–4]; for this reason, we have provided instruction on creating a personal life safety plan, how to identify colleagues at risk, and how to act when risk is apparent. Healthcare professionals have always been exposed to death in a way that warrants a structured approach to developing skills in grief management, and even more so since the COVID-19 pandemic. This is offered in two chapters; the first involves coping with grief due to patient death. These basic principles of grief management can also be applied to grieving the loss of "the way things were," a problem we have all faced as a result of the COVID-19 pandemic. Delving deeper, the final chapter addresses the need to prepare for and cope with the death of a patient or colleague due to suicide.

Given the range of topics covered, a wellness director or leader might wonder where to start. What should we address first? Which of these ideas should we offer? The answer is certainly that wellness offerings need to be balanced to meet the diverse needs of the workforce. Doctors, nurses, pharmacists, therapists, and chaplains work as teams. Therefore, integrating offered services (instead of offering separate services to physicians vs. others) is indicated to foster an understanding of each other and build stronger teams. One approach might be to align wellness assessments and services to Maslow's hierarchy of needs [5]. The five hierarchical layers of needs are physiologic, safety, love and belonging, esteem, and self-actualization (Fig. 1). When applied to healthcare professionals, physiologic needs may take the form of breaks, available water and nutrition, and scheduling. Safety

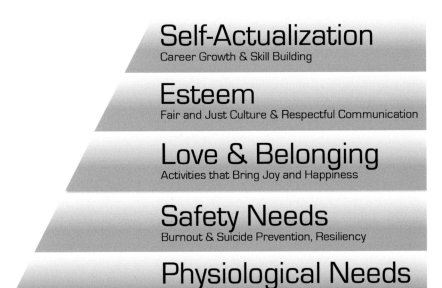

Fig. 1 Hierarchy of needs. Adapted from: Maslow, A.H., 1943. A theory of human motivation. Psychological review, 50(4), p. 370

needs include freedom from harassment, incivility, moral distress, violence, and prevention of injury. Love and belonging might include feeling cared for, feeling a sense of belonging, inclusion and engagement in activities that bring joy and happiness. Esteem is optimized through operating within a fair and just culture, respectful communication, and structured processes for input into decision-making. Self-actualization may be exhibited through opportunities for career growth and skill-building, creation of ideas that change practice, or creation of art that informs practice.

Though originally it was thought that it was important to establish attainment of needs in order from the lowest (physiologic) to the highest order (self-actualization), this premise has been challenged, and for good reason. Take for example, people in impoverished areas who find wellness benefits in engaging in the arts [6]. Tailoring activities to fit the physical and spiritual needs of the team is crucial to providing meaningful implementation. Every class, clinic, or department will have unique needs, and each individual within those discrete units will have individualized needs. For example, if the major workplace needs disclosed by the participants is incivility or workplace violence, focusing on that safety concern should not be ignored, and should receive priority. However, the sense of belonging generated through group activities can stimulate healing while dealing with the source of the core problem.

A basic needs assessment could be as simple as holding a focus group either virtually or in person and asking participants to disclose [anonymously] what they might find useful in creating a healthy work environment and wellness program. If the meeting is held in person this can be done through writing on post-it notes and attaching to a large pyramid depicting the pyramid drawn on a white board. Online interactive software is also available to achieve the same goal virtually (e.g., Mural). Gathering the input and stratifying according to the hierarchy of needs will provide a visual with which to prioritize efforts at the class, unit, or clinic level and then aggregate to identify organizational trends and needs.

Carrie Hudson, Medical Artist, created "As the flowers bloom" to conceptualize the work at hand with constructing wellness initiatives. The charcoal drawing depicted below symbolizes the contrast of emotions and experiences one can endure in a lifetime. Flowers have the ability to wilt or grow based on the environment they are in. The glass vase they are housed in can be seen as both supportive and strong yet vulnerable and fragile. In this textbook we hope to provide readers with evidence-based strategies to optimize the healthcare environment so that despite the fragility and complexity of the system, we can thrive throughout our careers together (Fig. 2).

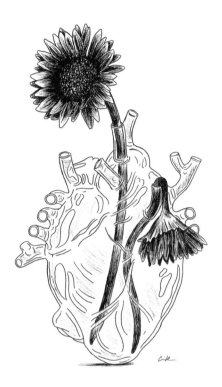

Fig. 2 "As the Flowers Bloom", Charcoal

References
1. Dzau VJ, Kirch DG, Nasca TJ. To care is human—collectively confronting the clinician-burnout crisis. N Engl J Med. 2018;378(4):312–314.
2. Davidson JE, Proudfoot J, Lee K, Terterian G, Zisook S. A longitudinal analysis of nurse suicide in the United States (2005–2016) with recommendations for action. Worldviews Evid Based Nurs. 2020;17(1):6–15.
3. Gordon YY, Davidson JE, Kim K, Zisook S. Physician death by suicide in the United States: 2012–2016. J Psychiatr Res. 2021;134:158–165.
4. Lee KC, Gordon YY, Choflet A, Barnes A, Zisook S, Ayers C, Davidson JE. Longitudinal analysis of suicides among pharmacists during 2003–2018. J Am Pharm Assoc (2003). 2022;62(4):1165–1171.
5. Maslow AH. A theory of human motivation. Psychol Rev. 1943;50(4):370.
6. Hale AJ, Ricotta DN, Freed J, Smith CC, Huang GC. Adapting Maslow's hierarchy of needs as a framework for resident wellness. Teach Learn Med. 2019;31(1):109–118.

La Jolla, CA   Judy E. Davidson
La Jolla, CA   Marcus Richardson
La Jolla, CA   Carrie Hudson Curcio

Contents

The Balance of Building Resilience

1

Isabel Gala Newton

Learning Objectives
1. Define resilience
2. Understand that balance is dynamic and requires daily intention setting
3. Describe three strategies for cultivating resilience

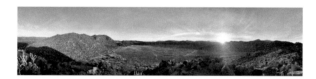

1.1 Presentation of the Science

Resilience refers to a kind of emotional flexibility that enables a person to bounce back after characteristically human difficulties, like loss, trauma, failure, hardship, or defeat [1]. A hallmark of resilience is the ability to turn these challenging

Focus: Maintaining resiliency is a constant effort with ebbs and flows, setting realistic intentions.

Supplementary Information The online version contains supplementary material available at https://doi.org/10.1007/978-3-031-16983-0_1.

I. G. Newton (✉)
Department of Radiology, University of California San Diego Healthcare System, San Diego, CA, USA

Department of Radiology, Division of Interventional Radiology, VA San Diego Healthcare System, San Diego, CA, USA
e-mail: inewton@health.ucsd.edu

experiences into opportunities for growth and evolution. Instead of retreating from adversity, resilient people tend to confront it in order to emerge as better versions of themselves. Although some people are more resilient than others, anyone can practice and strengthen it. Like any exercise, cultivating resilience requires a daily, mindful commitment that allows for shifting priorities and goals within the greater context of the human experience.

Resilience can be a constructive coping mechanism to deal with the daily barrage of human suffering, trauma, and loss inherent to the field of medicine. As it turns out, physicians tend to be more resilient than the general public, and this resilience confers some protection against burnout [2]. As discussed further in Chap. 24, burnout manifests as exhaustion, cynicism, and a sense of inefficiency that, together, can lead to emotional hardening [3]. This emotional varnish can provide insulation but also undermine the sort of compassion that enriches the therapeutic relationship and preclude the kind of camaraderie that can be so sustaining during challenging times. Most physicians, even the resilient ones, experience more symptoms of burnout, such as emotional exhaustion and depersonalization [2]. Trainees also experience burnout. The rate of burnout among medical students matches that of the general population at the beginning of training but increases with each passing year of training [4]. Nurses are also at high risk for burnout due to a lack of control, high volume, and low staffing [5]. Many of these issues reflect fundamental problems within hospital systems which must be addressed and for which resilience training is no substitute [6]. However, there is a growing recognition of the need to support resilience in trainees, nurses [7], and other healthcare providers. Just as resilience can partially mitigate burnout, burnout can deplete the emotional reserves necessary to fuel resilience. Part of the challenge of leveraging resilience in the face of increasing burnout is the unhealthy culture of healthcare.

Undermining the resilience of healthcare professionals is an inculcated expectation of the level of sacrifice required to care for others and succeed professionally. Apart from teaching the field of medicine, medical training also teaches self-abnegation at its most fundamental level. Medical and allied health students learn to ignore basic human needs such as hunger and fatigue. Self-care in the form of exercise, medical and dental check-ups, and time with loved ones is expressly or implicitly relegated to the realm of indulgences by leaders and peers alike. Residents pass down the advice to "Eat when you can, sleep when you can, and don't *mess* with the pancreas," an admittedly sanitized quip that reinforces the expectation of putting one's own needs last. Nonetheless, more robust self-care practices are associated with greater resilience and a lower risk of distress among trainees [8]. As promoted during the COVID-19 pandemic, well-meaning celebrations of healthcare workers as "heroes" create the expectation for superhuman contributions, sometimes without adequate compensation and almost always at the expense of one's own humanity. The natural learned reaction is the gradual loss of self and the ignoring of one's own needs. At the same time, trainees learn to regard as a sign of weakness any inclination to attend to these very human, universal requirements. This culture undermines a person's capacity for resilience and, instead, pushes individuals to snap (Fig. 1.1).

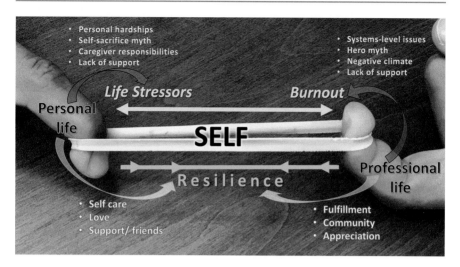

Fig. 1.1 Depiction of the clinician self as a frayed rubber band being pulled in two directions by personal life and professional life. Life stressors and burnout each stretch the self to the point of snapping. Resilience helps the self return to its original, relaxed state. Listed in each corner are contributing elements, both negative (*top*) and positive (*bottom*) to personal life (*left*) and professional life (*right*)

The fallacy of self-effacing self-sacrifice appears in Shel Silverstein's story *The Giving Tree* [9]. This widely loved story of selflessness is about a tree who loves a little boy and gives everything she has to him as he grows up—her apples, her leaves, her branches, her trunk—until all that is left is a stump for the little boy to sit on as an old man. After each sacrifice follows the mantra, "And the tree was happy." A five-year old once pointed out the stark reality of this story: "Why is he killing her?" she implored adamantly. Even in her childish self-centeredness, she did not buy into this warped story of terminal giving. Nonetheless, romanticized allegories of giving like this one drive healthcare workers to put all else first at all costs: patients, colleagues, trainees, research, institution. And while professional dedication certainly supports a robust healthcare system, it is not necessarily self-nihilistic. At the end of *The Giving Tree*, the stump repeats her feeble mantra as she serves as a place for the old man to sit. What about the other children who will never enjoy her leaves, apples, and branches? What about the birds and the squirrels? What about the tree, herself? Why does her story have to end there? *Does selfless giving really have to obliterate the self?* The answer is no.

Reinforcing these miscalibrated expectations are cultural norms surrounding caring for children and other family members, whose care needs tend to peak during medical training and practice. These cultural expectations normalize self-sacrifice at home, as in the workplace. This especially applies to women, who culturally bear a larger share of the responsibility as caregivers for the family. For these clinician/caregivers, home becomes the site of a second job rather than a place of respite and regeneration [10]. Very few workplaces offer accommodations to make the integration of family life and work more feasible and compatible, such as on-site childcare, sufficient parental leave, flexible hours, accommodations for nursing mothers, and fair and equitable part-time options. Unrealistic expectations and the lack of proper support and accommodations undermine talented healthcare professionals and make it difficult for them to thrive in these institutions. The workplaces that uphold these inhuman expectations shortchange themselves of the contributions of a talented and hard-working segment of their work force. Unfortunately, these institutions prove to be discouragingly difficult to change. Individuals often bear the burden of accommodating to or fixing a broken system rather than benefiting from improvements. This institutional intransigence further feeds feelings of burnout and hopelessness and leads to attrition. While resilience can certainly help, it is not the solution to pervasive problems for which systems-level changes are needed.

Romanticizing the medical profession creates an uncomfortable disconnect between an impossible ideal and the real experience. For example, where it may be possible to be a great clinician who teaches and engages in research while leading a fulfilling personal life, it is impossible to perform optimally in all these areas at the same time. Nonetheless, this expectation is not uncommon. A hallmark of resilience is the ability to assess and toggle among priorities and to adjust the level of effort and focus to what is required rather than ascribing to the delusion that everything must always be performed with the same high level of focus and achievement in order to be acceptable. One day may call for intense focus in the clinical arena, with resulting loss of performance in other areas of importance. The real challenge is to ensure that one priority does not get inadvertently sacrificed to another priority in the long run. Resilience affords the flexibility to negotiate a new balance when needed without disregarding values and long-standing priorities. What cannot be sacrificed is the daily exercise of self-reflection and the setting of intentions.

1.2   Application of Principles into Wellness Practice

Resilience is not a goal to be reached and then rested upon—it is a daily practice, one that is as dynamic as it is relative. This practice requires negotiating the various demands of life with one's own goals, priorities, and sources of joy. Balance does not mean that all important elements must be represented equally and constantly (Fig. 1.2). Not only do different elements have different weightings, but also these weightings can change in a lifetime, a year, a month, and even in a day. What it takes to be balanced on one day may be the opposite of what is required on another day (Fig. 1.3). An apparent imbalance may represent a new, temporary balance, if it is intentional and serves one's overall goals, such as meeting a deadline (Fig. 1.4). Balance is the conscious toggling among priorities in order to direct energy and resources where it most serves one's overall goals.

Healthcare professionals can employ strategies to help recognize, align, and balance priorities in order to foster greater resilience and fulfillment. To aid in remembering these seven strategies, they all include the letter P: Perception, Permission, Perspective, comPassion, emPowerment, Priorities, and People. Each is discussed in detail below.

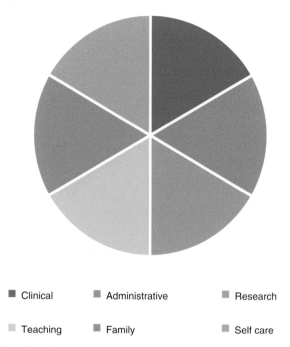

Fig. 1.2 Equal time allocation to one's priorities is unrealistic and unsustainable

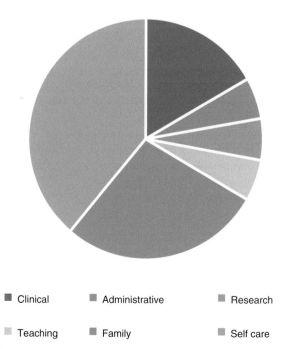

Fig. 1.3 Unequal allocation of time can adequately serve goals on one day (e.g., focus on personal goals) but represent a gross imbalance on another

Fig. 1.4 Gross imbalances
may be acceptable for
short periods if pursued
intentionally to meet
long-term goals (e.g., grant
deadline)

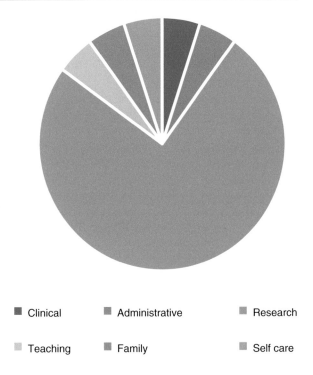

■ Clinical   ■ Administrative   ■ Research

■ Teaching   ■ Family   ■ Self care

- *Perception* refers to recognizing, acknowledging, and admitting what is really happening, especially when something is wrong. Often, the tendency is to discount or minimize one's perception of a challenging experience. Allowing uncomfortable situations to persist unchecked can lead to chronic stress. Honoring one's own perceptions helps to avoid the tendency to pretend everything is fine when it is not. Denial, putting forth a happy face, or projecting a tough façade can give the appearance of resilience, but it does not facilitate growth and can delay healing. Conversely, taking a moment to recognize and acknowledge when things are going well can fuel resilience and mitigate burnout.
- *Permission* refers to allowing oneself to feel one's true feelings during difficult times, whether they be grief, pain, anger, fear, disappointment, embarrassment, confusion, guilt, or loss of control. These feelings can be fraught with stigma or be confounded as signs of weakness when, in fact, they are signs of being human. Negotiating this permission is an exercise in balance to avoid falling prey to wallowing in negativity and becoming paralyzed by it. In resilience, some of these negative feelings can be reframed and redirected: Anger can drive purpose. Grief can add depth through layers of meaning. Embarrassment can inspire renewed focus.
- *Perspective* refers to recognizing one's own situation within its context and as it relates to the bigger picture. Perspective has the potential to remind one that

adversities are common to the human experience. The challenge of having perspective is to avoid belittling one's own grief or pain or comparing it to others' pain or experience. The risk of these tendencies is either to inflate the importance of one's situation or to discount its impact. Honesty, humility, and humor can help to recalibrate one's perspective.

- *ComPassion* in this context refers to a willingness to recognize one's own humanity—including one's capacity for flaws and mistakes—and to accept or even forgive these rather than regard them as signs of lack, of unworthiness, or of tarnish. Compassion is also the capacity to recognize the humanity in others, even in adversaries, and to let go off resentment and anger.
- *EmPowerment* is to actively take control of that which one can control and to be decisive in doing so. Indecision breeds further psychological stress. Informed decisiveness should include the recognition that making the best choice at one moment in time may not represent the same choice in a future moment. If that choice ends up being a mistake, regarding it as another learning opportunity rather than a source of regret is emblematic of resilience. Empowerment is also recognizing the stressors that one chooses to inflict on oneself and letting them go. Finally, empowerment is recognizing and accepting those things that one cannot control and letting them go, as well.
- *Priorities*: Each person gets to set their own priorities. These priorities will differ among people but also for the same person at different times. Setting priorities does not happen magically or naturally. Individuals must consciously decide how to spend their time. This requires taking a moment to choose and then own that choice. Inaction or indecision cannot be blamed on a lack of time or competing pressures. Aligning priorities during a challenging time requires stopping and consciously putting first those things that matter most. Sometimes it helps to have a touchstone to remind one of one's values. This can be a loved one, a pet, a special place, a poem, a religious passage, a piece of art, or an activity. Being able to return to one's touchstone can be a helpful way of honestly reassessing and reshuffling priorities during challenging times.
- *People*: Finally, the key to growing from a challenging or traumatic experience rather than snapping or collapsing under the weight of it is to lean on others. Loved ones, colleagues, mentors, neighbors, and friends can offer help. They can listen, offer acceptance, share their experiences, or just offer silent companionship. Love can fuel resilience. It is critical not to forget to offer the same to others, even when one's own plate feels too full to consider anyone else. Even as one is amid a difficult time, every surrounding person is experiencing their own wins and losses, big and small. Without diminishing one's own struggle, it can help to recognize the experiences of others. It can be immensely cathartic to offer support to a loved one and to be sympathetic. It shifts the focus away from oneself and offers context and perspective. There is strength that comes from sympathy and shared experiences.

Together, these strategies represent tools for cultivating resilience, aligning priorities, setting realistic expectations of oneself, and negotiating hardship.

1.3   Opportunities for Future Research

With the growing recognition of the prevalence of burnout and its toll on trainees and healthcare professionals, programs have begun efforts to address wellness and burnout and provide opportunities for resilience. Studies should assess whether the recent integration of wellness initiatives into residency programs is successful in creating a culture that is focused on professionalism, education, and performance rather than on nonsensical grit and inhuman self-abnegation. Similar research could assess wellness efforts led by national and international societies to determine whether these programs are effective or simply constitute lip service to these hot topics. Another area of future research could assess whether institutions are recognizing the moral, ethical, and financial arguments to mitigating burnout. These studies should also explore whether institutions that claim to champion wellness in fact promote more supportive work environments that offer flexibility, autonomy, and opportunities for healthcare professionals to perform at the top of their license. Finally, a rich opportunity for research is the short- and long-term impact of the COVID-19 pandemic on healthcare professionals. Both negative and positive effects could be anticipated, as the ability to work from home has afforded some healthcare workers greater flexibility while being a source of added stress for others.

In conclusion, mitigating burnout and developing resilience are not easy. It is about *balance*. Each day each person must face reality honestly. Each day each person must choose to reinvent, practice, and cultivate resilience. Honesty about trauma and its effects can breed awareness and creativity. Humor can offer context. Community, friends, and family can fuel empowerment and healing.

Glossary

Balance A dynamic state that requires self-reflection and intention to prioritize areas of focus based on changing needs, priorities, and values; what constitutes a balanced life on one day could represent gross imbalance on another day.

Burnout A syndrome arising from prolonged work-related stress and characterized by cynicism or detachment, physical and mental exhaustion, and feelings of decreased professional accomplishment. Institutions that do not recognize the systems that deplete the emotional reserves of their workers or make efforts to improve them contribute to burnout. Burnout leads to errors, low work performance, and attrition and can exacerbate depression.

Intention A conscious decision based on one's own priorities and goals. When a person sets an intention but does not follow through, they must examine what real or fabricated barriers are standing in the way and whether they wish to remove them. This iterative process can lead to the refinement of intentions and the elimination of wishful intentions that are not backed by true motivation.

Resilience A coping mechanism characterized by emotional flexibility that permits a person to approach a life challenge as an opportunity for growth and evolution.

Work-Life Balance A dynamic state where one's own goals and priorities of work life and those of their personal life both receive the same respect and primacy. These highly personal priorities co-exist without one eclipsing the other, though not always co-synchronously.

Discussion Scenarios and Questions

- One of your longtime patients is a middle-aged woman who received a new diagnosis of stage 4 colon cancer. She has two young children. You are particularly saddened by her plight and cannot stop thinking about it.
  - How would someone with a high capacity for resilience cope with this situation?
  - What can you do to cope with your responses?
- You have full clinical obligations that you struggle to balance with the demands of your three children. You regret having to miss picking them up from school in the afternoon. You also feel guilty for not being as involved administratively (in leadership roles) as your peers because you lack the time.
  - What would you do?
  - What advice would you give someone you care about?
- You arrive at work expecting to have a full case load, but there is a facilities problem with your work space, so your patients must be rescheduled to another day. You find yourself with an unexpected wide-open calendar for the day.
  - You have no obligations or deadlines. What do you do with your day?
  - You told a co-author you would have your revisions done on a manuscript by the end of the week, but you have not started. Does this change what you would do?
  - Your loved one has a soccer game today. Does this change what you would do?
- You have a busy clinical practice and pride yourself in being able to carry a large patient load efficiently. Recently, however, you have found it difficult to keep up because you are dealing with several personal issues, including a divorce and increasing obligations to care for your aging parents. You could really use some time off, but you feel an obligation to your patients and your mentees. You also worry about looking weak to your colleagues and the leadership.
  - What do you do?
  - What would a resilient person do?
- You are a caring, accomplished healthcare professional with a good reputation. You are taking care of a complicated patient in the hospital and miss an important diagnosis. As a result, your patient ends up in the ICU and goes on dialysis. You feel terrible sadness and guilt.
  - What do you do?
  - What would a resilient person do?
- You have dedicated the last 7 years to a research project, and its continuation depends on receiving a larger grant. Your last two grant applications have been

rejected, and you were anxiously waiting for a third. It just came back—rejected. You are worried about the future of your research and about paying the salaries of those in your lab.

- How do you think a resilient person would respond?
- How would you respond?

• For the past decade, you have been a respected member of key committees in your department. Recently, a new person was invited by leadership to join several of the committees you are on, and he has been harassing and bullying you. Finally, you report the behavior, but nothing happens. Instead, that person gets promoted. You are worried that if you complain more, you will be targeted even more.

- What do you do?
- What would be the best outcome?

Discussion Leader Guide

Video for Discussion - Instructional Video: The online version contains supplementary material available at https://doi.org/10.1007/978-3-031-16983-0_1

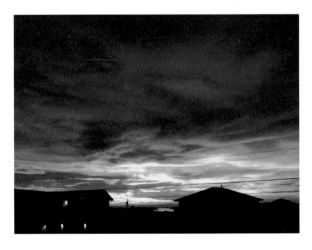

References

1. Sisto A, Vicinanza F, Campanozzi LL, Ricci G, Tartaglini D, Tambone V. Towards a transversal definition of psychological resilience: a literature review. Medicina (Kaunas). 2019;55(11):745. https://doi.org/10.3390/medicina55110745.
2. West CP, Dyrbye LN, Sinsky C, Trockel M, Tutty M, Nedelec L, Carlasare LE, Shanafelt TD. Resilience and burnout among physicians and the general US working population. JAMA Netw Open. 2020;3(7):e209385. https://doi.org/10.1001/jamanetworkopen.2020.9385.
3. Maslach C, Schaufeli WB, Leiter MP. Job burnout. Annu Rev Psychol. 2001;52:397–422. https://doi.org/10.1146/annurev.psych.52.1.397.
4. Dyrbye L, Shanafelt T. A narrative review on burnout experienced by medical students and residents. Med Educ. 2016;50(1):132–49. https://doi.org/10.1111/medu.12927.
5. Dall'Ora C, Ball J, Reinius M, Griffiths P. Burnout in nursing: a theoretical review. Hum Resour Health. 2020;18(1):41. https://doi.org/10.1186/s12960-020-00469-9.
6. Goroll AH. Addressing burnout-focus on systems, not resilience. JAMA Netw Open. 2020;3(7):e209514. https://doi.org/10.1001/jamanetworkopen.2020.9514.
7. Wei H, Roberts P, Strickler J, Corbett RW. Nurse leaders' strategies to foster nurse resilience. J Nurs Manag. 2019;27(4):681–7. https://doi.org/10.1111/jonm.12736. Epub 2019 Jan 21
8. Ayala EE, Winseman JS, Johnsen RD, Mason HRC. U.S. medical students who engage in self-care report less stress and higher quality of life. BMC Med Educ. 2018;18(1):189. https://doi.org/10.1186/s12909-018-1296-x.
9. Silverstein S. The giving tree. New York: Harper Collins; 2002.
10. Hamilton BN. Save lives, enjoy your own: finding your place in medicine. Fairfax: Stealth Intervention, Inc.; 2020.

Using Cognitive-Behavioral Therapy-Based Skills to Enhance Mental Health Resiliency and Outcomes in Clinicians

2

Bernadette Mazurek Melnyk, Jacqueline Hoying, and Andreanna Pavan Hsieh

Learning Objectives

By the end of this chapter, readers will be able:

- Formulate an evidence-based approach for enhancing mental health resiliency and outcomes in clinicians.
- Justify the importance of and evidence behind using cognitive-behavioral therapy-based skills for building mental resiliency in clinicians.
- Offer solutions for improving clinicians' mental health and well-being.
- Demonstrate a general understanding of CBT.
- Describe how MINDBODYSTRONG© is used in the academic, clinical, and leadership settings and the evidence behind the program.
- Outline the key content in MINDBODYSTRONG©.

Declaration of Interest: Dr. Melnyk is the creator of MINDSTRONG© and has a company, COPE2Thrive, LLC, that disseminates the original versions of this program for children, teens, and young adults, which are entitled COPE© (Creating Opportunities for Personal Empowerment). The remaining authors have no other conflicts to disclose.

B. M. Melnyk (✉)
University Chief Wellness Officer, The Ohio State University, Columbus, OH, USA
e-mail: melnyk.15@osu.edu

J. Hoying · A. P. Hsieh
College of Nursing, The Ohio State University, Columbus, OH, USA
e-mail: hoying.80@osu.edu; hsieh.336@osu.edu

2.1   Presentation of the Science

Even before the COVID-19 pandemic, rates of burnout, depression, anxiety, post-traumatic stress, and suicide were declared a public health epidemic by the National Academy of Medicine (NAM) [1]. Rates of burnout alone have ranged between 30 and 65% in clinicians with suicide rates higher than the general population [2, 3]. As a result, the NAM Action Collaborative on Clinician Well-being and Resilience was launched to provide evidence-based solutions to this alarming epidemic. Since the COVID-19 pandemic, mental health conditions among healthcare clinicians have skyrocketed even further along with declines in healthy lifestyle behaviors (e.g., increases in alcohol use, drops in physical activity and healthy eating, and adverse impacts on sleep) [4–7]. There is now a mental health pandemic inside of the COVID-19 pandemic. Healthcare system failures, including inadequate staffing and personal protective equipment shortages as well as having to be the primary support person to dying patients have contributed to clinician distress during the pandemic [8, 9]. Findings from research have indicated that poor mental and physical health of clinicians negatively impacts healthcare quality, safety, and patient outcomes as well as leads to high turnover rates and costs for hospitals and healthcare systems [6, 10–13].

Solutions to improve clinicians' mental health and well-being must be focused on fixing system problems (e.g., inadequate staff–patient ratios, lengthy shifts, problems with the electronic medical record) and equipping them with skills that build mental resiliency, which are known to be protective against both mental and physical health problems [14]. Evidence-based interventions also must be targeted along the continuum, from prevention to treatment and recovery [15]. Indeed, building and sustaining a wellness culture in healthcare systems is imperative because how clinicians perceive their worksite culture affects their emotions and lifestyle behaviors [16, 17].

Although *cognitive-behavioral therapy* (CBT) is the gold standard first-line treatment for mild to moderate depression and anxiety, few individuals receive it due to the shortage of mental health providers across the United States, lack of mental health screening in primary care, and persistence of mental health stigma [18–20]. CBT is based on the cognitive theory of depression and psychotherapy, which was developed by Aaron Beck [21], and behavioral theories developed by Skinner [22–24] and Lewinsohn [25]. Beck proposed a negative cognitive triad that is comprised of a negative view of oneself, one's environment, and the future. Cognitive theory focuses on becoming aware of or catching one's cognitive automatic distortions or unhelpful negative thoughts, checking them by asking whether the thoughts are helpful or true, and changing them into positive ones to feel emotionally better and engage in healthy behaviors (i.e., Catch, Check, and Change). This is often referred to as the *thinking, feeling, and behaving triangle* (Fig. 2.1). Negative or unhelpful patterns of thinking lead to anxiety, depression, and hopelessness.

Behavior theory contends that the lack of positive reinforcement from pleasurable activities and other people leads to negative thought patterns. Thus, engaging in activities that one enjoys even when the feeling to do so is not present is vital for feeling better later. It also emphasizes that individuals get depressed or anxious because they lack skills to achieve positive reinforcement from others or terminate negative reactions from them.

Fig. 2.1 The thinking, feeling, and behaving triangle [26]. From Melnyk, B.M. (n.d.) The Creating Opportunities for Personal Empowerment (COPE) Program

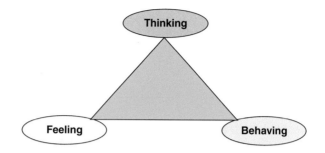

CBT consists of cognitive restructuring (i.e., understanding the connection between thoughts and feelings as well as behaviors, and reducing negative thoughts), increasing pleasurable activities when one does not feel like doing them, and enhancing assertiveness and problem-solving skills. Homework or skills building is an essential component of CBT so people can practice what they are learning to develop new habits.

A systematic review of 29 randomized controlled trials that tested interventions designed to improve mental health and healthy lifestyle behaviors in physicians and nurses found that mindfulness, CBT-based programs, gratitude practices, health coaching, and deep breathing were effective in reducing depression, anxiety, and stress and improving healthy lifestyle behaviors [27]. MINDSTRONG© is a targeted mindfulness integrated CBT-based intervention, also known as Creating Opportunities for Personal Empowerment (COPE)© in the literature, which has been shown to be effective in decreasing depression, suicidal ideation, stress/anxiety, and increasing healthy lifestyle behaviors and performance in 20 studies with culturally diverse children, adolescents, college-age youth/young adults, and Air Force cadets [27–44]. Created by Bernadette Melnyk over two decades ago, this CBT-based seven-session weekly program with skills-building activities is manualized in the form of a workbook so it can be delivered by non-psychiatric providers (e.g., primary care providers, teachers, nurses, social workers, health promotion professionals), thereby bringing evidence-based prevention and treatment to many who would not otherwise receive it. All key components of CBT are integrated into the COPE program and weekly skills-building activities. Versions of COPE© exist for young children 7–11 years of age, adolescents 12–18 years of age, and young adults 18–24 years of age. COPE© is being used in primary care settings with reimbursement; elementary, middle, and high schools; universities; community health settings; and private mental health/counseling practices [38]. A 4-h online training is available for individuals who desire to implement COPE©.

The COPE© program, also known as MINDSTRONG©, has been adapted for nurses and other healthcare clinicians and is entitled MINDBODYSTRONG©. A two-group randomized controlled trial was conducted to test the adapted program with 89 newly licensed registered nurses at a large, Midwestern academic medical center [27, 45]. Participants were racially and ethnically diverse. The group that received MINDBODYSTRONG© had better mental health outcomes (i.e., less depression and anxiety), more healthy lifestyle behaviors, and higher job satisfaction than the control group. Significant improvements were found for depressive symptoms and job satisfaction. There were moderate to large positive effects for the MINDBODYSTRONG© program on all outcomes and the program sustained its positive effects 6 months after the intervention ended.

MINDBODYSTRONG© is scaling to hospitals and health systems throughout the United States. It also has been piloted with nine Ohio Association of Community Health Centers (OACHC) primary care providers (including physicians, nurse practitioners, licensed social workers, and pharmacists) at one of their partner Federally Qualified Health Centers with promising findings [47]. Outcomes measured in this pilot study were current health, depressive symptoms, anxiety symptoms, burnout, perceived stress, and job satisfaction. At baseline, providers screened positive for mild depression, burnout, and stress. After participating in the MINDBODYSTRONG© program, clinicians no longer screened positive for depression, burnout, or stress.

Content of the seven MINDBODYSTRONG© program sessions is listed in Table 2.1. Each session is followed by skills-building sessions (i.e., homework) that help participants put the content that they are learning into practice, which is an essential component of CBT-based programs. Completion of the skills-building activities is critical as it typically takes 30–60 days to form a new habit. The program can be delivered by any health professional after a four-hour training.

Table 2.1 Content and skills in the seven-session MINDBODYSTRONG© program

Session	Key content	Put it into practice skills-building activities with weekly self-monitoring logs
1	• Thinking, feeling, and behaving • The ABCs of CBT • Mindfulness	• Positive self-talk/the ABCs
2	• Self-esteem and positive self-talk • Intentional gratitude • Managing change	• Self-esteem and positive self-talk
3	• Stress • Healthy coping • Abdominal breathing	• Managing stress
4	• Problem solving • Setting goals • Steps to problem solving	• Strategies to overcoming barriers
5	• Dealing with emotions in healthy ways • Using guided imagery • Coping strategies • Effective communication	• Dealing with emotions
6	• Coping with stressful situations/valuable sleep	• Coping with stressful situations
7	• Putting it all together for a health YOU!	

2.2   Application of Principles into Wellness Practice

2.2.1   Pre-licensure Application in the Academic Environment

MINDBODYSTRONG©/MINDSTRONG© has been used effectively with nursing and health sciences students as well as other undergraduate and graduate students across The Ohio State University (OSU) and other universities throughout the country. It has been integrated into a wellness onboarding program for OSU health sciences students for the last 7 years. Within 2 weeks of beginning their health sciences professional programs (e.g., medicine, nursing, pharmacy, veterinary medicine), students complete a personalized wellness assessment and are then paired with a nurse practitioner student who delivers the program. Studies have supported the positive outcomes of reduced depression, anxiety, and suicidal ideation as well as improvements in healthy lifestyle in students who receive this CBT program [45, 46, 48]. Peer delivery of the program also has resulted in similar positive outcomes. The program also is successfully offered as a one-credit course. The OSU Colleges of Nursing and Veterinary Medicine now require MINDSTRONG© in their entering students to enhance their mental resiliency and prevent mental health disorders.

2.2.2   Clinical Application Post-Licensure

MINDBODYSTRONG© is currently being delivered to clinicians in hospitals and healthcare systems across the United States. The seven-weekly session program, typically delivered in small groups, improves overall mental health and supports positive adaptation to stress, anxiety, and depression as well as enhances healthy lifestyle behaviors. Each session is 40 min and is led by a trained MINDBODYSTRONG© facilitator in a manualized format. All sessions provide in-between practice to establish and support healthier behavior patterns covered during the program. The MINDBODYSTRONG© program approaches well-being and mental health in two ways, providing preventive techniques and evidence-based strategies for those who have anxiety and depressive symptomatology.

2.2.3   Leadership Application (Structural and Organizational Considerations)

To date, the successful implementation of MINDBODYSTRONG© has occurred in over 48 healthcare institutions across 20 states. The logistics of the program delivery are reviewed in planning conferences with the MINDBODYSTRONG© team and interested organization. The organization identifies MINDBODYSTRONG© facilitators to attend a four-hour workshop that addresses the evidence behind the program as well as the fidelity and delivery of the program to achieve outcome efficacy. When identifying facilitators, consideration is given to program sustainability and facilitator engagement. In addition, program execution includes how to set up and select the cohorts, sequential program delivery of the seven-weekly sessions, make-up session administration, and delivery format. The healthcare institution determines program evaluation and outcome measurements in follow-up of program delivery.

2.3   Opportunities for Future Research

Plans exist to digitalize MINDBODYSTRONG© program in order to be able to scale the program more widely to reach a larger number of clinicians throughout the United States and globe. After digitalization, it will be necessary to conduct research to determine short- and long-term outcomes of the online program. Cognitive-behavioral therapy-based interventions have shown positive short-term outcomes; however, studies also have shown that non-completion of all online modules in digitalized programs tends to be challenging [49–51]. Therefore, research that tests self-administration of a digitalized program versus self-administration with a coach/ mentor who touches base with the participants at certain intervals along the course of the program is needed.

Since the current research to practice time gap is 15 years [52, 53], it is critical that we accelerate the pace at which evidence-based interventions are translated into real-world settings to improve outcomes. Clinicians deserve wellness cultures, system fixes, and evidence-based programs that are effective in improving their mental health and well-being. Only then will population health and well-being be improved and the quality and safety of healthcare be enhanced.

Glossary

Cognitive-Behavioral Therapy (CBT) The gold standard first-line treatment for mild to moderate depression and anxiety.

Cognitive Theory of Depression and Psychotherapy The basis of CBT. Focuses on becoming aware of or catching one's cognitive automatic distortions or unhelpful negative thoughts, checking them by asking whether the thoughts are helpful or true, and changing them into positive ones to feel emotionally better and engage in healthy behaviors (i.e., Catch, Check, and Change).

MINDSTRONG©/MINDBODYSTRONG© Targeted mindfulness integrated CBT-based interventions for youth/young adults (MINDSTRONG©) and healthcare clinicians (MINDBODYSTRONG©). These programs have been shown to be effective in decreasing depression, suicidal ideation, stress/anxiety, and increasing healthy lifestyle behaviors in the intended populations.

Thinking, Feeling, and Behaving Triangle The cycle of how one's thoughts affect one's feelings and subsequently one's actions. In turn, one's actions can affect one's thoughts and feelings.

Discussion Questions

1. Why is it important for hospitals and healthcare systems to promote and support clinician wellness and well-being?
2. What interventions have been shown to improve clinicians' mental and physical health?
3. What are the main concepts in cognitive-behavioral therapy?
4. What is the evidence behind MINDBODYSTRONG©?
5. In what settings can the MINDBODYSTRONG© program be used?

Discussion Guide

1. Findings from research have indicated that poor mental and physical health of clinicians negatively impacts healthcare quality, safety, and patient outcomes as well as leads to high turnover rates and costs for hospitals and healthcare systems.
2. Mindfulness, CBT-based programs, gratitude practices, health coaching, and deep breathing are effective in reducing clinician depression, anxiety, and stress and improving healthy lifestyle behaviors.
3. CBT emphasizes the thinking, feeling, and behaving triangle—that is, how one thinks directly affects how one behaves and feels.
4. MINDBODYSTRONG© decreases stress, and depressive and anxiety symptoms in clinicians as well as improves job satisfaction.
5. The program can be applied in academic, clinical, and leadership settings.

References

1. Dzau VJ, Kirch DG, Nasca TJ. To care is human—collectively confronting the clinician-burnout crisis. N Engl J Med. 2018;378(4):312–4. https://doi.org/10.1056/NEJMp1715127.
2. Davidson JE, Proudfoot J, Lee K, Terterian G, Zisook S. A longitudinal analysis of nurse suicide in the United States (2005–2016) with recommendations for action. Worldviews Evid-Based Nurs. 2020;17(1):6–15. https://doi.org/10.1111/wvn.12419.
3. Duarte D, El-Hagrassy MM, Couto T, Gurgel W, Fregni F, Correa H. Male and female physician suicidality: a systematic review and meta-analysis. JAMA Psychiat. 2020;77(6):587–97. https://doi.org/10.1001/jamapsychiatry.2020.0011.
4. Czeisler MÉ, Lane RI, Petrosky E, et al. Mental health, substance use, and suicidal ideation during the COVID-19 pandemic—United States, June 24–30, 2020. MMWR Morb Mortal Wkly Rep. 2020;69(32):1049–57. https://doi.org/10.15585/mmwr.mm6932a1.
5. Kirzinger A, Kearney A, Hamel L, Brodie M. KFF. The Washington Post frontline health care workers survey. KFF (Kaiser Family Foundation). April 6, 2020. https://www.kff.org/coronavirus-covid-19/poll-finding/kff-washington-post-health-care-workers/. Accessed 1 Dec 2021.
6. Melnyk BM, Hsieh AP, Tan A, et al. Associations among nurses' mental/physical health, lifestyle behaviors, shift length, and workplace wellness support during COVID-19: important implications for health care systems. Nurs Adm Q. 2022;46(1):5–18. https://doi.org/10.1097/NAQ.0000000000000499.

7. Pappa S, Ntella V, Giannakas T, Giannakoulis VG, Papoutsi E, Katsaounou P. Prevalence of depression, anxiety, and insomnia among healthcare workers during the COVID-19 pandemic: a systematic review and meta-analysis. Brain Behav Immun. 2020;88:901–7. https://doi.org/10.1016/j.bbi.2020.05.026.

8. Shechter A, Diaz F, Moise N, et al. Psychological distress, coping behaviors, and preferences for support among New York healthcare workers during the COVID-19 pandemic. Gen Hosp Psychiatry. 2020;66:1–8. https://doi.org/10.1016/j.genhosppsych.2020.06.007.

9. Shreffler J, Petrey J, Huecker M. The impact of COVID-19 on healthcare worker wellness: a scoping review. West J Emerg Med. 2020;21(5):1059–66. https://doi.org/10.5811/westjem.2020.7.48684.

10. Han S, Shanafelt TD, Sinsky CA, et al. Estimating the attributable cost of physician burnout in the United States. Ann Intern Med. 2019;170(11):784–90. https://doi.org/10.7326/M18-1422.

11. Melnyk BM, Orsolini L, Tan A, et al. A national study links nurses' physical and mental health to medical errors and perceived worksite wellness. J Occup Environ Med. 2018;60(2):126–31. https://doi.org/10.1097/JOM.0000000000001198.

12. Melnyk BM, Tan A, Hsieh AP, et al. Critical care nurses' physical and mental health, worksite wellness support, and medical errors. Am J Crit Care. 2021;30(3):176–84. https://doi.org/10.4037/ajcc2021301.

13. Shanafelt T, Goh J, Sinsky C. The business case for investing in physician well-being. JAMA Int Med. 2017;177(12):1826–32. https://doi.org/10.1001/jamainternmed.2017.4340.

14. National Academies of Sciences, Engineering, and Medicine. Taking action against clinician burnout: a systems approach to professional well-being. The National Academies Press (US); 2019. https://doi.org/10.17226/25521

15. The Ohio State University College of Nursing, Helene Fuld Health Trust National Institute for Evidence-Base Practice in Nursing and Healthcare, and Health Policy Institute of Ohio. A call to action: Improving clinician wellbeing and patient care and safety. 2020. https://www.healthpolicyohio.org/a-call-to-action/. Accessed 1 Dec 2021.

16. Melnyk BM, Amaya M, Szalacha LA, Hoying J. Relationships among perceived wellness culture, healthy lifestyle beliefs, and healthy behaviors in university faculty and staff: implications for practice and future research. West J Nurs Res. 2016;38(3):308–24. https://doi.org/10.1177/0193945915615238.

17. Melnyk BM, Szalacha LA, Amaya M. Psychometric properties of the perceived wellness culture and environment support scale. Am J Health Promot. 2018;32(4):1021–7. https://doi.org/10.1177/0890117117737676.

18. Bhattacharjee S, Goldstone L, Vadiei N, Lee JK, Burke WJ. Depression screening patterns, predictors, and trends among adults without a depression diagnosis in ambulatory settings in the United States. Psychiatr Serv. 2018;69(10):1098–100. https://doi.org/10.1176/appi.ps.201700439.

19. Chekroud AM, Foster D, Zheutlin AB, et al. Predicting barriers to treatment for depression in a U.S. national sample: a cross-sectional, proof-of-concept study. Psychiatr Serv. 2018;69(8):927–34. https://doi.org/10.1176/appi.ps.201800094.

20. Health Resources & Services Administration. Shortage areas [Data set]. U.S. Department of Health and Human Services. 2021. https://data.hrsa.gov/topics/health-workforce/shortage-areas. Accessed 1 Dec 2021.

21. Beck J. Cognitive therapy: basics and beyond. 3rd ed. New York: Guilford Press; 2021.

22. Skinner BF. Two types of conditioned reflex and a pseudo type. J Gen Psychol. 1935;12:66–77.

23. Skinner BF. Beyond freedom and dignity. Cambridge: B.F. Skinner Foundation; 1971.

24. Skinner BF. The origins of cognitive thought. Am Psychol. 1989;44:13–8.

25. Lewinsohn PM. A behavioral approach to depression. Essential papers on Depression 1974. p. 150–72.

26. Melnyk BM. The creating opportunities for personal empowerment (COPE) program. Columbus, Ohio: COPE2Thrive, LCC. https://www.cope2thrive.com/.

27. Melnyk BM, Hoying J, Tan A. Effects of the MINDSTRONG© CBT-based program on depression, anxiety and healthy lifestyle behaviors in graduate health sciences students. J Am Coll Health. 2020;70:1–9. https://doi.org/10.1080/07448481.2020.1782922.
28. Buffington BC, Melnyk BM, Morales S, Lords A, Zupan MR. Effects of an energy balance educational intervention and the COPE cognitive behavioral therapy intervention for Division I U.S. Air Force academy female athletes. J Am Assoc Nurse Pract. 2016;28(4):181–7. https://doi.org/10.1002/2327-6924.12359.
29. Hart Abney BG, Lusk P, Hovermale R, Melnyk BM. Decreasing depression and anxiety in college youth using the creating opportunities for personal empowerment program (COPE). J Am Psychiatr Nurses Assoc. 2019;25(2):89–98. https://doi.org/10.1177/1078390318779205.
30. Hoying J, Melnyk BM. COPE: a pilot study with urban-dwelling minority sixth grade youth to improve physical activity and mental health outcomes. J Sch Nurs. 2016;32(5):347–56. https://doi.org/10.1177/1059840516635713.
31. Hoying J, Melnyk BM, Arcoleo K. Effects of the COPE cognitive behavioral skills building TEEN program on the healthy lifestyle behaviors and mental health of Appalachian early adolescents. J Pediatr Health Care. 2016;30(1):65–72. https://doi.org/10.1016/j.pedhc.2015.02.005.
32. Kozlowski J, Lusk P, Melnyk BM. Pediatric nurse practitioner management of child anxiety in the rural primary care clinic with the evidence-based COPE. J Pediatr Health Care. 2015;29(3):274–82. https://doi.org/10.1016/j.pedhc.2015.01.009.
33. Lusk P, Hart Abney BG, Melnyk BM. A successful model for clinical training in child/adolescent cognitive behavior therapy for graduate psychiatric advanced practice nursing students. J Am Psychiatr Nurses Assoc. 2018;24(5):457–68. https://doi.org/10.1177/1078390317723989.
34. Lusk P, Melnyk BM. Decreasing depression and anxiety in college youth using the creating opportunities for personal empowerment program (COPE). J Am Psychiatr Nurses Assoc. 2018;25(2):89–98. https://doi.org/10.1177/1078390318779205.
35. Lusk P, Melnyk BM. COPE for depressed and anxious teens: a brief cognitive-behavioral skills building intervention to increase access to timely, evidence-based treatment. J Child Adolesc Psychiatr Nurs. 2013;26(1):23–31. https://doi.org/10.1111/jcap.12017.
36. Lusk P, Melnyk BM. COPE for the treatment of depressed adolescents. Lessons learned from implementing an evidence-based practice change. J Am Psychiatr Nurses Assoc. 2011;17(4):297–309. https://doi.org/10.1177/1078390311416117.
37. Lusk P, Melnyk BM. The brief cognitive-behavioral COPE intervention for depressed adolescents: outcomes and feasibility of delivery in 30-minute outpatient visits. J Am Psychiatr Nurses Assoc. 2011;17(3):226–36. https://doi.org/10.1177/1078390311404067.
38. Melnyk BM. Reducing healthcare costs for mental health hospitalizations with the evidence-based COPE program for child and adolescent depression and anxiety: a cost analysis. J Pediatr Health Care. 2020;34(2):117–21. https://doi.org/10.1016/j.pedhc.2019.08.002.
39. Melnyk BM, Amaya M, Szalacha LA, Hoying J, Taylor T, Bowersox K. Feasibility, acceptability and preliminary effects of the COPE on-line cognitive-behavioral skills building program on mental health outcomes and academic performance in freshmen college students: a randomized controlled pilot study. J Child Adolesc Psychiatr Nurs. 2015;28(3):147–54. https://doi.org/10.1111/jcap.12119.
40. Melnyk BM, Jacobson D, Kelly SA. Twelve-month effects of the COPE Healthy Lifestyles TEEN program on overweight and depression in high school adolescents. J Sch Health. 2015;85(12):861–70. https://doi.org/10.1111/josh.12342.
41. Melnyk BM, Jacobson D, Kelly S. Promoting healthy lifestyles in high school adolescents: a randomized controlled trial. Am J Prev Med. 2013;45(4):407–15. https://doi.org/10.1016/j.amepre.2013.05.013.
42. Melnyk BM, Kelly S, Jacobson D, Arcoleo K, Shaibi G. Improving physical activity, mental health outcomes and academic retention of college students with freshman 5 to thrive: COPE/healthy lifestyles. J Am Assoc Pract. 2013;26(6):314–22. https://doi.org/10.1002/2327-6924.12037.

43. Melnyk B, Kelly S, Jacobson D, et al. The COPE healthy lifestyles TEEN randomized controlled trial with culturally diverse high school adolescents: baseline characteristics and methods. Contemp Clin Trials. 2013;36(1):41–53. https://doi.org/10.1016/j.cct.2013.05.013.
44. Melnyk BM, Kelly S, Lusk P. Outcomes and feasibility of a manualized cognitive-behavioral skills building intervention: group COPE for depressed and anxious adolescents in school settings. J Child Adolesc Psychiatr Nurs. 2014;27(1):3–13. https://doi.org/10.1111/jcap.12058.
45. Sampson M, Melnyk BM, Hoying J. Intervention effects of the MINDBODYSTRONG cognitive behavioral skills building program on newly licensed registered nurses' mental health, healthy lifestyle behaviors, and job satisfaction. J Nurs Admin. 2019;49(10):487–95. https://doi.org/10.1097/NNA.0000000000000792.
46. Sampson M, Melnyk BM, Hoying J. The MINDBODYSTRONG intervention for new nurse residents: 6-month effects on mental health outcomes, healthy lifestyle behaviors, and job satisfaction. Worldviews Evid-Based Nurs. 2020;17(1):16–23. https://doi.org/10.1111/wvn.12411.
47. Ohio Association of Community Health Centers. [Provider resiliency training test data]. Unpublished raw data. 2020.
48. Melnyk BM, Hoying J, Hsieh AP, Buffington B, Terry A, Moore RM. Effects of a cognitive-behavioral skills building program on the mental health outcomes and healthy lifestyle behaviors of veterinary medicine students. J Am Vet Med Assoc. 2022;260(7):789–95. https://doi.org/10.2460/javma.21.03.0142.
49. Baumel A, Muench F, Edan S, Kane JM. Objective user engagement with mental health apps: systematic search and panel-based usage analysis. J Med Internet Res. 2019;21(9):e14567. https://doi.org/10.2196/14567.
50. Fleming T, Bavin L, Lucassen M, Stasiak K, Hopkins S, Merry S. Beyond the trial: systematic review of real-world uptake and engagement with digital self-help interventions for depression, low mood, or anxiety. J Med Internet Res. 2018;20(6):e199. https://doi.org/10.2196/jmir.9275.
51. Wasil AR, Gillespie S, Patel R, et al. Reassessing evidence-based content in popular smartphone apps for depression and anxiety: developing and applying user-adjusted analyses. J Consult Clin Psychol. 2020;88(11):983–93. https://doi.org/10.1037/ccp0000604.
52. Khan S, Chambers D, Neta G. Revisiting time to translation: implementation of evidence-based practices (EBPs) in cancer control. Cancer Causes Control. 2021;32(3):221–30. https://doi.org/10.1007/s10552-020-01376-z.
53. Melnyk BM. The current research to evidence-based practice time gap is now 15 instead of 17 years: urgent action is needed. Worldviews Evid-Based Nurs. 2021;18(6):318–9. https://doi.org/10.1111/wvn.12546.

Art as a Wellness Initiative

3

Bliss Masiarczyk

Abbreviations

CAT   Creative art therapy
HCP   Healthcare professional

Learning Objectives
1. Identify the importance of art as a wellness initiative for healthcare professionals.
2. Explain various options and opportunities to engage in art as a form of therapy and creative expression.
3. Describe the benefits of creative expression and art as a form of therapy for overall well-being and building resilience.

3.1   Presentation of the Science

Throughout this chapter, terms such as "art as a form of therapy," "art therapy," and "creative art therapy (CAT)" are used in reference to activities facilitated by a professional therapist, psychologist, or psychiatrist with specialized training. Creative art therapy (CAT) is a practice in self-expression, essentially the ability to release

Supplementary Information The online version contains supplementary material available at https://doi.org/10.1007/978-3-031-16983-0_3.

B. Masiarczyk (✉)
Manatee Memorial Hospital, Saint Petersburg, FL, USA

emotions and feelings without verbalization [1]. This process can help the individual understand that any trauma can be held, seen, and ideally healed within the therapeutic relationship.

Alternatively, "creative expression" is the individual practice in expression using art that is not facilitated by a professional art therapist. Creative expression has essentially nothing to do with one's artistic ability or the perceived quality of the outcome. The value of this exercise in self-care is found more in the process than in the product. Creative expression is simply the mental capacity to use your imagination and find joy through personal expression, allowing us the freedom to let go and see what happens. The use of art for healing has global application because the expressive arts intervention can be culturally tailored and implemented in a variety of settings [2].

The key point is that creative expression is something that anyone can do anywhere and anytime. We do not need to be an artist or have any particular skill set. Neither do we need a lot of time or energy to engage in creative expression. My ultimate goal is that each of you reading this will try several methods mentioned and try to find your outlet of choice to promote self-healing. Practicing creative expression as a form of self-care can have a multitude of benefits. Self-care was defined by the World Health Organization (WHO) first in 2009 as, "The ability of individuals, families and communities to promote health, prevent disease, maintain health, and cope with illness and disability with or without the support of a healthcare provider" [3]. We are all different in the ways in which we express emotions. There are a multitude of ways in which we can perform creative expression. Success is often found simply in the attempt itself and the push to continually make it part of our self-care routine. The goal is not to have a masterpiece or a finished product, as there are no defined limits on time or materials. Simply put, we know we have succeeded because we tried something new and became vulnerable while using art as an outlet for these feelings to be expressed.

There are a plethora of studies surrounding CAT facilitated by a trained professional [4]. Less is studied about independent creative expression. Research results demonstrate that independent, non-clinical engagement in arts, culture, and creative activities can increase mental health well-being of individuals who are experiencing mental health problems [3]. Some of the effects reported with creative expression were improved ability to cope, less negative feelings, increased quality of life, increased well-being, reduction in anxiety, better understanding of one's own body, reduced agitation, positive distractions, increased social interaction, reduced stress, increased self-confidence, increased sense of self-worth, lower levels of depression, increased sense of hope, and increased ability to connect with valuable parts of oneself [3].

Art activities such as workplace interventions have been found to promote well-being and psychological health, manage occupational stress and health risk at work, and strengthen organizational well-being [1]. Creative arts therapy can be helpful in reducing depression and trauma-related symptoms such as alexithymia, dissociation, anxiety, nightmares, and sleep problems [5].

A review of 27 recent studies on art activities found the majority of reported staff outcomes were positive, with arts activities in healthcare settings being perceived to have an impact on patients as well as staff health and well-being [6]. A review article summarizing the data on creative art therapy found that participants chose 50% art-based, 29% music-based, and 21% storytelling or narrative as their preferred form [2]. Improved outcomes were found in 13 of the 14 studies assessed with greatest improvements seen in burnout, stress, and emotional outcomes. Music and art-based interventions had greater impact on well-being than storytelling or narrative [2].

For many, creative expression helps us process events and feelings that are too difficult to put into words. According to a 2016 study published in the *Journal of the American Art Therapy Association*, less than an hour of creative activity can reduce your stress and have a positive effect on your mental health, regardless of artistic experience or talent [7]. Creative expression allows thoughts and feelings to be expressed visually rather than audibly. Creativity in various mediums of artistic expression can be used as a restorative self-care practice [3]. Art can be an extremely important tool to use, especially at a time when it can be difficult to discuss painful experiences and trauma with your colleagues when you know they are going through the same or similar situations. They may also be struggling and lacking empathy because they are suffering from burnout themselves. Many have also experienced increased difficulty discussing emotions with those who are not in health care as they are unable to relate or understand, with the pandemic creating an even greater divide. Those closest to me have admitted they feel at a loss of words because they cannot fathom enduring what we have and cannot even begin to comprehend the gravity of these events on our mental health. Yet we still continue to report to our shift and take care of those that need us. For some HCPs this inability to relate with loved ones leads further to the frustration of not being heard, understood, valued, or appreciated. Expressing yourself through art can overcome these barriers to processing emotions.

These feelings stem from many variables that differ based on our workplace environment and personal insights. A study among nurses found the risk factors for burnout were listed in prevalence of society, organization, interpersonal, community, and individual [4]. A study on the effectiveness of art therapy in the treatment of traumatized adults states that therapeutic art interventions provide the possibility to distance oneself from emotion and provide cognitive integration of emotion and stimulate meaning-making processes [2].

3.2   Testimony to the Benefits of Creative Expression

I have been participating in creative expression as a form of self-therapy for many years. I recognized in myself very early on that I was rapidly becoming burned out as an HCP. I had dreamed of becoming a pharmacist even years before I was accepted into school. After I had my first experience in an ICU, I knew where home was for me. I thought my resilience was great enough that I would not be affected by this burnout syndrome I heard discussed by others. It took some time to come to terms with the fact that I was indeed burned out within a year of professional practice. I knew the possibility existed that this could happen, but I felt I was too positive and optimistic to be affected. I was able to establish friendships and bonds with my coworkers, network outside of my institution and continued to achieve my professional goals. I had no idea how naive and arrogant I was to think I would not be affected by burnout. I remember thinking this is something I just need to push through, I did not feel I needed any interventions, assistance, or techniques—only to be strong. After all, healthcare professionals are deemed among the most resilient of career paths. I was still very good at my job and continued helping my patients, coworkers, and colleagues. However, I knew something within me had changed. I no longer felt the same drive, empathy, and passion as when I first started. I doubted my decision to choose this career path but after deep self-reflection, realized that I could not imagine myself doing anything else than what I was doing.

I have always loved working with my hands and painting or drawing throughout my early adulthood. Upon entering college and throughout the process of obtaining my doctorate and 2 years of residency, I felt I no longer had the time. When discussing with others, they also felt they did not have time for hobbies around their jobs, kids, or other social obligations. I was spiraling and searching for answers. Yoga and meditation were often suggested as many have found wondrous benefits and results, but I could not see this as something I personally would find joy in doing. I have tried yoga and meditation among many other experiences in my journey to find my personal outlet, but nothing felt quite as right as creative expression art to me. I initially practiced creative expression art a few times a month when I was really stressed out or felt like I had the time. Once the pandemic erupted, I knew I needed to commit myself to completing creative expression art on a much more frequent basis than I had ever imagined if I was going to survive this. At the height of the pandemic, I was indulging in art as a form of self-care nearly every day I worked. Examples of expressive arts intervention are defined as visual arts, storytelling, dance, music, imagery, chanting, poetry, drama, writing, drawing, movement imagery, photography, or any other creative process used for self-expression [8]. These have been shown to improve psychosocial functioning, spirituality, and meaning-making in numerous populations [2]. The more I engaged in creative expression, the more interested I became in its benefits.

Getting through each workday was difficult as I would be exhausted mentally, emotionally, and physically but felt I was able to hold myself together until I got home. I saw my fellow HCPs' behavior and attitude shift around me. The atmosphere of the unit was completely altered. Our unit was always full and busy with high acuity patients, but this was different. I have read many studies, blogs, and self-help books and have pondered how can I participate in a creative expression exercise at work in this tumultuous and hustling environment. What could I do to support my colleagues who are enduring tasks I could never imagine doing to get the help they need and deserve? A recent study of 39 healthy adults found that participant's cortisol levels significantly decreased after 45 min of art- making [2]. There is a positive correlation between the number of suffering patients seen daily and a reduced emotional well-being for the healthcare worker [5]. Every healthcare department will have their own challenges but during this pandemic working in the

ICU, there was a continual feeling of anxiety, fear, and sorrow in the air—the restraint of emotions being overwhelmed by alarms and calls for assistance, with different members of the team constantly being pulled into the isolation rooms. There is no time for anything outside of patient care it seems, so where do we go from here? Creative expression through art can be the answer.

3.3   Application of Principles into Wellness Practice

3.3.1   Individual Creative Expression at Home

The following list of ideas can be used for creative self-expression in the home:

- Journaling—helps you express what you are going through and dealing with on paper; by getting these emotions and feelings out, you can cleanse your mind
- Listening to or writing music
- Dancing or creative body movement expression
- Creative writing such as writing a play
- Taking photographs
- Needle work, sewing, knitting, or crocheting
- Sculpting with clay
- Painting such as watercolors, oils, finger-paints, acrylics, or even painting your nails
- Drawing with color or different instruments and mediums
- Woodworking
- Working with epoxy resin
- Digital art and graphic design
- Creating a collage
- Working with textiles

There is a wide selection of products and kits that can be purchased at a crafts store. They may also be purchased online by searching for "art therapy" or "DIY art kit." Coloring books for adults and paint by number kits are useful start-up tools. If you find it easier to order a kit than starting from a blank canvas, keep a sample of kits in the home to use after a particularly rough day when an outlet for stress is needed.

3.3.2   Pre-licensure Application in the Academic Environment

All the ideas presented in this chapter can be adapted to the academic environment. However, students may specifically explore techniques to practice creative expression of art during breaks while studying for exams and preparing for presentations [9]. Incorporate creative expression into your transition from the clinical rotation to home through music or poetry. Add creative expression as a transition between clinical time and homework. Use artwork in presentations. Use the assignment of a presentation as a vehicle for creative expression by focusing on use of color and design, use of role-playing, or adding music to set tone. Formulate a strategy to incorporate a habit of creative expression into daily life before becoming a healthcare professional. This life pattern can bolster your resilience throughout your career [10].

Academicians can encourage students to create art of any nature as a form of reflection given the events that have occurred during a clinical rotation. Use of art in presentations and assignments can be encouraged. Whenever poster presentations are used to culminate learning, art submissions can be encouraged to teach a concept [7].

3.3.3   Clinical Application Post-Licensure (at Work)

One of the main opportunities for creative expression on the job is to transform break times into times for creative expression. Limit yourself from engaging in stressful situations during your break time such as the news or the unit gossip/drama. Know that it is necessary and important to use your break time daily [11]. Creative expression in daily practice can promote the continued development of both empathy and innovation [3]. Art activities such as workplace interventions have been found to promote well-being and psychological health, manage occupational stress and health risk at work, and strengthen organizational well-being [12]. Therefore, by bringing in something that helps you in your efforts to help another coworker or college will strengthen the department.

Listed below are some ideas that could give you benefit in the short time you may be given during your workday.

1. Bring a sketch pad to work to doodle and draw during your break times.
2. Bring a journal to work to use during your break time or as a means of processing after a traumatic event.
3. Listen to music during your break time instead of watching television.
4. Explore music on your commute to and from work. Perhaps you find benefit in listening to something other than your typical type of music. You may find that house music, old country ballads, or classical or nature sounds is what gets you in the best frame of mind to tackle your day or unwind afterward.
5. Watch videos of baby animals, puppies and kitties, children laughing, your favorite sport, or hobby.
6. Watch videos of waves or flames to practice focused meditation while listening to calming music.
7. Bring in coloring books or sketch pads with necessary instruments and leave in the break room to encourage others to practice some self-care on their break in creative expressive art.

It has been shown that music can calm neural activity in the brain, which may lead to reductions in anxiety and help restore effective functioning in the immune system parity via the actions of the amygdala and hypothalamus [13]. In addition to using the break time for creative expression, song or live music led by staff can be infused into the clinical environment while working. The impact of live music in the environment can be beneficial to the person performing the music, the patients, and the balance of the staff in the work environment. During the pandemic there were multiple cases reported as exemplars of singing nurses who helped patients to heal while singing at work [14]. Teams can choreograph short dance routines and perform as "pop ups" to lift spirits and promote comradery. The nurses at Northwell Nurse Choir from Northwell Health used choreographed dance during the pandemic to generate hope and positivity. Their performances that started as a team-building exercise made national attention [15]. Providing a short story, song, or poem as a reflection at team huddles or start of a meeting can elevate the mood.

3.3.4 Leadership Application (Structural and Organizational Considerations) in the Workplace

In addition to promoting independent non-clinical engagement in art, leaders can develop a Creative Art Therapy (CAT) program as a wellness benefit. A CAT program can serve as an intervention to prevent burnout and promote resilience among healthcare professionals. Hiring artists to facilitate poetry, photography, drawing, and music can be part of a holistic wellness program much the same as many organizations offer fitness programs.

If CAT were incorporated into project days, training days, nurse residencies, retreats, orientation, lunchtimes, or before/after work, those interested could learn skills of creative expression to build resiliency. Visual arts developed during CAT could be displayed in supply closets, break rooms, bathrooms, hallways, and other areas where art could elevate the mood of the environment. An art exhibit could be held yearly to celebrate the use of creative expression as a wellness initiative.

When the pandemic started, makeshift walls were built in my unit to separate the COVID-positive patients, assuming we would never have a large enough census to require a full unit. These walls were soon decorated with inspirational quotes, funny sayings, cutouts of memes, hilarious photos of each other and funny memories, and pictures of our pets and our loved ones. These walls were the most comforting thing that we had, and everyone contributed and put up what they felt. These walls were truly a work of art and when they were able to take down the walls about a year and a half later, management took detailed pictures of these walls, enlarged them, and framed them. They hang in the break room so we could always see and remember the time we all came together and how we overcame these stressful and uncertain times as a team. At a time when there is great strife to keep up with staffing shortages and the overwhelming amount of patient cases with high levels of acuity, it can easily be made a priority to trial different workplace interventions to assess their effectiveness on staff well-being and morale.

One way leadership can promote creative expression is to foster the idea of being able to take a time out to decompress after a traumatic event. Creative expression can be used in conjunction with these decompression breaks if the person who is being offered a break for tranquility and relaxation also has access to tools for expression. While it is common for health systems to have a chapel or space for quiet and contemplation, leaders may also want to consider space and supplies dedicated for artistic expression. Meditation or break rooms often include things such as massage chairs, relaxing music, and segregated spaces to provide an environment free of distraction and socialization. Initiatives can easily be instituted to promote individual creative expression at work such as having coloring books with colored pencils, drawing pads, or a sand garden in the break or meditation room.

Examples that could incorporate the entire unit to be completed over a period of time include making a collage, sculptures, completing a scrabble game, puzzles, or large wall-sized coloring posters. Posting notes, pictures, or photographs of what makes the team happy in life to dedicated space on a bulletin board is another example. These exercises are completely anonymous and would require minimal time, but the resulting display of happiness may have a positive effect on empathy. Themes can be altered to "pets," "places," or other inspirational topics. A drop-box can be used where staff can leave their thoughts and feelings, not subject to review, but instead discarded, as a way of processing feelings.

Organize events outside of work for team building with creative art therapy such as participatory dance, drama, painting, photography, or mindfulness exercise. When visual art in the form of poetry or drawings is created, it is important to allow the creator the option of keeping them private when they are too personal to share. There are many possibilities of organizing creative expression or facilitating CAT, even in a busy and high-acuity environment.

While group- and individual-type therapy sessions both have positive outcomes, group sessions allow for greater peer-to-peer interaction and individual sessions allow for greater adaptability and personalization [10]. Leaders could consider incorporating an art therapist into the wellness team and schedule offerings through wellness benefits. Group-type CAT led by a trained facilitator would require event planning for when an HCW is not providing direct patient care. Another alternative is to have the CAT leader come to the unit or floor for a few hours every few days with materials provided and allow the HCW to participate when time allowed. Leadership can also support staff by providing short-term coverage while the staff member takes a mental health break.

3.4   Opportunities for Future Research

Further research is needed to demonstrate the impact of independent creative expression on the mental health of HCPs. Feasibility data are needed to see whether "art space" in the built design of healthcare systems would be used by employees to optimize mental health and well-being. The impact of a structured CAT program in addition to traditional wellness initiatives warrants future study. Most studies completed on art as a form of therapy among healthcare workers have focused on nurses. Expanding the research to other disciplines is indicated (Fig. 3.1).

Fig. 3.1 Author Bliss
Masiarczyk pictured with
wood burning created as a
personal wellness strategy

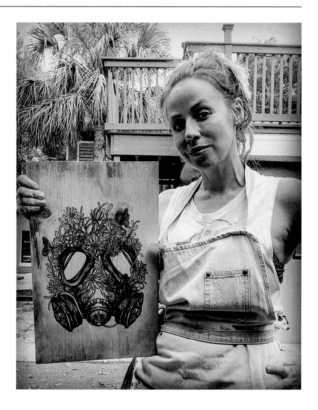

Glossary

Creative art therapy (CAT) The act of using creative art as a form of therapy such
as art therapy, dance/movement therapy, drama therapy, music therapy, writing
therapy, and poetry therapy, facilitated by a trained art therapist.

Creative expression The act of using art independently to express and process
thoughts, emotions, and feelings.

Discussion Questions

- Choose one form of creative expression (e.g., writing poetry, drawing, coloring
  from coloring pages, creating a collage from magazine clippings).
- Provide the supplies, give the group brief instructions, and encourage "expression" for 15 min.
- Play music in the background.

  Set the tone by describing what you would like them to reflect in the expression:
  (e.g., happiness, peace, emotions stimulated from a recent patient encounter)
  Afterward, share the output and use the discussion questions below:

1. What did this experience show you that you did not know before about yourself?
2. Do you feel creative art therapy helped you acknowledge or recognize any new feelings?
3. Do you feel this exercise was a healthy outlet for expressing your feelings and fears?
4. After having completed a self-guided exercise in creative expression or creative art therapy, do you feel any less stress, anxiety, or depression?
5. Describe how you could continue to complete self-guided creative expression or creative art therapy on a consistent basis?
6. What challenges do you currently foresee in continuing to complete creative expression on a consistent basis?
7. How may you overcome these challenges to empower yourself to have creative expression in any environment?

Discussion Leader Guide

• Enable participants in a creative art therapy session to recognize the team-building process and self-care elements that are embodied in the exercise. Establish how art therapy can be one means toward strengthening resilience.

Video for Discussion - Instructional Video: The online version contains supplementary material available at https://doi.org/10.1007/978-3-031-16983-0_3

References

1. Reed K, Cochran KL, Edelblute A, Manzanares D, Sinn H, Henry M, Moss M. Creative arts therapy as a potential intervention to prevent burnout and build resilience in health care professionals. AACN Adv Crit Care. 2020;31(2):179–90. https://doi.org/10.4037/aacnacc2020619.
2. Phillips CS, Becker H. Systematic review: expressive arts interventions to address psychosocial stress in healthcare workers. J Adv Nurs. 2019;75(11):2285–98. https://doi.org/10.1111/jan.14043. Epub 2019 June 6
3. Self-achievement through creativity in critical care. Crit Care Nurs Clin North Am. 2020;32(3):465–72. https://doi.org/10.1016/j.cnc.2020.05.004. Epub 2020 June 20.
4. Vaartio-Rajalin H, Santamäki-Fischer R, Jokisalo P, Fagerström L. Art making and expressive art therapy in adult health and nursing care: a scoping review. Int J Nurs Sci. 2020;8(1):102–19. https://doi.org/10.1016/j.ijnss.2020.09.011.
5. Jensen A, Bonde LO. The use of arts interventions for mental health and well-being in health settings. Perspect Public Health. 2018;138(4):209–14. https://doi.org/10.1177/1757913918772602. Epub 2018 Apr 30. Erratum in: Perspect Public Health. 2018 Sep;138(5):288
6. Schouten KA, de Niet GJ, Knipscheer JW, Kleber RJ, Hutschemaekers GJM. The effectiveness of art therapy in the treatment of traumatized adults. Trauma Violence Abuse. 2014;16(2):220–8. https://doi.org/10.1177/1524838014555032.
7. Kaimal G, Ray K, Muniz J. Reduction of cortisol levels and participants' responses following art making. Art Ther. 2016;33(2):74–80. https://doi.org/10.1080/07421656.2016.116683.
8. Jun J, Costa DK. Is it me or you? A team approach to mitigate burnout in critical care. Crit Care Nurs Clin North Am. 2020;32(3):395–406. https://doi.org/10.1016/j.cnc.2020.05.003.

9. Beans C. Science and culture: searching for the science behind art therapy. Proc Natl Acad Sci U S A. 2019;116(3):707–10. https://doi.org/10.1073/pnas.1821297116.

10. Chiang M, Reid-Varley WB, Fan X. Creative art therapy for mental illness. Psychiatry Res. 2019;275:129–36. https://doi.org/10.1016/j.psychres.2019.03.025. Epub 2019 Mar 16

11. Dijxhoorn AQ, Brom L, van der Linden YM, Leget C, Raijmakers NJ. Prevalence of burn-out in healthcare professionals providing palliative care and the effect of interventions to reduce symptoms: a systematic literature review. Palliat Med. 2021;35(1):6–26. https://doi.org/10.1177/0269216320956825.

12. Uttley L, Stevenson M, Scope A, Rawdin A, Sutton A. The clinical and cost effectiveness of group art therapy for people with non-psychotic mental health disorders: a systematic review and cost-effectiveness analysis. BMC Psychiatry. 2015;15:151. https://doi.org/10.1186/s12888-015-0528-4. Erratum in: BMC Psychiatry 2015;15:212.

13. Krout RE. Music listening to facilitate relaxation and promote wellness: integrated aspects of our neurophysiological response to music. Arts Psychother. 2006;34(2):134–41.

14. Singing nurses keep going viral. Could their music actually help patients heal? Advisory Board. 2020. https://www.advisory.com/daily-briefing/2020/02/18/singing-nurse. Accessed 1 Apr 2022.

15. Northwell Health Nurse Choir. Northwell. 2021. https://www.northwell.edu/choir. Accessed 1 Apr 2022.

The Impact of Art on the Workplace: Constructing an Aesthetically Soothing Workplace through Art

4

Hannah Saarinen and Kyle Broxterman

Abbreviations

EBD	Evidence-based design
IgA	Immunoglobulin A
IV	Intravenous (line)
Or	Operating room
PNI	Psychoneuroimmunology

Learning Objectives
1. Summarize and describe the benefits of arts in healthcare programs.
2. Apply the knowledge of how art can be used as a tool for healing. Create "Arts in Health" programs within healthcare organizations to promote health and well-being in patients and healthcare professionals.
3. Design hospitals and healthcare facilities around the basis of utilizing art to its fullest potential, through architectural design, permanent displays of art, landscaping, access to windows and healing garden areas.
4. Evaluate and justify the use of arts in healthcare programs within the organization using qualitative and quantitative data. Formulate a conclusion on the impact art in healthcare initiatives has on the physical and mental health of patients, healthcare professionals, family members, caregivers, employee satisfaction, and hospital costs. Interpret the information to formulate a conclusion on the success of the programs and revise the programs if unsuccessful.

H. Saarinen (✉)
Art Haz Energy, Reno, NV, USA

K. Broxterman
Brox Media, Reno, NV, USA

© The Author(s), under exclusive license to Springer Nature
Switzerland AG 2023
J. E. Davidson, M. Richardson (eds.), *Workplace Wellness: From Resiliency to Suicide Prevention and Grief Management*, https://doi.org/10.1007/978-3-031-16983-0_4

4.1   Presentation of the Science

4.1.1   Arts in Healthcare

Art is defined as the expression or application of human creative skill and imagination, typically in a visual form such as painting or sculpture, producing works to be appreciated primarily for their beauty or emotional power [1]. When considering art as it applies to healthcare, the definition becomes more complex and encompasses the ability art has to heal the mind and body of people suffering from a physical or mental illness. It also involves the power art has to bring positivity, light, and life into an environment that most often is cold, chaotic, and associated with pain and suffering. Since the 1970s, arts in health programs have been incorporated into hospitals, clinics, and community centers in the United States. There has even been an increase in government support for this work [2]. When art is implemented into an environment like the hospital, patients have more opportunities to feel connected to a part of themselves that lives outside of the hospital. Art can be used to promote feelings of safety, socialization, and connection [3]. This new wave of creativity is giving rise to a positive shift in healthcare.

The arts are integrated into healthcare for therapeutic, educational, and expressive purposes and have proven benefits to patients, their families, their caregivers, as well as healthcare professionals, staff, visitors, and volunteers, in various healthcare settings. "Arts in Health" is a broad term encompassing a range of practices primarily occurring in healthcare settings, bringing together the skills and priorities of both artists and health professionals [2]. A Department of Health working group on Arts and Healthcare reported a strong potential for the arts to create a better working environment for staff as well as increased well-being and health for patients [4]. Art as an intervention is contagious in its ability to positively affect everyone around it.

Coupled with an expanding global population, the increasing aging population presents a perfect opportunity for the implementation of arts programs into long-term care facilities. Elderly people often feel a profound sense of loss when they are required to move out of their homes and into a long-term care facility. Their new residence becomes a generic room, with mundane art. The control they once had over their daily routine and personal space is greatly altered. By using art-based interventions to provide color, life, and engagement, healthcare professionals can more easily begin to combat the loneliness, depression, lack of self-worth, and boredom commonly experienced during these major moments in people's lives. They will enjoy their living space more and be given inspiring opportunities to socialize with others. These changes create an overall uplifted environment and considerable improvements in quality of life. A major collaborative advantage of arts in health programs is its inclusivity for all. People from every walk of life can be captivated and positively influenced by art. From a young child to a patient on hospice care, art in health has no borders and exists to serve humankind. Hamist McDonald, an artist and cancer patient, wrote "I am a firm believer in the power that art has to inspire and help alleviate suffering and that it can play a key role in lessening the burden that illness brings" [4]. Art is a way for people to connect to a part of themselves that is raw, truthful, and expressive. It can be used to communicate thoughts and feelings in beautiful displays of colors, lines, shapes, or patterns.

It is important to note that while still aligned with arts in health, creative art therapies are part of a different discipline. Art therapists, for example, are mental health professionals who use art-based methods to improve health and wellness in patients suffering from illness. In comparison, the field of arts in health is made up of trained professional artists who facilitate and use the arts to promote healing in healthcare settings and communities. This field includes, and is not limited to, literary, performing, and visual artists, designers, architects, musicians, storytellers, dancers, and writers [5]. Because the arts are such a diverse field, there are endless possibilities for their impact on the world of health.

4.1.2   The Science of Art

Art is a fascinating complement to medicine. Although not traditionally taught in collaboration with each other, evidence supports the success of harmonizing art and medicine. Take into consideration the uplifted feelings experienced when observing a beautiful painting, connecting with a compelling photograph, listening to moving music, or watching a dramatic movie. This is a representation of art's influence on the human mind and emotions. The physiological processes taking place reveal a relationship between experiencing art and relieving stress. Images are linked to human emotions and the unconscious powers of comprehension; they also have the ability to communicate feelings that otherwise may not be understood by a conscious mind. Images and artwork have the ability to move someone in a way they cannot explain [6]. The experiences people go through in hospitals can be painful and traumatic. They are far removed from the comforts of their normal life and are constantly confronted with serious personal situations, afraid of what their healthcare providers might tell them next; another pill, another blood draw, another IV, another overnight stay. The arts offer a non-pharmaceutical, non-painful, and almost subconscious way to ameliorate discomfort.

In an early study in 1980, researcher Goldstein described "thrills" or tingling sensations people experience when exposed to emotionally arousing stimuli. This physiologic process can take place when experiencing certain forms of art, like a masterful painting. His findings show a relationship between the "tingles" and the release of endorphins in the body. Endorphins are known to help alleviate pain, relax the body, and boost mood [6]. When the body has less pain, less stress, and is in a better mood overall, the healing process is improved. Therefore, there is evidence to support that experiencing art can fundamentally benefit people in the healing process, or those undergoing stress.

Specific research related to this theory is called psychoneuroimmunology (PNI). PNI is a theoretical concept involved in scientifically explaining the associations between a person's participation in activities such as reading, writing, films, music, and paintings and alterations in their coping strategies and ability to handle stress [7]. This concept involves the correlation between stress and health, the study of the interactions between psychological processes and the nervous and immune systems [6]. There is not always an explanation for the powerful things experienced in life, but with steady research and advancements in medicine, sometimes explanations are uncovered. The science of art and how it influences human health is an intriguing subject that pushes the boundaries of both disciplines.

In a study cited by Lankston et al. [4], the effects of visual art on anxiety and depression were recorded in patients undergoing chemotherapy. Patients exposed to visual art compared to patients who were not, had lower levels of both depression and anxiety. In another fascinating study by Kettwich and colleagues, they created and tested stress-reducing medical devices and assessed their effects on needle phobia in adult and pediatric chemotherapy patients. The stress-reducing medical devices had colorful images of flowers, butterflies, and music notes on syringes, butterfly needles, and IV bags. In using them with children and adults with cancer, they discovered the rates of aversion, anxiety, fear, and overall stress were significantly reduced: 76% effective in preventing overt needle phobia in the children and 92% effective with the adults. Approximately two-thirds of children and over one-half of adults in the general population are needle phobic [8]. This simple intervention had a powerful effect on both adults and children and is a representation of what art can do for the world of medicine.

4.1.3 Maslow's Hierarchy of Needs Theory

As humans evolve, the complexity of medicine does as well. In Maslow's Hierarchy of Needs Theory, he separates human needs from basic to advanced and arranges them into levels on a pyramid. He states that every person can move up the pyramid to satisfy their self-actualization needs. He also theorized that humans may fluctuate between various levels of the pyramid, depending on their life experiences [9]. This provides evidence to support that people's higher levels of functioning should not be disregarded while in a hospital. In fact, it could be a great place for people to have profound experiences that expand their mindset and provide them with a broader understanding of their life and its purpose. "Many complex factors are known to influence health and wellbeing, and as levels of care improve, the importance of less easily quantifiable factors will likely increase…As more basic needs are met, for example by new drugs and treatments, those needs higher up the hierarchy, which include the visual environment, will assume greater importance" [4]. When surrounded by art, people can become inspired to create as well. This creation process strengthens one's connection to themselves, increases self-esteem, and allows emotions to be expressed.

In their current state, hospitals focus primarily on basic needs: food, water, warmth, safety, and security. Basic needs are the most important and require the most observation and treatment when the body is in critical condition. However, not all patients are in critical condition and require more attention and a more supportive environment to meet higher-level needs like psychological and self-fulfillment needs. Healthcare professionals, although not all licensed psychologists, attempt to satisfy a patient's psychological needs through active listening, compassion, empathy, and being an advocate. Nurses and nurse assistants spend the most time at the bedside and often find themselves caring for their patients on more than just a physical level, but this becomes challenging when the hospital environment alone causes patients unavoidable feelings of stress, anxiety, and isolation. Time pressures, caring for multiple patients at a time, and needing to prioritize physiological patient care, often leaves the psychological and emotional needs of a patient unmet.

Integrating art into this stressful environment can help patients feel more relaxed and engaged, instead of feeling reduced to a diagnosis or a number. Arts in Health programs, such as permanent displays of art, healing gardens, music, and nature photography, provide a more supportive healing environment using positive distraction. Creative design, architecture, and visual art integrated throughout a healthcare facility offer patients the freedom to think about something other than their worries. These interventions are proven to decrease stress in patients, which will improve their healing process.

Psychological needs include belongingness, love, respect, dignity, and esteem [8]. Visual art can inspire and cause positive emotional responses in people, which can help them achieve these higher levels of functioning and needs. While it is unrealistic to ensure all patients are meeting needs of self-actualization before discharge, healthcare organizations can still provide an opportunity for people to think about themselves in a broader sense, beyond their diagnosis, and beyond their medical record number, so that they leave the hospital with an expanded sense of self in addition to having their physical needs met.

While this is all known for patients, the same could be possible for healthcare professionals. By integrating art into the stressful environment, wouldn't we be more relaxed, engaged, and able to cope with the stressors of the day? Could we promote positive adaptive emotional responses to our work using art? Could we open our minds to the patient's experience and be more empathetic through their experience with the use of art?

4.1.4   Physical Design and Architecture and their Impact on the Workplace

The physical environment plays a major role in mood and reactions to experiences within an environment. This is particularly true in a healthcare setting. Stine et al. [3] uncovers research on how the physical environment affects health-related outcomes in hospitals. These studies revealed a new field that exists under the umbrella of arts in health programs called Evidence-Based Design (EBD). This area of focus supports that physical design and architecture have positive effects on both the treatment process and clinical outcomes for patients. To share this new understanding and to contribute to better health for all, there are now evidence-based design guidelines for arts in healthcare programs that use theoretical approaches including the Biophilia Hypothesis, Congruence Theory, and Distraction Theory in their design process [3]. These theories offer a glimpse into the psychology of art and the potential of creating comfortable healing spaces for patients.

There is a belief that environmental features can elicit positive feelings, and hold attention and interest, and therefore, are believed to reduce stressful thoughts. This belief is defined as "positive distraction." In contrast, in an environment that lacks positive distraction, patients may end up focusing on their worries, fears, or pain [4]. This can increase the impact of these emotions and in turn dramatically increase levels of stress. When compared to a hospital room with blank white walls, a hallway or wall painted colorfully and decorated with artwork gives a sense of life to a place that was once bare. When people are in the hospital for days, weeks, or months, a blank wall gives them no relief from the stressful thoughts and decisions they are faced with. A blank wall rebounds their thoughts back to them. An abstract painting, they have no connection to, could make them feel lost. When artwork is thoughtfully placed in places like this, patients are given a chance to breathe, to take a moment and escape from the stress and pain, and to think about things beyond the white walls and beyond the redundant thoughts in their heads. It is time for us, as healthcare providers, to intentionally take the same advantage of the art around us to ease our pain, ease our suffering, and ground ourselves.

Use of the arts fosters a supportive safe and useful healthcare environment [6]. When healing-focused attention is given to the architectural design, with permanent displays of artwork and access to natural lighting, and nature is incorporated through creative landscaping, the colorful living atmosphere helps create a safe place and a sense of relaxation and peace. These factors contribute to an overall decrease in patient and caregiver stress and anxiety. When considering the health and well-being of individuals in the healthcare setting, whether it be the providers or the patients, decreasing stress and anxiety plays a major role in the healing process. When stressed, healing is hindered, which creates a bigger challenge in treating life-threatening diseases or making life-altering decisions. Through incorporating art into the design and function of a healthcare facility, the overall well-being of patients and staff is improved, leading to better quality of care and reduced costs to the organization [6]. By creating an environment that promotes healing and relaxation, the process of bringing people back to health becomes much easier.

4.1.5 Visual Art in Healthcare

Hospital art in its current state often lacks a certain element of emotion and intention. In many cases, the chosen paintings blend in, as if to exist only as a rectangular picture on the wall. The traditional art on many hospital wards has not seemed to have any purpose of engaging its viewers to spark insight. With abundant evidence to support that displays of visual art, especially images of nature, can have positive effects on health outcomes including shorter length of stay in the hospital, increased pain tolerance, and decreased anxiety, it is time to start taking action [4]. There are endless possibilities for how this intervention can be creatively incorporated into healthcare—hundreds of hallways and even more patient rooms where visual art could be incorporated to support the healing of patients and resilience of healthcare professionals.

Not all art promotes feelings of calm, however. A study compared images of nature, abstract images, and no images at all. They found that while the images of nature proved to have the most positive outcomes in patients, the group exposed to abstract images had more anxiety than the group with no images [4]. The limitations of this study are related to the fact that different artwork has different effects on different people, but it is an important observation, nonetheless.

The Arts in Health field of study aims its research at uncovering why patients frequently express a preference for landscape and nature scenes. This discovery is explained with an evolutionary psychological theory called the biophilia hypothesis. The biophilia hypothesis predicts that people show positive emotional responses to images of flourishing natural environments because recognizing healthy natural environments was a survival advantage during human evolution. Flourishing natural environments provided early humans with the best resources and were positively reinforced by natural selection through positive emotional responses [4]. There is also evidence to support that patients prefer pictures dominated by blues and greens because these colors evoke more pleasure and calm emotions rather than reds and yellow, which elicit more emotions of arousal and stress [4]. When it comes to choosing paintings for healthcare, there are several factors to be considered. Visual art for the purpose of healing is not a one-fits-all intervention and requires more research to clarify the boundaries of what works and what does not work.

4.2   Application of Principles into Wellness Practice

4.2.1   Pre-licensure Application in the Academic Environment

In the academic environment, the idea of art soothing the workplace can be accomplished through the utilization of permanent displays of art that is educational, inspiring, and beautiful. Hanging artwork in medical educational organizations with relatable subject matter is a great way to inspire young students seeking a career in medicine. Giving students an opportunity or assignment, which requires them to speak with each other about the artwork, can allow for a deeper connection to their goals and their personal contribution to health. Incorporating medical humanities into the medical curriculum can increase a young physician's ability to understand and communicate with their colleagues and their patients.

Imagine a new medical student called to the field of medicine, but with no specific sense of direction regarding which specialty they should dedicate themselves to. Traditionally, through their years of training, physicians are eventually called to a specific field of medicine, but some may struggle with this decision, especially in the beginning of their journey. This is where art has the potential to inspire. In a space they frequently walk through, have class in, or study in, the walls could display art that represents different medical specialties or diseases; one image representing the cardiovascular system, another representing the nervous system, another representing the respiratory system, so on and so forth. Students would be provided with numerous opportunities to think about how these images make them feel and allow themselves to be inspired by the artwork.

Research in arts and medicine can lead to impressive and unusual discoveries. In a study by Naghshineh et al., medical students were instructed by museum experts on how to examine the skin of naked bodies in paintings. Following the instruction, the students examined the skin of real patients and, compared to the control group, the students who received the instruction by museum experts scored better on "sophistication in their descriptions of artistic and clinical imagery" [10]. Creative minds think outside the box, and they respectfully deserve a place in the world of medicine which is more linear and logically defined.

The arts also offer a highly effective way to educate people on difficult topics. Drama is a branch of the arts that has been successfully used in medical education programs. Take for example the 1999 Pulitzer Prize-winning play called *Wit*, written by Margaret Edson. It tells an emotional story of a woman diagnosed with metastatic ovarian cancer and her experiences with her treatments and medical team. The play portrays complex humanistic knowledge that would otherwise be hard to teach with conventional methods. Because plays like this evoke such strong emotions, they have a profound impact on the viewers and are more likely to promote understanding. This leads to an adaptation of positive behavior changes while caring for patients undergoing a similar diagnosis or going through a similar experience. In the Arts in Healthcare State of the Field Report, authors write about the Wit Educational Initiative which organized on-site readings of *Wit* at medical centers throughout the United States and Canada for medical students and staff. The play was followed by a structured discussion of the play's themes. The creators of the initiative attributed the success of the program to two factors. One, the realistic portrayal of terminal illness helped viewers better understand the strong emotions that accompany end-of-life experiences, and two, it gave viewers an opportunity to express their emotions in a supportive and noncritical environment. They concluded that strong emotional experiences are inevitable in medicine and can act as powerful motivators of behavior change [6]. There are certain experiences in medicine that are difficult to prepare healthcare professionals for thorough traditional training and education. However, the community would benefit greatly if staff were already exposed to the importance of acquiring strong empathy and communication skills. Drama serves as a tool for inexperienced practitioners to understand and communicate the difficult emotions that come with their role as a physician.

In summary, the academic environment offers many opportunities to introduce and utilize art. It can be used to bring positivity and light into the study space, as well as offer a potential connection to a specific focus in the field. Art can be a source of inspiration, motivation, clarity, and it can strengthen students' understanding of the complex emotional experiences of their patients.

4.2.2   Clinical Application Post-Licensure

Post-licensure clinical application of the arts in healthcare includes the use of permanent displays of art in hospitals and healthcare facilities. Meaningful, intriguing, and relatable works of art in the halls of hospitals can spark thought, emotion, and open communication between a patient and himself, a patient and his doctor, or a patient and his friend or family member. Take for example a patient who is hospitalized for several weeks due to a treatment regimen that restricts him from leaving. Day after day, he walks the same empty halls, watching the nurses run back and forth, listening to the beeps, alarms, and chatter of medical teams flowing through the halls. He has no visitors and only the TV for entertainment, which he gets bored of after a week. He misses his life, his friends, his dog. He walks past the same paintings day after day and never stops to look at them. His thoughts race as he circles the unit; he wonders if his illness is getting better, he wonders how many more needle sticks he will have to get, how many more tests, how many more conversations with the doctors. He wonders what he did to deserve this, and he worries about how he will be able to pay for all of his medical bills. His doctors and nurses do their best to give him moments of hope, positivity, and connection, but their jobs are demanding, and quickly they leave his room and tend to the next patient. The patient is alone again, walking the halls again.

Healthcare providers have an opportunity to change this patient's experience. There are several ways his experience could be improved through using various methods of art. Instead of hanging art that camouflages into the atmosphere of the hospital space, the hospital can hang artwork that is relatable and inspiring to the patient and his experiences—something the patient can get lost in, allowing his mind to take a break from his cycling thoughts and worries (Fig. 4.1). The use of permanent displays of artwork is one of the most common methods of using art in healthcare to promote healing [6]. Visual artwork holds the potential to spark powerful emotions in people. It can also be used to help people feel connection, belonging, purpose, happiness, freedom, relaxation, and acceptance. Art is a tool for communication when other forms of communication may be hindered or inaccessible due to being hospitalized. Without having to speak to anyone, a patient can have a conversation with a work of art and learn something new about themselves. Alternatively, art can also be used as a vehicle for shared contemplation between healthcare professionals and patients—sharing emotions or responses to the art that is passed during assisted ambulation or while in a procedure room.

Permanent displays of artwork can also be applied to the surgery setting. This includes Operating Rooms (ORs) in hospitals, surgery centers, and procedural units. Patients enter these rooms either half-awake or sleeping, so the audience for the art in this setting is mostly directed at the staff, although some patients, if awake upon entrance into the room, may benefit from it as well. Staff members working in an OR are trained to work in a fast-paced environment that also demands precision and razor-sharp focus. The surgeons, anesthesiologists, nurses, first assists, and scrub techs work together as a team to ensure each procedure is done perfectly, so the patient recovers without any complications and is pleased with the outcomes. Unfortunately, however, mistakes do occur.

There are about 4000 surgical errors that occur each year in the United States. Human error whether due to stress, inattention, time pressures, distractions, or increased workload can lead to these mistakes [11]. Reducing rates of surgical

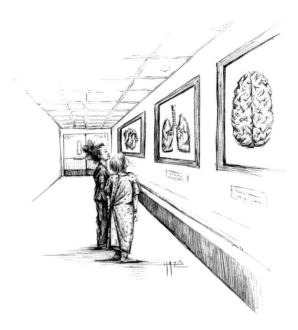

Fig. 4.1 "Art Creates Connection," 2021 (Created with black sumi brush ink on heavyweight Bristol paper). When integrated into healthcare settings, art can be used as a tool to educate, uplift, and improve communication between healthcare providers and patients. A nurse ambulating a patient in the hallway reflecting upon the images on the wall of the post-surgical floor of the hospital. Each image represents a body part usually worked upon in surgery. The artwork provides motivation for ambulation, an essential component of postoperative care

errors requires a diverse range of analytics and intervention that art-based therapies alone cannot achieve, but in considering the positive effects and variety of art-based interventions used throughout healthcare settings, the Operating Room should not be excluded. Observing surgery staff as both people and medical professionals connects these dots.

A large aesthetically pleasing image of a brain in a neurosurgery operating room, for example, can serve as an inspiring piece of art for the operative team members to enjoy. The first thing they see when they enter the room is an image that reminds them of how much they love what they do. It reminds them of why they chose to become a neurosurgeon, or a neuro-nurse, or scrub technician. It makes the space more enjoyable and memorable to those who spend 10–12 h working inside of it each day. Operating rooms are not always designated to a specific team of surgeons, but many of them are grouped. One OR might be for urology and OB/GYN, another for GI, and a different one for cardiothoracic surgery. Adding an inspiring image for each discipline that uses the OR would only increase the value and illumination of the room. Images like this can lift the spirits of the people they were created for. Displaying specific artwork chosen for the healthcare professionals who operate inside this sterile environment is a non-life-threatening way to add a bit of metaphorical life back into the room.

Music is a form of art used to soothe the workplace and can be easily integrated into the day-to-day flow of a healthcare facility. Music can be used to help patients cope with their illness, reduce stress levels, reduce the amount of analgesia and sedation required in the OR, and even improve recovery after surgical procedures. One way for hospitals to utilize the power of music is by including a variety of calm music and visual art channels on the television for patients to choose from. So rather than watching television shows and commercials all day and night, they can have the option of choosing from a list of calm music and art channels to help them achieve better rest and relaxation. In an article on art informing health psychology by Kaptein et al., two systematic reviews evaluate the effects of music in the operating room and recovery room, respectively. The first study revealed reduced stress levels in adults and children, which lead to a reduction in analgesia and sedation requirements while having patients listen to music in the operating room [7]. The other review and meta-analysis indicated that post-procedure recovery is improved using music in the postoperative period by reducing levels of pain and anxiety [12]. The positive influence of music can impact family members and visitors of patients as well. With one click of a button, the atmosphere changes from chaos to calm. This calmness in the environment will also transfer similar benefits to healthcare professionals.

Studies also suggest that a surgeon's heart rate, blood pressure, and muscle efficiency are also enhanced by music in the OR and that ambient music serves to increase the accuracy with which surgical tasks are performed [7]. Music proves to significantly increase salivary immunoglobulin A (IgA), an antibody that plays a crucial role in immunity and fighting infections. Music is also linked to infants' oxygen saturation levels, which measures respiratory regularity that is directly affected by their behavioral state and level of discomfort or pain [6]. The appropriate use of tranquil music in the workplace could have a powerful effect on the mood and stress levels of patients, visitors, doctors, nurses, ancillary staff, and anyone else who enters the building. It can act as a subconscious reminder that the hospital is a place for healing.

4.2.3 Leadership Application (Structural and Organizational Considerations)

If art is an integral part of hospital design, the health benefits and financial benefits will be maximized [4]. Bringing art into healthcare settings has exponential effects on both the people and the organization itself. It creates a strong culture of care, expanded thinking, and a love for diversity in life. This allows for people to connect to themselves as well as each other. The medical field is no longer solely focused on the physical health of humans, but psychological and soulful health as well. While the main goal of healthcare organizations remains the same, adding programs to help soften the difficulties of being a patient can help with the growth, development, and continued success of an organization.

This process begins in the blueprints. Place careful attention to the layout, design, and flow of the entire space during the construction phase of a healthcare facility. In creating a space with exceptional design as a core consideration, the organization will be providing patients and visitors with a high-quality environment and supportive healing experience [4]. Allowing both artists and healthcare providers to provide input on the incorporation of visual art from the beginning is a smart way to create a perfect balance of the two. Creating a hospital that incorporates art into its foundation means having space for art on the walls specifically targeted to the people around it the most. This includes working with artists to create work for the hospital and assist in the design process. Looking to the community for volunteers and local artists is a great way to create a space that is full of culture and a spectrum of creative healing methods.

Along with the physical design space, art can be integrated into an organization through Art in Healthcare departments that provide evidence-based therapies and programs for patients and healthcare providers. Leadership in governance would make this most effective. Having governance in leadership is the willingness and ability to take ownership in a part of an organization and to continually do what is best for the organization [13]. An integrated Arts in Healthcare program would be integral to the success of the organization and leadership would recognize it as such, supporting the department with staff, funding, artists, and designers. A great reference for information, policies, best practice guidelines, research, and developments in the field of arts in healthcare is an international online resource called artsandhealth.ie.

4.3 Opportunities for Future Research

Arts in health research has made impressive discoveries in recent decades, but there is more to be uncovered. The field of art in medicine is promising for the success and growth of healthcare organizations as well as the people in them. In a broad sense, the discoveries about how art impacts the workplace have revealed that art can heal and deserves a permanent place in healthcare. The spectrum of art is expansive and multidirectional, so the demand for further research is present.

There is great promise in investigating more about the economic benefits of arts in healthcare programs. Healthcare spending and quality of medical care are current areas of concern in the United States, and creative arts in healthcare interventions have many prospective benefits to combating financial battles while simultaneously improving quality of care and patient satisfaction [14]. Because arts in healthcare programs are so effective in their ability to decrease pain, anxiety, length of stay, amount of medication, and sedation requirements during procedures, the economic benefits to a healthcare organization can be significant. Americans for the Arts and the Society for the Arts in Healthcare conducted a survey of about 800 programs in 2008 to evaluate the financial benefits of arts in healthcare programs on healthcare organizations. Their findings revealed extensive evidence supporting various health benefits of their programs; however, it lacked quantitative evidence supporting the economic and cost benefits of arts in healthcare programs on costs to patients and healthcare organizations. At most, findings in this area of study were based on qualitative and anecdotal evidence

[6]. To drive home the potentially significant economic benefits creative arts programs have on healthcare organizations, more thorough research and investigation needs to be done.

While some exploration has started to develop in understanding the physiological processes taking place upon observation of art, further investigation would provide a more detailed and concrete understanding. It would also be important to determine if certain subject matter correlates with stronger health benefits to its viewers. Is there any subject matter that should be avoided? Should art with specific subject matter be placed on its corresponding area of the hospital or clinic? For example, what are the effects of displaying cardiac-based artwork on a cardiology floor, or neuroscience artwork on a neurosurgery floor? Do patients and healthcare providers have a positive or negative reaction to viewing the artwork of disease or illness displayed in a way that is aesthetically pleasing as a work of art? Does it help them understand their diagnosis and help them heal? There are countless questions to be answered regarding this particular field of study and uncovering them may lead to more satisfied patients and happier working environments for healthcare professionals. Most previous research has been conducted to measure patient outcomes. Though results are logically transferrable, all these past studies have potential for replication with a focus on how art in the healthcare environment affects healthcare professionals.

Potential research questions to be investigated include the following:

1. What are the effects of arts in health programs on the costs of healthcare organizations after they have been successfully implemented and adapted by patients and staff within the facility?
   (a) What are the effects of arts in health programs on employee retention rates?
   (b) What are the effects of arts in health programs on employee satisfaction rates?
2. When provided with an opportunity to do so, what percentage of healthcare providers are interested in creating employee-initiated artwork for the healthcare organization they work at?
   (a) What are the reactions of patients and healthcare providers to displays of artwork created by employees?
      • What conversations are being had?
      • How does this intervention affect professional relationships between healthcare providers and patients?
3. What are the effects of implementing a healing garden available to staff, patients, and visitors on employee satisfaction scores and patient satisfaction scores?
   (a) How often are patients, staff, and visitors utilizing the healing garden?
      • What are their reactions?
   (b) What are the effects of the healing garden on the mental health of healthcare providers who utilize the space during appropriate break times throughout their shifts?
   (c) What are the effects of the healing garden on the mental health of patients who are able to utilize the space during their hospital stay?

- What are the effects of the healing garden on patients' levels of stress, anxiety, and depression?
4. What is the impact of displaying artwork that contains cardiac-based subject matter on a cardiology unit or throughout a cardiology center?
   (a) How is this intervention received by patients, nurses, physicians, ancillary staff, and management?
   (b) Does this intervention increase a connection to the viewer's self or body?
   (c) Does the cardiac-inspired artwork appeal to patients who are suffering from cardiac diseases? Or does this artwork cause an unpleasant reaction?
   (d) Does this intervention have a similar effect for neurology? Pulmonary? Internal medicine? Dermatology? Ophthalmology? Orthopedics? etc.

My name is Hannah Saarinen. I am an artist and a nurse. Working as a bedside nurse since 2014, I have witnessed the negative impact that prolonged hospitalizations have on patients. I have worked on different units with many different patients, heard their stories, felt their pain, and held their hands through many difficult moments. As an artist, my inspiration comes from these people. Their experiences and their resilience inspire me to create artwork for hospitals. One of my paintings hangs in the University of California San Diego Hospital. It is of Esophageal Varices, a condition that causes enlarged veins in the esophagus, and frequently occurs in patients with advanced liver disease. *Esophageal Varices* is a deep purple and yellow oil painting displayed on the wall across from the nurses station (Fig. 4.2). On this floor, I cared for a great deal of people with liver failure, many of them with irreversible damage to their bodies. When I showed my painting to these

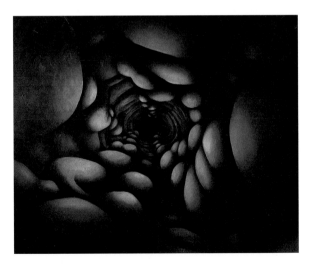

Fig. 4.2 "Esophageal Varices," 2018 (Oil paint on canvas). This painting was designed by artist and nurse, Hannah Saarinen. She cared for many patients suffering from chronic liver failure while working as a nurse at the University of California San Diego Hospital. Contemplating their fears, thoughts, worries, pains, and journey toward acceptance as they neared the end of their lives, this painting was created with a strong balance of good and bad, ugliness and beauty

patients, they reacted with intrigue, fascination, and a feeling of understanding and appreciation. A lot of them were even unfamiliar with what "esophageal varices" meant. It was just a word they knew they were associated with. The use of art in this situation opens a door for elevating awareness and connection, creating a stronger bond between the healthcare professionals and the patients. My coworkers also connected with the painting as they loved that I created something unique for our floor and were always proud to share it with patients. I aim to see these profound effects of art in healthcare replicated in healthcare organizations around the world. Healthcare professionals, patients, and artists have the ability to think creatively and utilize the arts to relieve stress, express emotions, and feel elevated in their workplace. Let us bring about the positive changes art brings into the world of healthcare.

4.3.1 Employee-Initiated Art in the Work Environment

Art gives me a soulful purpose in life, especially when paired with my role as a caregiver. It helps me communicate difficult emotions. I have been lucky enough to have my work displayed at hospitals, and, through this experience, learned about the exciting potential of employee-initiated art in the workplace. It builds a strong connection with coworkers and a more trusting and expansive relationships with patients. It reveals a depth of humanistic appreciation in the organization, uncovering who we are as people outside of the hospital. I know that I am not alone in my love for both art and medicine. Many caregivers are artistically talented and use art to cope with the intensity of being a healthcare professional, but there is not always an outlet for them to display their work. I hope to see employee-initiated art become an essential piece of arts in health programs throughout the country and even the world. Art exhibited in this way visually and creatively communicates compassion to patients with diverse diagnoses.

Warm-hearted nurses and healthcare professionals from all disciplines each have a unique voice. They have all witnessed different experiences and connected with many people throughout their careers. When given an opportunity to creatively express themselves and share their experiences through art, healthcare professionals are able to connect with and inspire others through their work. Because of this intervention, artwork displayed in hospitals could have a more profound and meaningful impact on its audience. The application of employee-initiated art in the workplace could add a deeply humanistic element to healthcare facilities that inspires universal love and care in an environment that needs it the most.

Glossary

Art The expression or application of human creative skill and imagination, typically in a visual form such as painting or sculpture, producing works to be appreciated primarily for their beauty or emotional power [1].

Biophilia hypothesis It suggests that the ability to recognize healthy natural environments is a survival advantage, since these environments provide the best resources [4].

Governance Leadership in governance is the willingness and ability to take ownership in a part of an organization and to continually do what is best for the organization. Effective corporate leaders stand on a foundation of solid governance principles [13].

Immunoglobulin A An antibody that plays a crucial role in immunity and fighting infections [6].

Positive distraction The belief that environmental features can elicit positive feelings, hold attention and interest, and, therefore, reduce stressful thoughts [4].

Psychoneuroimmunology (PNI) A theory that is concerned with the correlation between stress and health. Specifically, PNI is the study of the interaction between psychological processes and the nervous and immune systems of the human body [7].

Discussion Questions

1. Have you ever felt emotionally impacted by a work of art?
   (a) What was it and what was your reaction?
2. Have you ever felt emotionally impacted by a work of art in a healthcare facility?
   (a) What was it and what was your reaction?
3. Have you ever worked in a facility that had medically based artwork?
   (a) Did it make you feel more connected to your profession? To your body?
4. If you were a patient with a lung condition, how would an illustration of healthy lungs make you feel?
5. If you had a disease, how would an illustration of it make you feel?
6. Are there any negative effects of putting more energy and effort into integrating the arts into healthcare?
7. What is stopping hospitals and healthcare facilities from getting started?

Discussion Leader Guide

- The discussion questions are aimed at understanding peoples' relationship to art, especially as it relates to the medical field.
- A person's "emotional reaction" to a work of art is something that can only be fully understood by the individual, unless spoken or written about to others.
- The discussion questions are meant to start an open conversation about something new, and something they have possibly never spoken about.
- Conversations about art in health can lead to a deeper understanding of the field. It can also lead to a deeper understanding of one another, which creates a healthier work environment.

References

1. Oxford University Press. 2021. Art. Oxford Languages. Accessed 10 September 2021.
2. Artsandhealth.ie. 2021. http://artsandhealth.ie. Accessed 5 Sept 2021.
3. Nielsen SL, Fich LB, Roessler KK, Mullins MF. How do patients actually experience and use art in hospitals? The significance of interaction: a user-oriented experimental case study. Int J Qual Stud Health Well-being. 2017;12(1):1267343. https://doi.org/10.1080/17482631.201 6.1267343.
4. Lankston L, Cusack P, Fremantle C, Isles C. Visual art in hospitals: case studies and review of the evidence. J R Soc Med. 2010;103(12):490–9. https://doi.org/10.1258/jrsm.2010.100256.
5. College of the Arts & University of Florida. Center for Arts in Medicine. 2021. https://arts.ufl.edu. Accessed 15 Sept 2021.
6. State of the Field Committee. State of the field report: arts in healthcare 2009. Washington, DC: Society for the Arts in Healthcare; 2009.
7. Kaptein AA, Hughes BM, Murray M, Smyth JM. Start making sense: art informing health psychology. Health Psychol Open. 2018;5(1):2055102918760042. https://doi.org/10.1177/2055102918760042.
8. Kettwich SC, Sibbitt WL, Brandt JR, Johnson CR, Wong CS, Bankhurst AD. Needle phobia and stress-reducing medical devices in pediatric and adult chemotherapy patients. J Pediatr Oncol Nurs. 2007;24(1):20–8. https://doi.org/10.1177/1043454206296023.
9. McLeod S. Maslow's hierarchy of needs. Simply Psychology. 2020. https://www.simplypsychology.org/maslow.html. Accessed 5 Sept 2021.
10. Naghshineh S, Hafler JP, Miller AR. Formal art observation training improves medical students' visual diagnostic skills. J Gen Med. 2008;23:991–7.
11. Shouhed D, Gewertz B, Wiegmann D, Catchpole K. Integrating human factors research and surgery: a review. Arch Surg. 2012;147(12):1141–6. https://doi.org/10.1001/jamasurg.2013.596.
12. Hole J, Hirsch M, Ball E, et al. Music as an aid for postoperative recovery in adults: a systematic review and meta-analysis. Lancet. 2015;386:1659–71.
13. Price NJ. The importance of recognizing strong governance leaders. Diligent Insights 2019. https://insights.diligent.com. Accessed 20 Sept 2021.
14. Americans for the Arts. 2015. http://www.americansforthearts.org. Accessed 4 Sept 2021.

Mindfulness and the Mind

5

Aran Tavakoli, Marta Patterson, Jody Atkinson, and Hannah Saarinen

Abbreviations

ANS	Autonomic nervous system
HCPs	Healthcare professionals
JKZ	John Kabat-Zinn
MBSR	Mindfulness-based stress reduction
PMS	Parasympathetic nervous system

Acknowledgements for vignettes: Melissa Forde, BSN, RN, RYT and Health McCain, BSN, RN, Test

Supplementary Information The online version contains supplementary material available at https://doi.org/10.1007/978-3-031-16983-0_5.

A. Tavakoli (✉)
UC San Diego Health, San Diego, CA, USA
e-mail: atavakoli@health.ucsd.edu

M. Patterson
UC San Diego Center for Mindfulness, San Diego, CA, USA
e-mail: mpatterson@health.ucsd.edu

J. Atkinson
Sharp Grossmont Hospital, La Mesa, CA, USA
e-mail: Jody.Atkinson@Sharp.com

H. Saarinen
Art Haz Energy, Reno, NV, USA

J. E. Davidson, M. Richardson (eds.), *Workplace Wellness: From Resiliency to Suicide Prevention and Grief Management*, https://doi.org/10.1007/978-3-031-16983-0_5

Learning Objectives

1. Implement tools that empower HCPs to perform mindfulness or self-compassion skills to address the stress response in the moment.
2. Describe why the term empathetic distress needs to be adopted instead of compassion fatigue.
3. Identify when mindfulness practices or programs are not useful and consider other interventions to reduce potential harm.

5.1   Presentation of the Science

5.1.1   Physiology of Stress: Why We Need Mindfulness?

Stress has become common in our fast-paced, complex society and is a normal reaction that affects every human being. Due to many factors, healthcare professionals (HCPs) are particularly vulnerable to prolonged and chronic stress. A little stress helps us function better, but ongoing stress can be detrimental to physical and mental well-being.

Stress was originally described as the fight-or-flight response by Walter Bradford Cannon in the 1920s. Cannon developed the theory to explain the physiology of an animal's evolutionary survival mechanism when faced with a threat. The activation of the sympathetic portion of the autonomic nervous system (ANS) prepares the animal to fight or flee [1]. During this reaction, the amygdala, the portion of the brain that registers threat, is activated and hormones like adrenaline and cortisol are released. This accelerates the heart rate, slows digestion, directs blood flow to major muscle groups, and changes various other autonomic nervous functions, giving the body both strength and energy [2].

Dr. Hans Selye was the first to use the term stress to refer to anything that threatens homeostasis—the dynamic balance between the two ANS branches. A real or perceived threat to an organism is called the "stressor" and the response of an organism is the "stress response." Selye observed that the stress response is an evolutionary adaptive process, but chronic, grievous stress responses may cause tissue damage and disease [3].

Lazarus and Folkman [4] defined stress as a relationship between the individual and the environment that is appraised as significant enough to exceed the resources available for coping. Whether stress is an external event like encountering a patient in acute distress, or an internal event such as the fear of giving a big presentation, the reaction is the mobilization of the fight-or-flight response.

The counterpart to the sympathetic nervous system is the parasympathetic nervous system (PNS), which is responsible for returning the body to baseline after a stress response. Referred to as "rest and digest," the PNS calms the nervous system allowing the mind to become clearer, slowing the heart rate, deepening the breath, and relaxing the muscles [2].

In times of stress, the practice of mindfulness can induce calming effects by shifting our nervous system from the fight-or-flight response to the parasympathetic mode. In other words, we calm down. Research demonstrates that when mindfulness meditation is practiced, it helps slow down the heart rate and promotes feelings of safety. When we are calm, we have a greater ability to control attention, be more self-aware, and regulate our emotions [5]. According to Gross, emotion regulation refers to the ability of individuals to decide when, how, and for how long they want to experience and express emotions [6].

5.1.2 Mindfulness and Mindfulness-Based Practices

Mindfulness is a mental training that has its roots in Buddhist meditation and has become a popular secular practice to deal with stress and promote well-being. Mindfulness can be cultivated by engaging in meditation, mindful movement, and other practices that increase the ability to focus on the present moment and achieve a heightened level of attention [7].

Jon Kabat-Zinn (JKZ) who has been credited with bringing mindfulness to the mainstream and medicine defines mindfulness as, "What arises when you pay attention, on purpose, in the present moment, non-judgmentally, and as if your life depended on it. And what arises is nothing other than awareness itself" [8].

Practice can be formal, which involves setting aside time to practice meditation or other exercises, and informal, which involves bringing mindful attention to everyday activities such as driving, eating, brushing your teeth, showering, and listening. When the mind wanders, gently bring attention back to the task at hand [7].

Mindfulness-based stress reduction (MBSR) was developed by JKZ and is considered one of the most widely accepted training courses in mindfulness. It has been thoroughly researched with numerous studies completed and has demonstrated effectiveness in reducing stress and alleviating stress-related symptoms [9, 10]. Studies of MBSR focusing on HCPs have shown promising results such as increased focus, attention, and calmness as well as reduced levels of fatigue, anxiety, depression, and stress [11, 12].

The research also suggests positive impact on the overall patient experience, including enhanced feelings of social connection, improved patient communication, increase in compassion when suffering was present, and more satisfied patients [13, 14]. The full MBSR program consists of a 2.5-h class lasting 8 weeks, plus a full retreat day and an expectation of daily home practice [7]. Due to the hectic schedules of most HCPs, it may be difficult to attend an entire MBSR program. Shorter, modified versions of MBSR have also proven to be effective for HCPs and others in the workplace and can be less of a burden for those with time constraints [15–18].

5.1.2.1 Being in Your Body
Working in an environment of constant stress can lead to the formation of emotions such as anger, frustration, guilt, feeling overwhelmed, and many others. It is important to note that emotions themselves are a natural phenomenon and are not

inherently "good" or "bad"; the actions that one chooses in response to these emotions have led our society at large to correlate these labels with certain emotion states. Over time, these emotions can lead to development of self-doubt, job dissatisfaction, and apathy, as the individual begins to associate and define themselves by the persistent existence of these emotions [19]. Mindfulness practices focused on body awareness may help to mitigate the immediate response as well as decrease the long-term impact that these emotions may impose.

One key concept of the methods described is that the intent is to simply recognize the presence of certain emotions, noting that their mere presence does not define the individual [20]. Mindfulness practices are intended to employ a non-judgmental awareness of the current situation and allow the individual to come to the realization that while they may not have the ability to change the situation at hand, they can change their response. This is described by some as a "bottom-up" mindfulness-based strategy by engaging with the current state of the body to describe and become aware of one's emotional state [21]. There are a wide variety of techniques and methods; two such methods that can easily be incorporated into a healthcare work environment are Mindful Handwashing and Soles of the Feet Meditation.

5.1.2.2 Mindful Handwashing

Handwashing has long been established as an effective infection control method and one in which every healthcare provider is well versed. This simple act can be taken a step further to allow the individual a moment to engage in a practice focused on body awareness to reduce feelings of stress, anxiety, or unease. This technique can be performed in a variety of ways. See Box 5.1 for one simple method of increasing basic body awareness while washing one's hands [22] (see Vignette 5.1).

5.1.2.3 Soles of the Feet Meditation

Anger and frustration are emotions that can be difficult to manage and may lead to verbal or physical aggressive reactions. There has been much research conducted to measure the effect of a mindfulness meditation titled "Soles of the Feet." These studies have found that use of this technique results in reduction in aggressive behavior and decreased feelings of anger [23]. This particular strategy holds many benefits in that it can be performed anywhere in any setting, sitting/standing/walking, is remarkably simple to follow, and does not require a significant amount of time to complete. The steps for this meditation are listed in Box 5.2 [24].

5.1.2.4 Structured Breathwork

Breathing is a natural process and often one which requires little thought or consideration. At its core, breathing is the body's regulatory mechanism responsible for maintaining appropriate gas exchange, ensuring adequate oxygen and carbon dioxide levels as well as a suitable pH to allow for proper system-wide functioning of the body as a whole [25]. As healthcare professionals (HCPs), we are also aware of the respiratory response in times of stress or perceived threat, inherent to the "fight or flight" response in which the body inherently increases the heart rate and respiratory rate, and sense of vigilance, to prepare one to fight or flee. It is well documented that a body in a constant or prolonged state of stress begins to exert negative effects on the overall functioning of the body's systems. Further research notes that the work of HCPs produces high-enough stress levels to result in mental health conditions, burnout, and leaving the profession [26]. Structured breath work has gained attention recently to reduce and/or mitigate the effects of an ever-increasingly stressful healthcare environment.

Meditative practices, such as Yoga, have long made use of intentional breathing and active modification of breathing patterns to increase relaxation and personal insight during one's practice [27]. Recent research on focused breathing techniques in healthy individuals has proven successful in stress and anxiety reduction as well as increased emotional awareness [25, 27, 28]. The body's inherent breathing pattern is controlled mainly by the brain to maintain adequate gas exchange, a top-down process. This process can also be reversed by focused or controlled breathing which affects processes in the brain such as mood and/or perception of the situation at hand, a bottom-up process. It is important to note that altering one's breathing pattern does not alter the environment but can help to reduce one's internal stress or anxiety while working in the current environment [25]. One such technique that can be utilized in a hectic healthcare environment is called Box Breathing or Square Breathing. See Box 5.3 for an example [29].

5.1.2.5 Scanning for Normalcy

Maintaining focus in a hectic, stress-inducing environment seems an overwhelming and unobtainable task. Yet this is what we ask of and expect from HCPs daily. Mindfulness-related research has discovered that tapping into one's senses can help one to regain focus in the midst of chaos [30]. It is important to note, as previously stated, that the intent of any Mindfulness practice is not to obtain control of a situation but to provide insight into the fact that one has control of their response to the situation at hand.

Practices utilizing a focus on the sense of sight can be especially helpful in allowing one to regain focus during trying times. One such practice is called "Scanning for Normalcy." This technique can be performed in just about any situation, though it is not recommended when one is driving, and takes little time to complete. This practice includes turning the head to help activate the Vagus nerve, which can be helpful in alleviating stress, while noting the ordinary objects in one's visual field helps to break the "fight or flight" response which cues the individual to scan for threats. This practice serves to ground the individual in the normalcy of the environment to allow for decreased levels of stress and regained focus [50]. Scanning for normalcy can be performed as suggested in Box 5.4.

5.1.2.6 Mindful Movement

Mindful movement premise can be applied to almost any activity where one practices being in, or mindfully inhabiting their body. Mindful movement brings together three powerful tools—the body, the breath, and the mind. Most often mindful movement is coupled with the practice of yoga or walking but called upon at any time.

Yoga improves flexibility, strength, and balance of the entire body, and contributes to feeling energized after the practice. There is a difference between exercise which focuses on what the body is doing, pushing and being goal (internal or external) driven, and Yoga, where space is created to lean about yourself without striving, forcing, or judging and to just practice being [7]. A systematic review performed by Jung and colleagues [31] found that mindfulness-based interventions did not make a statistical difference on burnout of HCPs, but yoga did, which has been validated by several recent studies [32–34] (see Vignette 5.2). Both mindfulness-based interventions and mindful movement are interventions that can support the HCP.

Walking meditation is an amazingly simple way to bring awareness into daily life, including movement throughout a hospital or within a unit from room to room or on a break. Meditation while walking brings attention to the experience of walking when walking. It is knowing that you are walking and focusing on the act of walking. Not walking, and thinking about all the things that need to get done or absorbed in one's own thoughts. By mindfully walking, one is concentrating on one movement of a step, at a time, with awareness, starting with the legs or feet first. With further practice one can increase their awareness to their body walking, breathing, sights, sounds, or the feel of air on the skin [7].

5.1.2.7 Body Check-Ins

Feeling hunger, thirst, or stress in the body and then mindfully responding to the body's cues reinforce a feeling of safety in the body. By stepping out of a fight-or-flight response, the HCP can step into the role of a caregiver that can create a healing environment, for ourselves and those we serve. When sitting at a computer, neck and shoulder rolls can be used as tension is acknowledged. Intuitive movement is listening to the body and its wisdom that informs what is needed, and then honoring that. For instance, drinking when thirsty or using the bathroom when prompted is a form honoring the body's needs that activates the parasympathetic nervous system (see Vignette 5.3).

5.1.3 Rethinking Compassion Fatigue

One of the main challenges facing HCPs is the emotionally demanding job of caring for people who are suffering. The continual exposure to another's suffering can cause HCPs to have similar feelings of distress and negative consequences of caregiving known as compassion fatigue and burnout [35]. Burnout, as defined by Maslach et al., is a prolonged response to chronic work-related emotional and relational stressors, identified by emotional exhaustion, depersonalization, and lack of perceived social accomplishments [36]. Burnout is not limited to a specific profession, while what is referred to as "compassion fatigue" is experienced only by those professionals who witness the suffering of others [37].

Compassion fatigue was first identified by Figley (1995) and described as personal suffering related to working with traumatic situations or being in the presence of another's distress and overly identifying with their negative emotions [37]. The term compassion fatigue is often used by HCPs to describe work-related physical and mental exhaustion. This shows up as emotional disconnection from patients, feelings of isolation, and lack of interest and ability to care for both self and others [38].

A frequent issue of the misunderstanding of compassion is the confusion with empathy. These terms are often used interchangeably [39]. When HCPs empathize with patients' distress, to some degree it is experienced as their own [40]. Neuroimaging studies show that the same sections of the brain are activated in both the person who is in pain and the person who is witnessing the pain [41]. These studies demonstrate empathy is directed by similar neural networks referred to as mirror neurons and shared neural networks [42, 43]. In general, empathy allows us to resonate with another's emotional state whether positive or negative. Empathic distress means "taking on" another's suffering as one's own, typically causing withdrawal from the painful situation. Exposure to suffering can lead to two outcomes: empathic distress and compassion [43].

A compassionate response toward another who is in pain activates the parts of the brain linked with reward, connection, and protection from stress [41]. This is due to having a compassionate, caring attitude instead of being overly identified with the experience of another's pain. The feelings of connection and caring generated by compassion are positive and fulfilling rather than negative and draining [44]. Additionally, there is motivation to engage in prosocial behavior and act with compassion to relieve suffering [40, 45].

5.1.3.1 Self-Compassion as a Buffer against Empathic Distress

It is essential that HCPs understand that empathic emotions are in response to witnessing another's suffering and is not their own suffering [42]. When applied during empathic distress, self-compassion provides an antidote for HCPs and allows for the delivery of authentic and compassionate care [46]. For self-compassion to be adopted to alleviate empathic distress, widespread compassion education is necessary [38] (see Fig. 5.1).

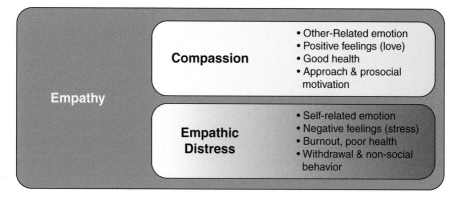

Fig. 5.1 Empathy. Adapted from: Singer T., Klimecki O.M. Empathy and compassion. *Curr. Biol.* 2014;24(18):R875–R878. https://www.sciencedirect.com/science/article/pii/S0960982214007702

Self-compassion can be learned and cultivated and may strengthen resilience as well as bring about increased attachment with self and others [47]. Compassion training does not decrease or eliminate negative emotions. Instead, it increases activation in the brain areas associated with connection, positive emotions, and reward. This is the reason compassion training is effective as a buffer against empathic distress [45].

Psychologist Kristin Neff was the first researcher to define and measure self-compassion. She describes self-compassion as being kind and supportive toward ourselves (particularly when we make a mistake) rather than being harsh and critical. Self-compassion means treating ourselves with the same kindness and understanding that we would offer a good friend in the same situation [48]. Studies show harsh self-talk and self-criticism activates the sympathetic nervous system that stimulates the threat response, harming our mental health and well-being [41].

According to Neff there are three components of self-compassion: self-kindness, common humanity, and mindfulness. The counterparts to self-compassion are self-judgment, isolation, and over-identification, respectively [48].

As summarized below, self-compassion has three components:

1. Self-Kindness vs Self-Judgment
   - Treat ourselves with kindness and understanding rather than harsh self-criticism and judgment, similar to how we would treat a good friend.
   - Compassion involves a concern to do something about suffering. This active component includes comforting, protecting, and supporting ourselves when we are in pain.
   - The word suffering is used to describe any mental, emotional, or physical discomfort.
2. Common Humanity vs Isolation
   - Seeing our imperfections as part of the human condition rather than feeling like we are alone in our suffering.
   - Often when we struggle or fail, we tend to feel isolated as if we are the only ones in that situation.
3. Mindfulness vs. Over-Identification
   - For us to give ourselves compassion, we have to first recognize that we are struggling in some way.
   - Mindfulness gives us the ability to see clearly what is happening and turn toward difficult feelings, making space for the emotions just as they are.
   - We do not get caught up in the drama about what is happening but understand what is here with a balanced state of awareness [48].

Self-compassion allows us to be with ourselves in a compassionate way—comforting, reassuring, and validating. This, in turn, prepares us to make self-compassionate choices when acting in the world, by protecting, providing for, and motivating ourselves to keep us safe and meet our needs [48].

5.1.3.2 Physiology of Self-Compassion

When we offer ourselves self-compassion, we are accessing the mammalian care-giving system. The care-giving system works by causing the release of oxytocin which increases feelings of safety, trust, calm, and connection with others. This in turn promotes warmth and compassion for ourselves. Oxytocin is released in various social situations such as when a mother breastfeeds her child, a tender touch is given or received, or when parents and young children interact [49]. The mammalian care-giving system is activated by two essential elements: gentle touch and soft vocalizations [50]. The extraordinary part about self-compassion is that it does not matter whether kind thoughts, emotions, or touch are offered to ourselves or others. The physiological effect is the same!

While self-compassion supports us, self-criticism has a distinctly different effect on our bodies. When a threat is detected in the environment by the amygdala, the fight-or-flight response is activated. Signals from the amygdala cause the release of hormones including adrenaline and cortisol. The body reacts physiologically, preparing itself to run away or confront the threat. This system evolved to deal with physical threats but is also activated by emotional attacks from others and ourselves. When we criticize ourselves, we activate the same response [48].

5.1.3.3 Benefits

Self-compassion de-activates the threat response and mobilizes the care-giving system. When applied in a moment of difficulty, this causes oxytocin and endorphins to be released, increasing feelings of safety and reducing stress. Comforting and soothing ourselves when painful emotions are present or when we notice self-criticism changes not only our emotional state but also our body chemistry [49]. Greater self-compassion promotes improved psychological health, such as reduced anxiety and depression [51]. Positive states including happiness, life satisfaction, and optimism are strongly associated with self-compassion [52]. Empirical data demonstrate that health care professionals who practice self-compassion have greater satisfaction with one's care-giving role [53].

5.1.3.4 Self-Care and Self-Compassion

What makes self-compassion so powerful is that it is so user-friendly. It can be accessed anytime and anywhere—in the midst of caring for a patient or when harsh self-criticism shows up. Self-care is often recommended for HCPs to alleviate emotional distress and burnout. Self-care is essential to well-being but is limited as far as accessibility is concerned. You cannot excuse yourself for a bubble bath, yoga practice, or a vacation while at work, but you can pause momentarily and practice self-compassion. See Box 5.5 for examples [54].

5.1.4 Gratitude

Gratitude has been a topic of note over the past several years and has been recognized to boost happiness and improve life satisfaction. It is fundamental to psychological health and general well-being throughout each stage of human life. A growing body of evidence demonstrates the many benefits associated with gratitude [55]. These benefits include a sense of general well-being [56], less depression and greater life satisfaction [57], greater levels of optimism [58], reinforcing positive emotions [59], and improved physical health [60]. Gratitude is an attitude of appreciation, of giving thanks for the things that we have in life, rather than complaining for the things we do not have. It can be expressed internally toward ourselves or externally toward others who have given us something of value or helped us in some way.

Harvard Medical School defines gratitude as "a thankful appreciation for what an individual receives, whether tangible or intangible. With gratitude, people acknowledge the goodness in their lives. In the process, people usually recognize that the source of that goodness lies at least partially outside themselves. As a result, being grateful also helps people connect to something larger than themselves as individuals–whether to other people, nature, or a higher power" [61]. Emmons states, "Gratitude has been conceptualized as an emotion, a virtue, a moral sentiment, a motive, a coping response, a skill, and an attitude. It is all of these and more. Minimally, gratitude is an emotional response to a gift. It is the appreciation felt after one has been the beneficiary of an altruistic act [56]. See Box 5.6 for the two key components of gratitude.

Gratitude has been held as a desirable trait throughout history in virtually all cultures. Like any practice, it must be learned and cultivated to become integrated into one's life [55]. See Box 5.7 for examples. Psychologists have identified several gratitude exercises that can be practiced to cultivate and strengthen gratitude. These practices invite people to pause and take a moment to notice, savor, acknowledge, and respond with gratitude to all that is around us in everyday life.

5.2 Application of the Principles into a Wellness Practice

Well-being and preventative mental health care must be built-in across the healthcare continuum and HCP continuum. The pandemic has only made the need for these programs and system changes more critical, as record numbers of HCPs are leaving the medical establishment from burnout, toxic work environments, and poor compensation. HCPs who are at risk for marginalization (such as, but not limited to, LGBQT+, Black, Latinx, Muslim, or female) deal with increased toxicity in the environments that must be addressed [62]. By incorporating mindfulness practices and self-compassion a person can move into a parasympathetic state allowing for more creativity, imagining and implementing innovative solutions to decades-old problems and habits.

Mindfulness and self-compassion are evidence-based ways to increase resilience, yet relying only on those for worker well-being without reforming systems will not help the HCP. Mindfulness practices can no longer be laid down at the feet of the individual HCPs to help them cope with stress without also addressing system issues. Mindfulness cannot be used in isolation to avoid changing toxic systems. HCPs in positions of leadership and power need to use these tools, but then acknowledge how the systems, hospitals, government, and insurance companies contribute to stress and address root causes. Later chapters within this text address many of the root causes of stress.

5.2.1 Pre-Licensure Application in the Academic Environment

Inclusion of mindfulness-based practices has been proven to translate to more compassionate healthcare practices. Intentional teaching of mindfulness practices including self-compassion and reflection can cultivate a state of self-compassion [65]. Multiple studies have already proven the benefits of utilizing self-compassion strategies to HCP curriculum to increase self-compassion and improve the confidence of students in providing grounded, calm, and compassionate care [65].

Though, the recent evidence discovered by neuroscientists on empathic distress has yet to be integrated into HCP education and research, compassion fatigue continues to be the dominant term. Leaders in the field have a duty to understand the cause of empathic distress to provide appropriate resources for students and HCPs [38]. Academics and educators have an important role in teaching healthcare students about empathic distress, emotion regulation, and empathy [66].

5.2.2 Clinical Application Post-Licensure

HCPs are often overwhelmed with tasks which can create a state of stress and anxiety. HCPs must also cope with extremely difficult situations that need timely and accurate decision-making. Those decisions affect human lives in insignificant or profound ways [67] . Mindfulness can be performed on the spot and calms the nervous system, which allows the HCP to be more present in mind and body. This promotes a safer, focused, and attentive interaction with patients at the bedside.

A research article, by Andrews et al. [68], described the phenomena that nurses need permission from others for self-care and self-compassion. Nurses and other HCPs waiting for permission, consider this your permission slip to care compassionately for yourself first, so that you can care compassionately for others and have a long, resilient career. But even better than a permission slip, you do not need permission, and independently engage in practices that support your well-being! It is crucial that HCP find and cultivate practices that benefit their well-being in a way that is personal to them and resonates with their uniqueness.

Context informs the experience of self-compassion such as system's issues, the work environment, and workload [69]. No amount of mindfulness can change the external situation, only help with the internal reaction to it and create a space between the external healthcare system and the patient interaction. Mindfulness does not excuse a toxic or dangerous work environment. In practice, it is important to foster a sense of discernment (is my response a reaction to issues of self, the situation, or a combination of the two?) to keep focused and be able to identify needed changes in either self and/or situation.

5.2.3 Leadership Application

When implementing mindfulness programs in the workplace, leaders must be clear on the intent. Is this program being launched to improve retention, metrics, or outcomes? Or is it a genuine, compassionate, and non-judgmental approach to supporting employees in whatever way the HCP needs, so they show up for themselves first and are able to care for others in a way that is fulfilling for them? Employees know the intention behind programs; as leaders it is crucial to be transparent with offerings, otherwise it will be met with suspicion or resentment. Slavin [62] recommends changing the focus from well-being programs to directly addressing problems and situations that HCPs are facing. This shifts the focus to the experience of work, rather than encouraging wellness practices outside of work as a way to "deal with" work [62]. It is inexcusable to limit wellness programs to responsibilities of the individual excluding addressing root causes of poor working conditions. When HCPs are unable to do their best due to system issues, it causes distress due to the care they know they can give versus the care they are able to give. Recognizing the limitations and addressing the barriers to providing care excellence in the eyes of the HCP will help decrease stress at an organizational level.

The COVID-19 pandemic has put more burden on HCPs as they are experiencing a level of stress much greater than at any other time in their career. The acute and then chronic, stress response increased the concern for long-term mental and physical health consequences. The traditional coping method of HCPs, "I am fine," is no longer sustainable and in retrospect should never have been acceptable. The time is now to develop and implement a clear approach for professional wellness in learning environments and in work [70]. It is also critical to know when to refer to other mental health professionals and have a clear scope on the programs. While developing, revising, or contemplating mindfulness and wellness programs, be aware of who is providing financial or time assistance for the work on these initiatives. Free up time or compensate the employees who will be working on this endeavor. Another option is to hire a Wellness Officer whose only job is staff wellness into a high-level leadership position, just like many organizations are doing for diversity, inclusion, and equity.

In this time of uncertainty, ongoing pandemic, and disruption, having emotional balance, clarity, vision, and fortitude with the help of self-compassion will assist those in leadership roles move forward with clear action and resiliency [71]. As a leader, have a strong mindfulness practice and be aware of the tone you set for those who work with you. Being an HCP leader is a difficult job; balancing a broken healthcare system with the needs of patients and HCP staff is complex. Having a grounded, present, and compassionate approach will go a long way in advocating, advancing, and changing the healthcare system while providing the needed support for HCPs.

5.3   Opportunities for Future Research

Mindfulness is not one-size-fits-all intervention, and the risk of harm needs to be addressed. Most studies to this point have focused on measuring the benefits of mindfulness. As with all interventions, there is risk for harm [63]. From the teacher, the method, to the participants, underlying life experience, trauma, and training can all play a role in possible negative side-effects of mindfulness. In a review of the literature, Baer [64] found that 1–10% of mindfulness practitioners experienced adverse effects such as negative emotions, anxiety, and depression, which can be even more exacerbated for participants with a history of trauma. When implementing mindfulness programs, teachers must be trauma-informed and know how and when to intervene and who to refer to when the risks outweigh the benefits.

The areas of mindfulness, compassion, and gratitude are strongly supported by scientific literature. Focus research on implementing a personalized approach to programming. The COVID-19 pandemic will be highly impactful on HCP's health, and research is needed to develop interventions for long-term resiliency in ongoing public health crisis. With a top-down approach, focus work on systems-level harm such as how the current state of the healthcare system (local and national) is a burden to providing safe, effective, and equitable care. With a bottom-up approach, mindfulness in the hands of the HCP can increase resiliency while the healthcare delivery system is being improved.

Glossary

Mindfulness The practice of purposely bringing one's attention in the present moment without evaluation.
Compassion A feeling of concern for another person's suffering, which is accompanied by the motivation to help.
Empathy General capacity to resonate with others' emotional states irrespective of their valence—positive or negative.
Empathic distress Strong aversive and self-oriented response to the suffering of others, accompanied by the desire to withdraw from a situation to protect oneself from excessive negative feelings.

Discussion Questions

1. Share a practice from this chapter that resonated with you. Explain why and how you can implement it in your life.
2. Describe signs of empathetic distress. What support could you give a colleague who might be experiencing empathetic distress?
3. Describe ways self-compassion can lead to increased capacity as a healthcare professional and be a buffer against empathetic distress.
4. Take a moment to be in your body. What feelings, sensations, or emotions can you identify, and just observe? No need to take any action.
5. Describe the physiology of self-compassion. What are examples of where you can use self-compassion in your life? Did you realize that your thoughts can change your body's chemistry?

Discussion Leader Guide

1. Guide participants to share their insights with each other while actively listening.
2. For signs of empathetic distress, see Fig. 5.1. Role-play how to approach someone who might be experiencing empathetic distress.
3. Some examples include: strengthen resilience, antidote for empathetic distress, positive feeling of connection and caring, delivery of authentic and compassionate care, treating ourselves with the same kindness and understanding that we would offer a good friend in the same situation, etc.
4. Can thoughts, sensations, emotions be identified without taking action? Was resistance noted or going into thinking or problem solving an engrained response? How could mindfulness help?
5. Lead a discussion with the group about the power of thoughts. Identify how participants can use self-compassion in their lives. Self-compassion de-activates the threat response and mobilizes the care-giving system. When applied in a moment of difficulty, this causes oxytocin and endorphins to be released increasing feelings of safety and reducing stress. Comforting and soothing ourselves when painful emotions are present or when we notice self-criticism changes not only our emotional state but also our body chemistry.

Video for Discussion: Mindfulness and Compassion Practice

Video for Discussion - Instructional Video: The online version contains supplementary material available at https://doi.org/10.1007/978-3-031-16983-0_5

Vignette 5.1 Hand Hygiene
Jody Atkinson, MSN, RN, CCRN

Working in a Med/Surg/Oncology ICU can be stressful. Add a pandemic involving a newly discovered virus with no known cure and consistently changing guidelines, addressing all aspects from standards of care to PPE recommendations, and you can easily cross from stress to panic. This was the state of my unit as we first started caring for COVID-19 patients. My coworkers and I often discussed our concerns in regard to how to safeguard ourselves from contracting the virus or worse, contracting it and carrying it to our families. Feelings of hopelessness and fear that we may not find effective treatment in time only grew with each patient who died. We held their hand and comforted them since their families were not allowed visitation. As the doors to the ICU opened, I could feel the heaviness and I seemed to assume that weight like a winter coat on my shoulders as I crossed the threshold. My colleagues often described the same sensation as we began our shifts each morning.

I had been a member of my organization's Holistic Practice Committee for some time. In the early days of the pandemic, our chair had the foresight to focus on opportunities for self-care to increase the mental health and well-being of our staff. Over the next months, we would meet with a variety of Holistic and Integrative Medicine practitioners and specialists who provided those in attendance with a variety of self-care strategies. While attending one of these meetings, we began to discuss how we could extend the reach of these practices to our colleagues who were not present and able to participate in the offerings. One of the committee members discussed how she had begun reciting mantras to herself as she washed her hands. A lightbulb went off in my head; I recalled the number of times that I had used handwashing as a cue to say a prayer or place an intention for friends or family members over the years. Every healthcare worker washes their hands multiple times daily; if we could couple that with an opportunity for self-care, imagine the impact we could have on levels of stress, anxiety, fear, and morale!

After gaining approval from my management, I found a few positive affirmations, meditations, and reflections that I felt would be appropriate. Over the next few months, I created a number of "Handwashing Meditations" and attached a copy to each of the paper towel dispensers located next to the sinks throughout the unit. Of course, some of my coworkers felt this a little too "touchy feely." Others though told me that having the visual reminder to refocus and re-center multiple times daily helped keep their spirits up. I felt a positive impact to my own well-being. While performing these handwashing meditations, a little bit of the heaviness left my shoulders and I felt ready and capable to move on to the next task after having taken the time to check-in. Taking the time to care for myself allowed me to become more clued into my own well-being and that of my colleagues. I spent more time checking-in on my coworkers, sitting down for just a moment to ask how they were doing instead of getting caught up in the never-ending tasks of the day. This simple practice has stayed with me, allowing me the opportunity to take a moment to be present both to myself and those around me.

As you wash your hands, follow this practice to ground yourself and your thoughts.......

Inhale deeply for a count of 4

As you exhale, repeat "**I am safe, I am safe, I am safe**"

Inhale deeply for a count of 4

As you exhale, repeat "**I am healthy, I am healthy, I am healthy**"

Inhale deeply for a count of 4

As you exhale, repeat "**I am strong, I am strong, I am strong**"

Inhale deeply for a count of 4

As you exhale, repeat "**I am safe, I am healthy, I am strong, I've got this!**"

Box 5.1 Mindful Handwashing
1. Take a deep breath (or two), in through the nose and out through the mouth. Throughout this practice, acknowledge and observe any thoughts or feelings that may arise but allow them to pass and redirect your focus to the present.
2. How does your body feel? Is there tightness in your neck or shoulders? If so, visualize the release of this tension.
3. Focus on the water temperature. Is it hot/cold/lukewarm? Does it need to be adjusted?
4. How does the soap in your hands feel? How do your hands feel as they glide past one another? Take the time to massage your palms and fingers; how does this feel?
5. As you rinse your hands, listen to the sound of the water; watch as it drains. How do your hands feel as compared to when you first started?
6. Before turning the water off, check-in again with your body. Is there any tension or tightness? Are there specific emotions or feelings that arise? If so, acknowledge and observe this in a non-judgmental manner.
7. While drying your hands, how does the towel/paper towel feel? How does it feel on your skin? Take one or two more deep breaths, in through your nose and out through your mouth.
    Telluride Regional Medical Center, 2020 [22].

Box 5.2 Soles of the Feet Mediation
1. Assume a relaxed, natural stance. Ensure feet are flat on the floor, arms uncrossed.
2. Think of the event or encounter that led to a feeling of anger. Relive the moments of this event or encounter.
3. Allow yourself to feel this anger; note if/where this anger displays as a physical response (tense shoulders/neck/back/jaw, increased heart rate, etc.). Let thoughts flow freely; do not push them away; sit with this anger.
4. Now shift your focus to the soles of your feet.
5. Slowly and deliberately begin to move your toes, feeling the inside of your shoes, the texture of your socks, flexing and extending the arch of your foot, and shift your heel to feel the back of your shoe.
6. Breathe naturally and maintain your focus on the soles of your feet until the feeling of anger is replaced with a feeling of calm.
7. Once calm, assess the best response to the situation and act accordingly.
   Positive Psychology, n.d [24].

Box 5.3 Box Breathing Example
Box breathing can be performed sitting or standing, though it is recommended that one sit upright in a comfortable chair with feet flat on the floor. The technique consists of four steps:

1. Inhale through the nose slowly and deeply for a count of four. Pay attention to how this feels to fill the lungs; imagine doing so section by section until the air reaches the abdomen.
2. Hold the breath for the same slow count of four.
3. Exhale through the mouth for the same slow count of four. Pay attention to how this feels to fully empty the lungs and abdomen.
4. Hold the breath for the same slow count of four.

Repeat this process for a total of four cycles as needed to achieve a sense of calm; it is important to note that beginners to this practice may become dizzy or lightheaded and may need to limit the number of cycles completed [29].

Vignette 5.2 Health
Heather McCain, RN, RYT

I was at a difficult time in my life, which led me to yoga. I was encouraged to take teacher training for personal growth. The training changed me in a positive way with each class. Teaching brings so much joy, confidence, and improved communication skills. I want to live the life I teach my students to live.

During COVID-19, the morale has been so low. I wanted to bring an activity to employees that would give them something to look forward to and a soul reboot during their shift. I implemented Yoga on the Lawn at my hospital and offer it twice a month. It gives employees a moment to practice self-care, which tends to be the last care humans provide. I want this experience to be the light in the middle of a rough and busy day. My main goal, as a yoga teacher and nurse, is to bring a smile or sense of peace to each HCP who practices with me.

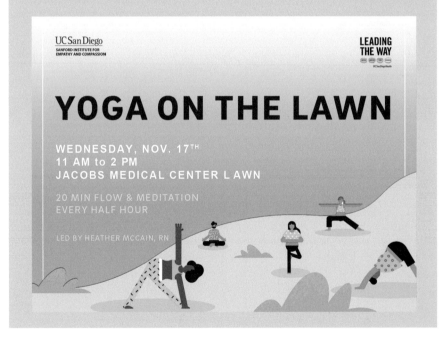

Box 5.4 Scanning for Normalcy
1. Turn the head to the left, keeping your eyes open.
2. Slowly turn the head to the right, keeping eyes open.
3. As you turn your head, note the "ordinary" or "normal" objects that are in your line of sight (i.e., pen, paper, computer, and desk) [65].

Vignette 5.3 Mindfulness Tools at Work
Melissa Forde, BSN, RN, RYT

When I was first learning to incorporate mindfulness into my daily life and work, the best advice I received was to use naturally occurring cues in my environment as a reminder to stop and check-in with my body. Even on really busy days, while working as a nurse in a hospital, I found ways to reclaim moments for myself by putting this advice to use. Every time I took a patient's vital signs, I would make a point of feeling my feet on the ground, deepening my breath, and centering myself in the present moment. Whenever I had to wait in line at the Pyxis to pull meds, I would notice the tension in my shoulders and stretch my neck. After repeating these things over and over, checking-in with my body became something I automatically did constantly throughout my day—and the more present I was able to be with myself, the greater capacity I had to be present with my coworkers and patients.

While working as a home hospice nurse, I had the honor of taking care of a terminally ill seven-year-old girl. Taking care of dying children is as heart wrenching as you might imagine. There is definitely a temptation to disconnect from the moment and dissociate from the painful emotions swirling around everything. While working on this case, I used my mindfulness muscles to return to my breath each time I felt overwhelmed. In the moments when everything inside me wanted to fix things for my patient's parents (who were facing the most devastating loss I can imagine), I took deep breaths and sat in silence with them instead. My willingness to witness their pain without trying to fix anything created a space where they felt safe to feel. At one point, while my patient was unconscious and actively dying, her dad commented that he would give anything to go back to when she could talk. Because we had built so much trust, we were able to have a conversation about how after she died, he would probably wish he could go back to the moment we were in, where he could still hold her warm body and feel her breath. In one of the most profound moments of my career, I watched this man come into complete presence with his daughter's death. He nods knowingly and we both gently traced her skin with our hands, appreciating the opportunity to be with her body, while tears ran down our faces.

Aside from supporting my own physical health and helping me be more connected to the people I have served, practicing mindfulness has instilled a radar in me that gives me undeniable information about when I have overextended myself and need to take a break. In the context of a system that does a very poor job of taking care of people who take care of people, I believe this is one of the most important tools I have as a nurse. I know the early signs that I am beginning to burn out and I feel confident in holding boundaries and leaving roles that do not support my well-being—because I know something that is making me sick is not helping anyone.

Box 5.5 Practicing Accessible Self-Compassion
1. Become aware of your inner critic—notice how you speak to yourself when you make a mistake, or something does not go well for you.
2. Acknowledge the pain non-judgmentally—e.g., "this hurts," "I am noticing sadness," and "this is difficult for me." Make space for these feelings rather than trying to push them away.
3. Act with kindness—take a kind, rather than harsh, action toward yourself:
   • Self-talk—talk to yourself kindly ("We are human, we all make mistakes"). Try thinking of how you would talk to a friend in the same situation.
   • Self-touch—lay a hand gently on the pain or on a soothing area such as your chest, abdomen, or face, or give yourself a gentle hug (experiment and find what works for you).
   • Self-soothe—find an activity you find soothing (music, yoga, meditation, bath, going for a walk in nature, cup of tea, call a friend, or reading).

Box 5.6 Two Key Components of Gratitude
Robert Emmons, one of the leading experts on gratitude has identified two key components of gratitude:

• Gratitude is an affirmation of the good things in the world we have received.
• Recognition that the source of this goodness is outside of ourselves. We acknowledge that other people, or even higher powers, have given us many gifts to help us along the way and get us to where we are now [58].

Box 5.7 Gratitude Practices
1. Gratitude journal. Write down 3–5 specific blessings on a daily or weekly basis. Focus on gratitude for people rather than material objects. Take time to savor each blessing, and remain open to the unexpected [58].
2. Gratitude letter. Write a letter to someone who you have not yet thanked that expresses what you are specifically thankful for [72].
3. Gratitude conversation. This gratitude practice occurs when people intentionally engage in conversation with others about positive experiences that happen each day. By openly expressing gratitude, people broaden and build up their social bonds with others [73].
4. Write down three things that went well today and identify the causes of those good things [72].
5. See more on Greater Good Gratitude Resource Link [74]: Gratitude Practice for Nurses | Greater Good Science Center (berkeley.edu).

References

1. Cannon WB. Bodily changes in pain, hunger, fear and rage; an account of recent researches into the function of emotional excitement. 2nd ed. New York: D. Appleton and Company; 1929.
2. McCorry LK. Physiology of the autonomic nervous system. Am J Pharm Educ. 2007;71(4):78. https://doi.org/10.5688/aj710478.
3. Selye H. The stress of life. New York: McGraw-Hill; 1956.
4. Lazarus RS, Folkman S. Stress, appraisal, and coping. New York: Springer Pub. Co.; 1984.
5. Tang YY, Hölzel BK, Posner MI. The neuroscience of mindfulness meditation. Nat Rev Neurosci. 2015;16(4):213–25. https://doi.org/10.1038/nrn3916.
6. Gross JJ. Antecedent- and response-focused emotion regulation: divergent consequences for experience, expression, and physiology. J Pers Soc Psychol. 1998;74(1):224–37. https://doi.org/10.1037//0022-3514.74.1.224.
7. Kabat-Zinn J. Full catastrophe living: using the wisdom of your body and mind to face stress, pain, and illness. Revised and updated edition. New York: Bantam Books Trade Paperback; 2013.
8. Kabat-Zinn J. Mindfulness for beginners: reclaiming the present moment—and your life. Boulder, CO: Sounds True; 2012.
9. Hofmann SG, Sawyer AT, Witt AA, Oh D. The effect of mindfulness-based therapy on anxiety and depression: a meta-analytic review. J Consult Clin Psychol. 2010;78(2):169–83. https://doi.org/10.1037/a0018555.
10. Ludwig DS, Kabat-Zinn J. Mindfulness in medicine. JAMA. 2008;300(11):1350–2. https://doi.org/10.1001/jama.300.11.1350.
11. Geary C, Rosenthal SL. Sustained impact of MBSR on stress, well-being, and daily spiritual experiences for 1 year in academic health care employees. J Altern Complement Med. 2011;17(10):939–44. https://doi.org/10.1089/acm.2010.0335.
12. Goodman MJ, Schorling JB. A mindfulness course decreases burnout and improves well-being among healthcare providers. Int J Psychiatry Med. 2012;43(2):119–28. https://doi.org/10.2190/PM.43.2.b.

13. Condon P, Desbordes G, Miller WB, DeSteno D. Meditation increases compassionate responses to suffering. Psychol Sci. 2013;24(10):2125–7. https://doi.org/10.1177/0956797613485603.
14. Beach MC, Roter D, Korthuis PT, Epstein RM, Sharp V, Ratanawongsa N, et al. A multicenter study of physician mindfulness and health care quality. Ann Fam Med. 2013;11(5):421–8. https://doi.org/10.1370/afm.1507.
15. Fortney L, Luchterhand C, Zakletskaia L, Zgierska A, Rakel D. Abbreviated mindfulness intervention for job satisfaction, quality of life, and compassion in primary care clinicians: a pilot study. Ann Fam Med. 2013;11(5):412–20. https://doi.org/10.1370/afm.1511.
16. Aikens KA, Astin J, Pelletier KR, Levanovich K, Baase CM, Park YY, et al. Mindfulness goes to work: impact of an online workplace intervention. J Occup Environ Med. 2014;56(7):721–31. https://doi.org/10.1097/JOM.0000000000000209.
17. Zeidan F, Johnson SK, Diamond BJ, David Z, Goolkasian P. Mindfulness meditation improves cognition: evidence of brief mental training. Conscious Cogn. 2010;19(2):597–605. https://doi.org/10.1016/j.concog.2010.03.014.
18. Ameli R, Sinaii N, West CP, Luna MJ, Panahi S, Zoosman M, et al. Effect of a brief mindfulness-based program on stress in health care professionals at a US biomedical research hospital: a randomized clinical trial. JAMA Netw Open. 2020;3(8):e2013424. https://doi.org/10.1001/jamanetworkopen.2020.13424.
19. Schuman-Olivier Z, Trombka M, Lovas DA, Brewer JA, Vago DR, Gawande R, et al. Mindfulness and behavior change. Harv Rev Psychiatry. 2020;28(6):371–94. https://doi.org/10.1097/HRP.0000000000000277.
20. Farb N, Daubenmier J, Price CJ, Gard T, Kerr C, Dunn BD, et al. Interoception, contemplative practice, and health. Front Psychol. 2015;6:763. https://doi.org/10.3389/fpsyg.2015.00763.
21. Guendelman S, Medeiros S, Rampes H. Mindfulness and emotion regulation: insights from neurobiological, psychological, and clinical studies. Front Psychol. 2017;8:220. https://doi.org/10.3389/fpsyg.2017.00220.
22. Center TRM: Turn Handwashing Into A Mindfulness Exercise. 2020. https://tellmed.org/news/mindfulhandwashing. Accessed 30 Aug 2021.
23. Fix RL, Fix S. The effects of mindfulness-based treatments for aggression: a critical review. Aggress Violent Behav. 2013;18:219–27. https://doi.org/10.1016/j.avb.2012.11.009.
24. Positive, psychology: positive psychology toolkit: meditation on the soles of the feet. https://positivepsychology.com/wp-content/uploads/Meditation-on-the-Soles-of-the-Feet.pdf. Accessed 8 Sept 2021.
25. Boyadzhieva A, Kayhan E. Keeping the breath in mind: respiration, neural oscillations, and the free energy principle. Front Neurosci. 2021;15:647579. https://doi.org/10.3389/fnins.2021.647579.
26. Reith TP. Burnout in United States healthcare professionals: a narrative review. Cureus. 2018;10(12):e3681. https://doi.org/10.7759/cureus.3681.
27. Zaccaro A, Piarulli A, Laurino M, Garbella E, Menicucci D, Neri B, et al. How breath-control can change your life: a systematic review on psycho-physiological correlates of slow breathing. Front Hum Neurosci. 2018;12:353. https://doi.org/10.3389/fnhum.2018.00353.
28. Brown RP, Gerbarg PL, Muench F. Breathing practices for treatment of psychiatric and stress-related medical conditions. Psychiatr Clin North Am. 2013;36(1):121–40. https://doi.org/10.1016/j.psc.2013.01.001.
29. Healthline: Box Breathing. 2020. https://www.healthline.com/health/box-breathing. Accessed 8 2021.
30. Ahmed M, Sipasuwanchai C, Niksirat K, Ren X. Understanding the role of human senses in interactive meditation. In: CHI '17: Proceedings of the 2017 CHI conference on human factors in computing systems 2017. p. 4960–5.
31. Jung SE, Ha DJ, Park JH, Lee B, Kim MS, Sim KL, et al. The effectiveness and safety of mind-body modalities for mental health of nurses in hospital setting: a systematic review. Int J Environ Res Public Health. 2021;18(16):8855. https://doi.org/10.3390/ijerph18168855.

32. Scheid A, Dyer NL, Dusek JA, Khalsa SBS. A yoga-based program decreases physician burnout in neonatologists and obstetricians at an Academic Medical Center. Workplace Health Saf. 2020;68(12):560–6. https://doi.org/10.1177/2165079920930720.
33. Patronis S, Staffileno BA. Favorable outcomes from an in-person and online feasibility mindful moment pilot study. Holist Nurs Pract. 2021;35(3):158–66. https://doi.org/10.1097/HNP.0000000000000443.
34. Hilcove K, Marceau C, Thekdi P, Larkey L, Brewer MA, Jones K. Holistic nursing in practice: mindfulness-based yoga as an intervention to manage stress and burnout. J Holist Nurs. 2021;39(1):29–42. https://doi.org/10.1177/0898010120921587.
35. Duarte J, Pinto-Gouveia J. The role of psychological factors in oncology nurses' burnout and compassion fatigue symptoms. Eur J Oncol Nurs. 2017;28:114–21. https://doi.org/10.1016/j.ejon.2017.04.002.
36. Maslach C, Schaufeli WB, Leiter MP. Job burnout. Annu Rev Psychol. 2001;52:397–422. https://doi.org/10.1146/annurev.psych.52.1.397.
37. Figley CR. Compassion fatigue: coping with secondary traumatic stress disorder in those who treat the traumatized Brunner/Mazel psychosocial stress series, vol. 23. New York: Brunner/Mazel; 1995.
38. Hofmeyer A, Kennedy K, Taylor R. Contesting the term 'compassion fatigue': integrating findings from social neuroscience and self-care research. Collegian. 2020;27:232–7. https://doi.org/10.1016/j.colegn.2019.07.001.
39. Mills J, Chapman M. Compassion and self-compassion in medicine: self-care for the caregiver. AMJ. 2016;9:87–91. https://doi.org/10.21767/AMJ2016.2583.
40. Klimecki OM, Singer T. Empathic distress fatigue rather than compassion fatigue? Integrating findings from empathy research in psychology and social neuroscience. In: Oakley B, Knafo A, Madhavan G, Wilson DS, editors. Pathological altruism. New York: Oxford University Press; 2012. p. 368–83.
41. Klimecki OM, Leiberg S, Ricard M, Singer T. Differential pattern of functional brain plasticity after compassion and empathy training. Soc Cogn Affect Neurosci. 2014;9(6):873–9. https://doi.org/10.1093/scan/nst060.
42. Singer T, Klimecki OM. Empathy and compassion. Curr Biol. 2014;24(18):R875–R8. https://doi.org/10.1016/j.cub.2014.06.054.
43. Vrticka P, Favre P, Singer T. Compassion and the brain. In: Gilbert P, editor. Compassion: concepts, research and applications. New York: Routledge; 2017. p. 135–50.
44. Goetz JL, Keltner D, Simon-Thomas E. Compassion: an evolutionary analysis and empirical review. Psychol Bull. 2010;136(3):351–74. https://doi.org/10.1037/a0018807.
45. Klimecki OM. The plasticity of social emotions. Soc Neurosci. 2015;10(5):466–73. https://doi.org/10.1080/17470919.2015.1087427.
46. Neff K, Germer CK. The mindful self-compassion workbook: a proven way to accept yourself, build inner strength, and thrive. New York, NY: Guilford Press; 2018.
47. Vachon MLS. Attachment, empathy and compassion in the care of the bereaved. Grief Matters. Grief Matters. 2016;19(1):20–5.
48. Neff KD. Self-compassion: the proven power of being kind to yourself. New York: Harper Collins; 2011.
49. Neff KD. The physiology of self-compassion: our bodies know how to feel care. 2012. https://www.psychologytoday.com/us/blog/the-power-self-compassion/201207/the-physiology-self-compassion. Accessed 20 Aug 2021.
50. Stellar JE, Keltner D. Compassion. In: Tugade MM, Shiota MN, Kirby LD, editors. Handbook of positive emotions. New York: The Guilford Press; 2014. p. 329–41.
51. Neff KD. The development and validation of a scale to measure self-compassion. Self Identity. 2003;2:223–50.
52. Neff KD, Rude SS, Kirpatick KL. An examination of self-compassion in relation to positive psychological functioning and personality traits. J Res Pers. 2007;41(4):908–16.

53. Raab K. Mindfulness, self-compassion, and empathy among health care professionals: a review of the literature. J Health Care Chaplain. 2014;20(3):95–108. https://doi.org/10.108 0/08854726.2014.913876.
54. Neff KD, Knox MC, Long P, Gregory K. Caring for others without losing yourself: an adaptation of the mindful self-compassion program for healthcare communities. J Clin Psychol. 2020;76(9):1543–62. https://doi.org/10.1002/jclp.23007.
55. Emmons RA, Mishra A. Why gratitude enhances well-being: what we know, what we need to know. In: Sheldon KM, Kashdan TB, Steger MF, editors. Designing. Positive psychology: taking stock and moving forward. New York: Oxford University Press; 2011. p. 48–62.
56. Emmons R, Crumpler C. Gratitude as a human strength: appraising the evidence. J Soc Clin Psychol. 2000;19(1):56–69. https://doi.org/10.1521/jscp.2000.19.1.56.
57. Wood A, Joseph S, Maltby J. Gratitude uniquely predicts satisfaction with life: incremental validity above the domains and facets of the five factor model. Personal Individ Differ. 2008;45(1):49–54. https://doi.org/10.1016/j.paid.2008.02.019.
58. Emmons R, McCullough M. Counting blessings versus burdens: an experimental investigation of gratitude and subjective Well-being in daily life. J Pers Soc Psychol. 2003;84(2):377–89. https://doi.org/10.1037/0022-3514.84.2.377.
59. Amin A. The 31 benefits of gratitude you didn't know about: How gratitude can change your life. 2014. https://www.happierhuman.com/benefits-of-gratitude/. Accessed 26 Sept 2021.
60. Hill PL, Allemand M, Roberts BW. Examining the pathways between gratitude and self-rated physical health across adulthood. Pers Individ Dif. 2013;54(1):92–6. https://doi.org/10.1016/j.paid.2012.08.011.
61. Harvard, Health Publishing, School HM: Giving thanks can make you happier. 2021. https://www.health.harvard.edu/healthbeat/giving-thanks-can-make-you-happier.. Accessed 14 Aug 2021.
62. Slavin S. Reimagining Well-being initiatives in medical education: shifting from promoting wellness to increasing satisfaction. Acad Med. 2021;96(5):632–4. https://doi.org/10.1097/ACM.0000000000004023.
63. Britton WB. Can mindfulness be too much of a good thing? The value of a middle way. Curr Opin Psychol. 2019;28:159–65. https://doi.org/10.1016/j.copsyc.2018.12.011.
64. Baer R, Crane C, Miller E, Kuyken W. Doing no harm in mindfulness-based programs: conceptual issues and empirical findings. Clin Psychol Rev. 2019;71:101–14. https://doi.org/10.1016/j.cpr.2019.01.001.
65. Hagerman LA, Manankil-Rankin L, Schwind JK. Self-compassion in undergraduate nursing: an integrative review. Int J Nurs Educ Scholarsh. 2020;17(1):2020–0021. https://doi.org/10.1515/ijnes-2020-0021.
66. Levett-Jones T, Cant R, Lapkin S. A systematic review of the effectiveness of empathy education for undergraduate nursing students. Nurse Educ Today. 2019;75:80–94. https://doi.org/10.1016/j.nedt.2019.01.006.
67. Pipe TB, Bortz JJ, Dueck A, Pendergast D, Buchda V, Summers J. Nurse leader mindfulness meditation program for stress management: a randomized controlled trial. J Nurs Adm. 2009;39(3):130–7. https://doi.org/10.1097/NNA.0b013e31819894a0.
68. Andrews H, Tierney S, Seers K. Needing permission: the experience of self-care and self-compassion in nursing: a constructivist grounded theory study. Int J Nurs Stud. 2020;101:103436. https://doi.org/10.1016/j.ijnurstu.2019.103436.
69. Barron K, Deery R, Sloan G. Community mental health nurses' and compassion: an interpretative approach. J Psychiatr Ment Health Nurs. 2017;24(4):211–20. https://doi.org/10.1111/jpm.12379.
70. Morrow E, Call M, Ransco M, Hofmann KM, Locke A. Sustaining workforce Well-being: a model for supporting system resilience during the COVID-19 pandemic. Glob Adv Health Med. 2021;10:2164956121991816. https://doi.org/10.1177/2164956121991816.
71. Fernandez F, Stern S. Self-compassion will make you a better leader. https://hbr.org/2020/11/self-compassion-will-make-you-a-better-leader. 2020. Accessed 19 Sept 2021.

72. Seligman ME, Steen TA, Park N, Peterson C. Positive psychology progress: empirical validation of interventions. Am Psychol. 2005;60(5):410–21. https://doi.org/10.1037/0003-066X.60.5.410.
73. Fredrickson BL. Gratitude, like other positive emotions, broadens and builds. In: Emmons RA, McCullough ME, editors. The psychology of gratitude. New York: Oxford University Press; 2004. p. 145–66.
74. Center GGS: Gratitude Practice for Nurses. 2021. https://ggsc.berkeley.edu/gratitudefor-nurses. Accessed 24 Sept 2021.

Animal-Assisted Activity for Clinicians

6

Heather L. Abrahim

Abbreviations

AAA Animal-assisted activity
AAI Animal-assisted intervention
AAT Animal-assisted therapy
HAI Human–animal interaction

Learning Objectives
1. Explain the difference between types of human–animal interaction.
2. Describe how service animals differ from pets and therapy animals.
3. Summarize the potential benefits of animal-assisted activities.
4. Identify ways to incorporate animal-assisted activities into self-care practice.

6.1 Introduction

The relationship between humans and animals has developed over thousands of years [1]. Initially, humans domesticated animals for labor and consumption, but as technology advanced and culture evolved, one of the primary roles of animals changed to that of companion [2]. More people than ever are sharing their homes with companion animals. In fact, worldwide, 57% of consumers report having

H. L. Abrahim (✉)
University of California San Diego Health, San Diego, CA, USA
e-mail: hlabrahim@health.ucsd.edu

© The Author(s), under exclusive license to Springer Nature
Switzerland AG 2023
J. E. Davidson, M. Richardson (eds.), *Workplace Wellness: From Resiliency to Suicide Prevention and Grief Management*, https://doi.org/10.1007/978-3-031-16983-0_6

pets [3]—totaling over 840 million cats and dogs kept as pets globally [4]. Seventy percent of American households—90.5 million homes—have pets; and it is estimated that Americans will spend approximately 109.6 billion dollars on their pets in 2021 [5]. As our knowledge, understanding, and compassion for animals grow, we are finding new ways to involve them in our everyday lives. We are also growing more interested in how our interactions with companion animals can benefit our physical and emotional health [2]. Over three decades ago, the National Institutes of Health held the workshop "The Health Benefits of Pets" which provided an examination and systematic review of the current knowledge in the field and identified areas for future research. Since then, a large body of knowledge has developed regarding the benefits of the human–animal bond [1, 2]. Studies have shown that interaction with animals can improve physical and emotional well-being, assist in management of stress, promote resilience, promote healthy aging, promote social engagement, and strengthen communities [7]. This chapter will explore (1) how the benefits of human–animal interaction can be harnessed to positively impact healthcare worker wellness, and (2) how the use of animal-assisted activity to intentionally stimulate oxytocin release can facilitate the difficult conversations often required in health care.

6.2   Presentation of the Science

Over the past 10–15 years, there has been significant growth in research on the benefits of various types of human–animal interaction (HAI) [6]. Pet ownership—simply living with and caring for a companion animal—has been shown to offer a wealth of benefits, from improved cardiovascular health to greater community engagement [6, 7]. Animal-assisted intervention (AAI)—a structured interaction with a companion animal—has also been shown to provide a breadth of benefits. In the healthcare setting, AAI has demonstrated effectiveness in improved pain relief, decreased anxiety and fatigue, and improved patient satisfaction scores [7]. AAI is provided not by the recipient's personal pet, but by a specially trained companion animal and handler dyad. Animal-assisted therapy is a more formal type of AAI, provided not by a volunteer, but by a trained health professional whose work is aided by a trained companion animal. AAT is based around specific treatment goals tailored to the individual patient. Progress toward these goals is measured and documented in the patient's clinical record [8]. Examples of AAT are an occupational therapist helping a patient improve their fine motor skills by grooming a dog [9] or a psychologist integrating groundwork with horses into a counseling program to enhance a client's positive affect [10]. Because it is a formal clinical intervention, AAT will not be addressed in this chapter.

Another type of HAI frequently utilized in the healthcare setting, and the focus of this chapter, is animal-assisted activity (AAA). AAA is usually provided by a companion animal and a volunteer handler to enhance quality of life by providing motivational, educational, and/or recreational benefits [11]. Examples of AAA are programs where children read to a dog visiting the library or a volunteer handler and

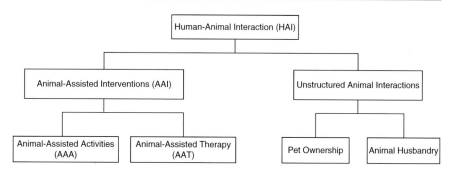

Fig. 6.1 Types of human–animal interaction frequently encountered

dog visit with patients and staff in a hospital. Dogs are the most commonly used companion animal in AAA.

Any discussion of AAI would be incomplete without touching on the role of service animals and emotional support animals. A service animal is a dog or minia- ture horse that has been specially trained to provide a service to an individual with a disability. The service that the animal has been trained to provide is directly related to the individual's disability. Service animal accessibility in public facilities and private businesses is governed by the Americans with Disabilities Act, which requires service animals be allowed to accompany people with disabilities in all areas of the facility where the public is normally allowed to go [12]. Emotional sup- port animals are prescribed by a mental healthcare professional for emotional sup- port of a patient because it is deemed the animal's presence will mitigate the individual's symptoms [13]. Unlike service animals, emotional support animals are not restricted to a certain species, but most are canines. Emotional support animal access is not protected by the Americans with Disabilities Act [12, 13]. Figure 6.1 provides a summary of the types of HAI frequently encountered.

6.2.1 Benefits of Animal-Assisted Activities

Animal-assisted activities have been shown to benefit many aspects of human well- being [14]. This state of the science review will focus on psychosocial variables such as: empathy and social interactions; human physical and mental health, includ- ing effects on hormones and the autonomic nervous system; and on the effects of companion animals in the workplace.

Comprehensive reviews by Beetz [15, 16] found evidence that AAA has positive effects on social interaction, empathy, and mood. Further, AAA was shown to lower stress as indicated by changes in biophysiologic parameters (hormone levels, heart rate, heart rate variability, and blood pressure). Recent studies have found similar outcomes from interaction with trained companion dogs. Unstructured time (15–20 min) with a therapy dog was found to decrease perceived stress [17–19], heart rate [19], and blood pressure [17] in university students and state anxiety levels in men in substance abuse treatment [20]. Women who watched a traumatic film clip reported lower state anxiety and negative affect scores than those who watched the clip alone or with a toy dog (though scores were not significantly different than those who watched the traumatic film clip with a friendly stranger) [21]. In another study, students in an undergraduate psychology class had decreased salivary cortisol levels, a biomarker that increases with stress, after a 20-min group interaction with a therapy dog [22].

In the work environment, the presence of a friendly dog has been shown to have positive impacts on employee interactions, job perception, and stress. In small workgroups, dog presence was found to increase prosocial behaviors (e.g., cooperation, friendliness, comfort, level of activity, enthusiasm, attention) [23]. Research has also looked specifically at healthcare work environments and the ability of AAA to positively affect burnout—a reaction to the chronic stress of the healthcare work environment that results in emotional exhaustion, depersonalization, and feeling of a lack of personal accomplishment [24]. A study published in 2021 examined the effect of a pediatric hospital's facility dog—a highly trained canine that provides services to hospital patients and their families—on the hospital's staff. Findings of the study revealed that even though the purpose of the dog was to assist patients and families, the positive impact of the dog's presence impacted hospital staff as well. Compared with matched controls in a hospital without a facility dog, staff in the hospital with a facility dog reported less burnout and depression and better mental health and more positive affect overall [25]. Similar findings were reported in a pilot study of AAA with staff of a hospital-based clinic. In the pilot study, clinic employees who participated in one-hour drop-in sessions with volunteer handler/therapy dog dyads reported improved mood and a decrease in burnout related to interaction with patients [26] (Fig. 6.2).

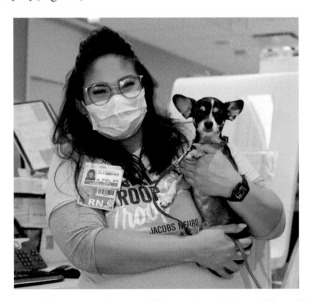

Fig. 6.2 You can see this nurse's smile even with her mask on! A dog visiting with hospital nursing staff improves the mood on the whole unit

6.2.2 Mechanism of Action

Several theories of how AAA exerts its positive influence have been presented in the literature. Some researchers propose that positive AAA outcomes are a result of increases in oxytocin, a hypothalamic hormone released into the brain and the circulation in response to sensory stimulation [15, 27]. Tactile stimulations such as warmth, stroking or petting, and hugging have been shown to increase oxytocin [28]. Oxytocin has a multitude of positive effects including facilitating social bonding and relationship building; increasing empathy; improving communication; decreasing depression, stress, and anxiety; and decreasing heart rate and blood pressure as a result of increased parasympathetic tone [28]. Oxytocin has been proposed as a way to "prime" healthcare providers for potentially difficult conversations (e.g., delivering a diagnosis with a poor prognosis, goals of care conversations) by enhancing the ability to "identify social cues and information in a patient's or caregivers' masked emotional expressions and decreased stress during communications with patients" [29, p. 49] (Fig. 6.3).

6.2.3 Risks Associated with AAA

AAA is generally safe but is not completely risk free. Risks can be broadly grouped into four categories: (1) fear of animals or animal dander allergies; (2) traumatic injuries; (3) zoonotic infection; and (4) animals acting as fomites [7]. Fortunately,

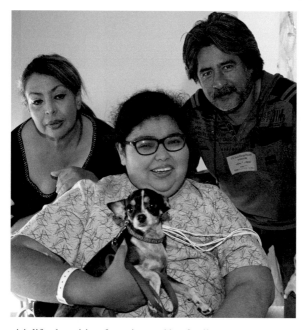

Fig. 6.3 A dog visit lifts the spirits of a patient and her family

most of these risks are easily mitigated. First, excuse those who are afraid of or allergic to animals from participating in AAA. Although not technically a risk, cultural preferences regarding animal interactions must also be considered and accommodated. Second, train and evaluate animals and handlers participating in AAA to assure they can safely interact with participants. Organizations such as Pet Partners, Therapy Dogs International, and Alliance of Therapy Dogs offer temperament evaluations and handler and animal training [7]. Traumatic injuries such as bites, accidental scratches, or trips and falls are unlikely to occur as a result of a well-mannered AAA animal if properly monitored and handled during activities [7].

The third category of risk, zoonotic infection, can be minimized through proper screening of animals participating in AAA. Zoonotic diseases are those that can be transmitted from animals to humans. Most animal diseases are species-specific or not contagious to humans; however, some infections and parasites are transmissible. As noted by Barchas and colleagues [7], in developed countries where mass vaccination of companion animals is combined with effective flea and tick preventative use, zoonotic infection is uncommon. Policy statements are indicated for animals participating in AAA regarding veterinary health screening evaluations, vaccinations, and maintaining a program of flea and tick prevention. Do not feed animals used in AAA a raw food diet. Since cooking kills bacteria and parasites, animals fed raw food diets are more likely to be exposed to and transmit gastrointestinal pathogens. Finally, animals can act as fomites, transmitting an infectious organism from one human to another. The use of universal precautions, especially proper hand hygiene before and after AAA interaction, minimizes this risk. In general, healthy and well-trained animals participating in AAA are unlikely to cause harm [7].

6.3   Application of Principles into Wellness Practice

6.3.1   In the Academic Environment

Programs in the health sciences are ideally suited to incorporate education about animal-assisted interventions in their curricula. With a wide variety of applications across the spectrum of a patient's interaction with the healthcare system, educators are remiss if they fail to expose future healthcare workers to the potential benefits of incorporating animal activities into a plan of holistic patient care and self-care.

Health sciences students can also directly benefit from stress reduction and mood lifting interactions with animals. Programs that prepare healthcare professionals (HCPs) are academically rigorous and notoriously stressful. Incorporating opportunities for AAA either directly in the classroom environment or as an extracurricular activity can provide a much-needed respite and emotional boost for students. Instructors may use an AAA intervention prior to providing feedback to students to promote empathic communication.

6.3.2 Clinical Application

Some healthcare organizations offer AAA for their employees; however, if AAA is not available specifically for employees, clinicians can seek out opportunities to interact with volunteer therapy animal/handler dyads that visit with patients and families. Even a few minutes of petting a therapy animal or engaging with the animal in a meaningful way can have positive physical and psychological effects for clinicians.

Research has found that AAA stimulates the release of oxytocin, which is known to decrease stress and improve communication. Clinicians could use this knowledge to facilitate difficult conversations. For example, if a goal of care conversation is planned with a patient and family, the clinician could arrange a volunteer AAA visit for the patient (if the patient were agreeable) before the meeting. The clinician could plan to spend 5–10 min with a therapy animal before the meeting as well. The animal visit may reduce stress hormones, heart rate, and blood pressure, while boosting oxytocin. With both patient and clinician optimally "primed" for more effective communication, even difficult conversations have potential to be made more comfortable.

6.3.3 Leadership Application

Leaders may benefit from AAA prior to attending difficult meetings, dealing with conflict resolution, or prior to coaching and counseling sessions. Healthcare leaders can support research and practice application of AAA by facilitating development of policies, procedures, and workflow guidelines that ensure not only facility access for AAA dyads, but also staff, volunteer, and patient safety. Include all stakeholders (e.g., nursing services, environmental services, risk management, infection control) in the development of structure and process to support AAA. Because handlers in AAA teams are volunteers, logistics of AAAs are generally managed by the volunteer services department in healthcare organizations. Providing adequate resources to the volunteer services department can facilitate implementation of AAA to promote staff wellness.

Supporting the implementation of AAA not only offers the opportunity to support the well-being of healthcare organization staff but can also serve to help recruit new talent. Formal and word-of-mouth advertising of employee AAA programs can result in people applying for employment because they share the values of holistic self-care the organization demonstrates by supporting AAA in the workplace as part of a well-rounded wellness program. Consider the presence of patient's own pets in addition to that of the trained AAA team (Fig. 6.4).

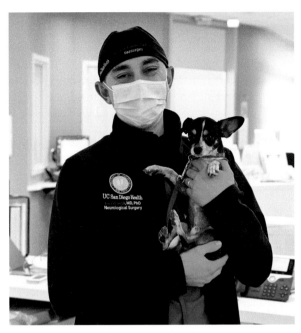

Fig. 6.4 "I think my blood pressure just dropped 20 points." A physician describes the stress-reducing power of animal-assisted activity

6.4 Opportunities for Future Research

"There is a conviction within healthcare professions, academia, and the community in general that animals, as social supports, provide benefits to humans" [30, p. 672]. However, until this century, there was little scientific evidence to support this conviction. The body of literature on HAI has grown significantly in the past 20 years, but there remains a plethora of opportunities for future research on the overall benefits of HAI, and, more specifically, AAA in the healthcare setting. To overcome limitations in prior studies, ensure future researchers examining the benefits of animal-assisted activities use rigor in both their methods and reporting. Research needs to be conducted using appropriate experimental design and statistical analysis to account for confounding variables. Include comprehensive descriptions of characteristics of both human and animal participants in reports of findings. Provide detailed descriptions of the type, duration, context, and structure of the human–animal interaction examined to assist others to replicate studies and confirm findings [31].

Despite limited studies to date, there are promising findings that can be expanded upon. Opportunities for future research include developing our understanding of the impact of animal interaction on: the physiology (e.g., stress hormones, cardiovascular parameters) of both human and animal participants; the perceived impact on a person's mood and stress level; academic or work performance; comfort having difficult conversations with patients/families or each other; and job stress, burnout, and employee turnover. Measuring the dose response to patient's own pets versus

AAA animals warrants investigation. Further research is also needed to confirm the acceptability and feasibility of AAA in the healthcare setting and best-practice strategies to overcome barriers to implementation.

Potential future research questions include:

1. Is AAA for healthcare workers more effective in individual or group settings?
2. What are the characteristics (e.g., gender, age, pet ownership status) of those who respond best to AAA?
3. What is the efficacy of AAA involving species other than canines?
4. What is the most effective "dose" (e.g., length of session, frequency of sessions) of AAA?
5. How long do the benefits of AAA last?

Glossary

Animal-assisted activity (AAA) Animal-assisted activities are informal interactions/ visitations often conducted on a volunteer basis by the human–animal team for motivational, educational, and recreational purposes. There are no treatment goals for the interactions. AAAs are generally facilitated by individuals who do not have a health, education, or human service degree. Human–animal teams have received at least introductory training, preparation, and assessment to participate in informal visitations.

Animal-assisted intervention (AAI) An animal-assisted intervention is a goal-oriented intervention that intentionally includes or incorporates animals in health, education, and human service for the purpose of therapeutic gains in humans.

Animal-assisted therapy (AAT) Animal-assisted therapy is a goal-oriented, structured therapeutic intervention directed and/or delivered by health, education, and human service professionals. Intervention progress is measured and included in professional documentation. AAT is delivered by a formally trained professional within the scope of the professionals' practice.*Above definitions from*: Jegatheesan B, Beetz A, Ormerod E, Johnson R, Fine A, Yamazaki K, Dudzik C, Garcia RM, Winkle M, Choi G. IAHAIO White Paper 2014: The IAHAIO Definitions for Animal Assisted Intervention and Guidelines for Wellness of Animals Involved. Seattle: International Association of Human-Animal Interaction Organizations.

Discussion Questions

1. What is your experience with companion animals? Have you or do you own any pets? If so, do you think companion animals can have an impact on physical or emotional wellbeing?

2. Have you ever participated in any type of structured animal interaction with an unfamiliar animal? If so, did you enjoy it? Why or why not?
3. What is your first reaction when you think about interacting with an unfamiliar companion animal at work? Why do you think you feel that way?
4. What is the best way to measure the impact of animal-assisted activity on a person? Do you think it is something that can be measured objectively?
5. Despite many people firmly believing that HAI benefits human wellbeing, research to support this assertion is difficult to conduct in a rigorous manner. Why might this be? Is rigorous scientific research needed to "prove" these benefits, or is anecdotal evidence enough to justify promoting HAI for wellbeing?

Discussion Leader Guide

Prior experience individuals have had with either their own or others' companion animals can impact the way they perceive animal-assisted activities. The first three questions provide an opportunity for self-reflection about those experiences and may help individuals appreciate the potential biases they bring to the discussion. The final two questions engage the learner to think about the challenge of quantifying the outcomes of an inherently complex interaction between a human and an animal.

References

1. Walsh F. Human-animal bonds I: the relational significance of companion animals. Fam Process. 2009;48(4):462–80.
2. Fine AH, Beck AM. Understanding our kinship with animals: input for health care professionals interested in the human–animal bond. In: Handbook on animal-assisted therapy. New York: Academic Press; 2015. p. 3–10.
3. Pet food industry. www.petfoodindustry.com/articles/5845-infographic-most-of-world-owns-pets-dogs-are-tops. Accessed 25 Sept 2021.
4. Statista. Dog and cat pet population worldwide. www.statista.com/statistics/1044386/dog-and-cat-pet-population-worldwide. Accessed 25 Sept 2021.
5. Pet industry market size & ownership statistics. American Pet Products Association. https://www.americanpetproducts.org/press_industrytrends.asp. Accessed 20 Sept 2021.
6. Barchas D, Melaragni M, Abrahim H, Barchas E. The best medicine: personal pets and therapy animals in the hospital setting. Crit Care Nurs Clin. 2020;32(2):167–90.
7. McCune S, Kruger KA, Griffin JA, Esposito L, Freund LS, Hurley KJ, Bures R. Evolution of research into the mutual benefits of human–animal interaction. Anim Front. 2014;4(3):49–58.
8. Nimer J, Lundahl B. Animal-assisted therapy: a meta-analysis. Anthrozoös. 2007;20(3):225–38.
9. Casey HM. A survey of occupational therapists using pet-facilitated therapy. J Home Health Care Pract. 1996;8(4):10–7.
10. Roberts H, Honzel N. The effectiveness of equine-facilitated psychotherapy in adolescents with serious emotional disturbances. Anthrozoös. 2020;33(1):133–44.
11. Jegatheesan B, Beetz A, Ormerod E, Johnson R, Fine A, Yamazaki K, Dudzik C, Garcia RM, Winkle M, Choi G, IAHAIO White Paper. The IAHAIO definitions for animal assisted intervention and guidelines for wellness of animals involved. Seattle: International Association of Human-Animal Interaction Organizations; 2014.

12. ADA National Network. Service animals. https://adata.org/factsheet/service-animals. Accessed 25 Sept 2021.
13. Gibeault S. Everything you need to know about emotional support animals. American Kennel Club. 2021. https://www.akc.org/expert-advice/news/everything-about-emotional-support-animals/ Accessed 25 Sept 2021.
14. Friedmann E, Son H, Saleem M. The animal–human bond: health and wellness. In: Handbook on animal-assisted therapy. New York: Academic Press; 2015. p. 73–88.
15. Beetz A, Uvnäs-Moberg K, Julius H, Kotrschal K. Psychosocial and psychophysiological effects of human-animal interactions: the possible role of oxytocin. Front Psychol. 2012;3:234.
16. Beetz AM. Theories and possible processes of action in animal assisted interventions. Appl Dev Sci. 2017;21(2):139–49.
17. Barker SB, Barker RT, McCain NL, Schubert CM. A randomized cross-over exploratory study of the effect of visiting therapy dogs on college student stress before final exams. Anthrozoös. 2016;29(1):35–46.
18. Wood E, Ohlsen S, Thompson J, Hulin J, Knowles L. The feasibility of brief dog-assisted therapy on university students stress levels: the PAwS study. J Ment Health. 2018;27(3):263–8.
19. Martos-Montes R, Ordóñez-Pérez D, Ruiz-Maatallah J, Martínez-Cobos M. Psychophysiological effects of human-dog interaction in university students exposed to a stress-induced situation using the Trier Social Stress Test (TSST). Hum Anim Interact Bull. 2019;8(2):36–50.
20. Scott TMT, Kirnan J. When are the dogs coming back? animal-assisted activities with men in residential substance abuse treatment. Humanist Psychol 2021. Advance online publication. http://dx.doi.org/10.1037/hum0000245.
21. Lass-Hennemann J, Peyk P, Streb M, Holz E, Michael T. Presence of a dog reduces subjective but not physiological stress responses to an analog trauma. Front Psychol. 2014;5:1010.
22. Joanna Tychowski BS, Gonzalez A, Boyd Z. Human-canine interaction: exploring stress indicator response patterns of salivary cortisol and immunoglobulin A. Res Theory Nurs Pract. 2012;26(1):25.
23. Colarelli SM, McDonald AM, Christensen MS, Honts C. A companion dog increases prosocial behavior in work groups. Anthrozoös. 2017;30(1):77–89.
24. Maslach C, Schaufeli WB, Leiter MP. Job burnout. Annu Rev Psychol. 2001;52(1):397–422.
25. Jensen CL, Bibbo J, Rodriguez KE, O'Haire ME. The effects of facility dogs on burnout, job-related well-being, and mental health in paediatric hospital professionals. J Clin Nurs. 2021;30(9–10):1429–41.
26. Etingen B, Martinez RN, Smith BM, Hogan TP, Miller L, Saban KL, Irvin D, Jankowski B, Weaver FM. Developing an animal-assisted support program for healthcare employees. BMC Health Serv Res. 2020;20(1):1–9.
27. Wells DL. The state of research on human–animal relations: implications for human health. Anthrozoös. 2019;32(2):169–81.
28. Uvnäs-Moberg K. Oxytocin may mediate the benefits of positive social interaction and emotions. Psychoneuroendocrinology. 1998;23(8):819–35.
29. Enck G. Pharmaceutically enhancing medical professionals for difficult conversations. J Ethics Emerg Technol. 2013;23(1):45–55.
30. Chur-Hansen A, Zambrano SC, Crawford GB. Furry and feathered family members—a critical review of their role in palliative care. Am J Hosp Palliat Med. 2014;31(6):672–7.
31. Rodriguez KE, Herzog H, Gee NR. Variability in human-animal interaction research. Front Vet Sci. 2021;7:1207.

The Chemistry of Nutrition

7

Jennifer Nemeth and Hannah Saarinen

Learning Objectives
1. Define the importance of combating preventable chronic diseases by incorporating the power of a plant-based diet.
2. Identify key steps that can be taken to implement strategies for successful employee wellness programs.
3. Recognize the current food system is unsustainable and action must be taken for the health of the planet, well-being of animals, and people's health.

"You are what you eat." It's a statement that has likely permeated your ears before but perhaps you haven't given much thought. We are what we eat. What we eat has a profound effect on the planet. As healthcare professionals, our brains are consumed with decision-making. That's not counting the complexity of home life and managing schedules with family and friends. Let's face it. Choosing what's easy is often the road most traveled because frankly, our cerebral cortex desires a break. But what if choosing the path of least resistance, such as the fast food drive-through or the pepperoni pizza at the hospital's cafeteria, isn't in our best interest? What would happen if we spent a bit more time in our kitchen, crafting meals that serve us rather than the doctor's office healing a malady caused by poor nutritional intake? We really are what we eat. Our bodies host more bacteria and viruses than our own

Supplementary Information The online version contains supplementary material available at https://doi.org/10.1007/978-3-031-16983-0_7.

J. Nemeth (✉)
University of California San Diego Health, La Jolla, CA, USA
e-mail: jlnemeth@health.UCSD.edu

H. Saarinen
Ridge Circle Sparks, NV, USA

cells and we eat to feed them. If we put junk in, the result is a cesspit of disease-promoting microorganisms. On the other hand, if we put nature's bounty in, we create vitality.

At the core of every healthcare professional's heart is the desire to promote the best quality of life for patients. Unfortunately, what is often lost in the process is the ability to care for ourselves. When one is running on empty, how can we adequately fill the cup of another? In this chapter, you'll learn the science behind the benefits of a plant-based diet and how to apply principles of nutrition that fuel a healthy body. Healthcare systems have the opportunity to provide this education as a matter of workplace wellness with a goal of improving employees' health. Taking an even deeper dive, we'll explore a way of eating that matches our deep-rooted ethical values of love and compassion, values that likely sparked our interest in healthcare.

7.1   Presentation of the Science

Most of our ancestors ate a non-processed, plant predominant diet up until about the 1970s. At that time, there was a revolution in the food industry that shifted gears to mass produce hyper palatable, addictive "food" laden with artificial flavors and preservatives [1]. This is a significant point in history when convenience replaced clean eating. One huge component that was lost was something that doesn't get much attention: fiber. In the Paleolithic Stone Age era, it was estimated our relatives were eating 100 g of fiber per day. The average American in the modern era consumes a mere 12–15 g per day [2]. Many worry about not getting enough protein but the real question should be: Are we getting enough fiber?

Fiber comes only from plants and is deficient in animal-based foods. Dietary fiber in the gastrointestinal tract lowers the pH of stool which inhibits pathogen adhesion and bacterial fermentation of harmful bacteria such as *E. coli* [3]. The gut lining covers about two tennis courts in surface area and is only half the thickness of a human hair. Simply put, the sole purpose of the gut lining is to let the good stuff in and keep the bad toxins out while building the immune system. Fiber also produces beneficial short chain fatty acids such as butyrate that lowers inflammation and reduces the risk for cardiovascular disease, colon cancer, diabetes, and obesity [4]. Cardiovascular disease continues to be the #1 cause of death for men and women in the United States so more fiber please! In addition, the gastrointestinal system is the primary producer of serotonin which regulates mood. When we eat fiber-rich plant foods, our body rewards us with that feel-good neurotransmitter.

Another factor contributing to poor health outcomes in America is the alarming amount of meat that is eaten. The average American eats around 200 pounds per year! The World Health Organization states that processed meats are "carcinogenic to humans." One hot dog or a few pieces of bacon eaten daily can increase cancer risk by 18% [5]. Americans are habitually obsessed with protein intake and that often means consuming protein from animal-based sources at most meals. A meta-analysis involving 715,128 participants within 32 studies saw that switching to plant-based protein reduces risk of an early death from any cause, including heart disease. It also showed that each additional 3% of calories that came from plant protein correlated with a 5% risk reduction in death [6]. Another study found that those who more often chose animal-based protein sources versus plant-based sources increased their risk of death from chronic disease by 23% [7].

According to the Physicians Committee for Responsible Medicine (PCRM), adults only need about 0.36 g of protein per pound of body weight. Thankfully this is easy to obtain with the abundant protein found in plants such as in beans, tofu, tempeh, seitan, whole grains, nuts, seeds, and even vegetables. A cup of broccoli has 3.7 g of protein. If one eats enough calories on a plant-based diet, they are almost certain to get enough protein. The awesome double benefit of plant-based sources of protein is they also contain health-promoting fiber.

The Adventist Health Study-2 correlated a vegetarian diet with reduction against cardiovascular disease, cardiometabolic risk factors, some cancers, and total mortality, but a vegan diet provided additional protection from obesity, hypertension, type 2 diabetes, and cardiovascular mortality [8]. Another comprehensive meta-analysis found a significant protective effect of a vegetarian diet with a reduction of mortality from heart disease by 25% and 8% decrease in incidence from total cancer. A vegan diet produced a significant reduced risk of 15% of incidence from total cancer [9]. A vegetarian diet includes eggs and dairy products whereas a vegan diet does not. Egg consumption increases risk for all-cause and cardiovascular disease mortality. A study published in the European Journal of Nutrition found that two to four eggs per week increased the risk for cancer mortality and all-cause and heart disease mortality by 22% and 43%, respectively [10]. An advantage to ditching the dairy is it is the top source of saturated fat in the American diet and it is linked to an increase risk of breast [11] and prostate cancer [12, 13].

Simply put, if it comes from a plant, it is likely a wise choice. Conversely, if the food is developed in a processing plant, steer clear. Foods that are high in refined carbohydrates, saturated fats, sodium, and animal proteins promote inflammation, obesity, diabetes, cancer, coronary disease and the list goes on. On the opposite end of the spectrum, filling the shopping cart with fruits, vegetables, whole grains, legumes, nuts, and seeds increases longevity.

Start the day with a green smoothie, overnight or cooked oats topped with nuts and berries or a tofu scramble with sautéed vegetables paired with a whole grain bread. The word tofu causes some to become frightened but give it a try in a scramble using extra firm tofu and adding turmeric for yellow coloring and black salt for an egg-like taste. A simple meal guide for lunch and dinner is "a bean, a green and a grain" with a sauce on top for additional flavoring. Examples include black beans, brown rice, and romaine greens with salsa on top (step it up a notch and add corn, cilantro, green onion, and avocado!). Or chickpeas, quinoa, and broccoli with BBQ sauce. Still another option is a barley bean chili with some kale or spinach tossed in it. Fruit makes for great dessert! Try freezing slices of banana and combining these with other frozen fruit such as blueberries or cherries with some plant-based milk in the high-speed blender for delicious nice cream!

Kitchen gadgets undeniably make our lives easier and there are two main ones to recommend. The Vitamix blender is an investment but well worth every penny as mine has been going for 11 years strong. A good blender makes it easy to make smoothies, creamy sauces, soups, nice cream, and even peanut butter! The Instant Pot makes cooking grains, beans, soups, and international cuisines such as curry effortless with a touch of a button.

For additional guidance, PCRM has a free, 21-day kickstart challenge where you'll receive meal plans, recipes, and advice from nutrition experts at kickstart. pcrm.org. Another free resource with similar guidance can be found at challenge22.com

This chapter would not be complete without mentioning the antibiotic resistance crisis, incredible resource use, emissions, and inefficiency of American's obsession with eating meat. About 60 billion animals are unnecessarily slaughtered every year to meet the demand of human consumption. Many turn a blind eye to deeply rooted ethics of love and compassion when it comes to sentient beings. Approximately 80% of the antibiotics sold in the United States are used for animal agriculture to prevent infection from overcrowding while marginally improving growth rates. There is evidence demonstrating that antibiotic resistance in humans is largely caused by the nontherapeutic antibiotic use in animals [14]. Think about the impact antibiotic resistance has on modern medicine and your role in decreasing the risk by consuming more plant-based nutrition.

Meat is also largely inefficient when compared to plant-based proteins such as legumes which take significantly less resources to cultivate. It takes about 9 calories of feed for chicken to get 1 calorie of chicken meat for human consumption or about 25 calories are required to get just 1 calorie of beef. Of the corn produced in the United States, 55% is fed to animals, 40% of the worldwide grain is fed to animals, and 85% of the worldwide soybeans end up as animal feed. The production of livestock globally is also responsible for about 18% of the greenhouse gas emission which is larger than all modes of transportation combined such as automobiles at 14% [15]. Switching to plant-based sources of protein will have a greater effect than if everyone in America purchased an electric car (Fig. 7.1).

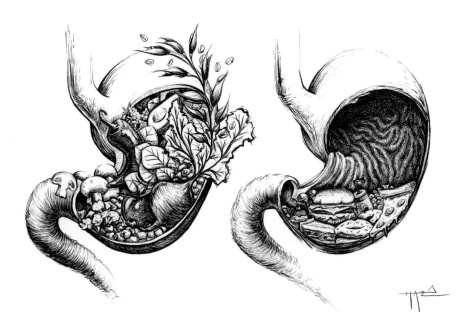

Fig. 7.1 "Whole food vs. junk food," 2021. A comparison between the effects of whole food and junk food on the stomach

7.2   Application of Principles into Wellness Practice

7.2.1   Pre-licensure Application in the Academic Environment

Dr. Michael Klaper is a physician making waves in the medical community after adopting a plant-based lifestyle in 1981 and never looking back. He asks a paramount question, "Why is the power of applied nutrition not taught in medical schools to physicians?" Medical students typically receive less than 20 h of nutrition education in 4 years. Dr. Klaper is working to change this by making applied nutrition part of every medical school's core curriculum. He offers a 12-unit master class in plant-based clinical nutrition, giving live presentations at medical schools and offering free monthly plant-based clinical nutrition forums (doctorklaper.com).

Dr. Michael Greger realized the same dilemma that medical students were graduating without receiving one of the most powerful tools available with nutrition education to prevent, treat, and even reverse chronic disease like heart disease: the #1 killer. As a labor of love to commemorate his grandmother who inspired him to go into medicine and healed herself through the Pritikin program, he and his team offer over 2000 free videos on peer-reviewed health and nutrition topics (nutritionfacts. org). There is an abundance of confusing and conflicting nutritional advice but he provides factual education in an easy-to-understand format free to everyone.

One additional resource is the Physicians Committee for Responsible Medicine (PCRM) that provides next generation physicians and current clinicians plant-based education tools, an annual International Conference on Nutrition in Medicine with 20 continuing medical education (CME) credits, free CME courses, and a mobile app providing evidence-based support to healthcare professionals on various topics called the Nutrition Guide for Clinicians (PCRM.org).

7.2.2 Clinical Application Post-licensure

Pivio, the complete health improvement program, is an exciting plant-based program producing positive morale and health outcomes for healthcare employees. It has been described by the American College of Lifestyle Medicine as "achieving some of the most impressive clinical outcomes published in the literature" [16]. One study looked at 442 employees from 6 healthcare worksites who simply watched the video program twice per week for 8 weeks. At baseline and at 8 weeks, demographic and biometric data were collected. All the sites individually and collectively demonstrated significant reductions in body weight, body mass index, total cholesterol including low density lipoprotein (LDL) cholesterol, triglycerides, and fasting glucose levels in 8 weeks. The program increased productivity by reducing sick calls and provided employees with a higher quality of life [17].

This scientifically proven intensive program has an added benefit to empower healthcare professionals to make meaningful lifestyle changes and reduce employer costs by potentially doubling their investment by the second year. Leaders in the healthcare system can find more information at piviohealth.com to greatly benefit their employees.

7.2.3 Leadership Application (Structural and Organizational Considerations)

There are some healthcare facilities that are practicing what they preach by striving to make their patients and employees healthier. One of these is Adventist Health Portland. Their hospital-based Garden Cafe embraces "practicing a vegetarian lifestyle to support the holistic nature of humankind." Another is Hayek Hospital in Beirut, Lebanon. They announced, "Starting today, March 1, 2021, our patients will no longer wake up from surgery to be greeted with ham, cheese, milk and eggs … the very food that may have contributed to their health problems in the first place. We believe it's well about time to tackle the root cause of disease and pandemics not just symptoms."

7.3   Opportunities for Future Research

The pharmaceutical giants have a lot more capital to publish research about their products than the broccoli farmer does. This may be one main reason research regarding plant-based foods is limited. More research is needed on the positive health outcomes of educating healthcare workers on the power of a plant-based diet and the downstream effects this education can have on their patient population. Healthcare systems have the opportunity to explore health outcomes, retention, and sick time before and after offering a lifestyle program such as Pivio. Most importantly, research has already shown that a plant predominate diet is beneficial for preventing, treating, and even reversing disease. As Dr. Michael Greger said, "There's only one diet ever been proven to reverse heart disease in the majority of patients: a plant-based diet. If that's the only thing a plant-based diet can do, reverse the number one killer, shouldn't that be the default diet until proven otherwise?" Research is indicated to evaluate the impact of making healthy food options available in the workplace on employee lifestyle changes.

Glossary

Dietary fiber The indigestible carbohydrates that come from a plant and aids in the reduction of chronic disease such as heart disease, diabetes, and cancer.

Plant predominate diet Choosing to receive all or a majority of caloric intake from fruits, vegetables, whole grains, legumes, nuts, and seeds.

Plant-based protein Protein that comes from a plant-based source such as beans, tofu, tempeh, seitan, whole grains, nuts, seeds, and vegetables.

Discussion Questions

1. What steps can you take today to commit to plant-based eating for at least 21 days to see how it can change your health for the better?
2. How can you encourage your patient population to eat in a way that improves their health and decreases antibiotic resistance?
3. How can you encourage your health-care organization to offer lifestyle programs such as Pivio and food service to offer plant-based meals to empower its employees?
4. How can you inspire faculty to offer substantial nutrition education in their curriculum?

Discussion Leader Guide

1. Discuss the health benefits of including more plants in the diet for yourself, colleagues, and patients.
2. Discuss the effect this will have on the environment and for animals.
3. Encourage conversation on how each person can take one step to eat more plants in their diet this week.
4. For a fun competition, see who can eat plant-based the longest. Use kickstart. pcrm.org as a resource.

Recipes
Peanut Sauce
1/2 cup peanut butter
1/2 cup light or full fat canned coconut milk
1 tablespoon rice vinegar
1 tablespoon maple syrup
1 tablespoon soy sauce or tamari
Blend in a high-speed blender until smooth.
Pesto Sauce
1/2 cup water
1/2 cup cashews
2 cups fresh basil
1/4 to 1/2 teaspoons salt, or to taste
Blend in a high-speed blender until smooth.
Chocolate Mousse
1 package of silken, shelf stable tofu (12.3 oz); drained of liquid
2 tablespoons cacao powder
1/3 to 1/2 cup maple syrup
1 teaspoon vanilla
1/4 teaspoon salt
Blend in a high-speed blender until smooth. Chill in the refrigerator before serving.

Video for Discussion - Instructional Video: The online version contains supplementary material available at https://doi.org/10.1007/978-3-031-16983-0_7

References

1. Greger M. How not to diet: the groundbreaking science of healthy, permanent weight loss. New York, NY; 2019.
2. Tuohy K, Gougoulias C, Shen Q, et al. Studying the human gut microbiota in the trans-omics era—focus on metagenomics and metabonomics. Curr Pharm Des. 2009;15:1415–27.
3. Zimmer J, Lange B, Frick J, et al. A vegan or vegetarian diet substantially altered the human colonic faecal microbiota. Eur J Clin Nutr. 2012;66:53–60.

4. Benus R, Van Dear Werf TS, Welling GW, et al. Association between faecalibacterium prausnitzii and dietary fibre in colonic fermentation in healthy human subjects. Br J Nutr. 2010;104:693–700.

5. Bouvard V, Loomis D, Guyton KZ, et al. Carcinogenicity of consumption of red and processed meat Lancet Oncol. Published online 2015 Oct 26. https://doi.org/10.1016/S1470-2045(15)00444-1.

6. Naghshi S, Sadeghi O, Willett WC, et al. Dietary intake of total, animal, and plant proteins and risk of all cause, cardiovascular, and cancer mortality: systematic review and dose-response meta-analysis of prospective cohort studies. BMJ. 2020;370:2412–29.

7. Virtanen HEK, Voutilainen S, Koskinen TT, et al. Dietary proteins and protein sources and risk of death: the Kuopio Ischaemic Heart Disease Risk Factor Study. Am J Clin Nutr. 2019;109:1462–71.

8. Le LT, Sabate J. Beyond meatless, the health effects of vegan diets: findings from the adventist cohorts. Nutrients. 2014;6:2131–47.

9. Dinu M, Abbate R, Franco Gensini G, Casini A, et al. Vegetarian, vegan diets and multiple health outcomes: a systematic review with meta-analysis of observational studies. Crit Rev Food Sci Nutr. 2017;57:3640–9.

10. Ruggiero E, Di Castelnuovo A, Costanzo S, et al. Egg consumption and risk of all-cause and cause-specific mortality in an Italian adult population. Eur J Nutr. 2021;60:3691.

11. Fraser G, Jaceldo-Siegel K, Orlich M, et al. Dairy, soy and risk of breast cancer: those confounded milks. Int J Epidemiol. 2020;49:1526–37.

12. Aune D, Rosenblatt DAN, Chan DSM, et al. Dairy products, calcium, and prostate cancer risk: a systematic review and meta-analysis of cohort studies. Am J Clin Nutr. 2015;101:87–117.

13. Song Y, Chavarro JE, Cao Y, et al. Whole milk intake is associated with prostate cancer-specific mortality among U.S. male physicians. J Nutr. 2013;143:189–96.

14. Martin M, Thottathil S, Newman T. Antibiotic overuse in animal agriculture: a call to action for health care providers. Am J Public Health. 2015;105:2409–10.

15. Grant J. Time for change. Benefits of a plant-based diet. Can Fam Physician. 2017;63:744–6.

16. Morton D, Rankin P, Kent L, et al. The complete health improvement program (CHIP): history, evaluation, and outcomes. Am J Lifestyle Med. 2014;10:64–73.

17. Aldana S, Greenlaw R, Diehl H, et al. Impact of the coronary health improvement project (CHIP) on several employee populations. J Occup Environ Med. 2002;44:831–9.

Fitness in the Workplace

8

Jansen Irving Pagal, Christie Lane, and Christina Dinh

Learning Objectives

1. Identify workplace fitness activities that can be incorporated during team huddles, breaks, and downtime in the healthcare setting.
2. Develop a workplace fitness program for the healthcare professionals.
3. Promote and create a culture of health and wellness in the workplace among healthcare professionals.

8.1 Presentation of the Science

Exercise and fitness are well known in promoting resilience and engagement in the workplace, mediating preventable disease, and enhancing cognitive functioning. Both healthcare employers and employees will benefit from implementing the proposed programs in their daily work routine.

It is evidenced that engagement and resilience in the workplace should be goals for both employers and employees. Improved workplace engagement can keep an

Supplementary Information The online version contains supplementary material available at https://doi.org/10.1007/978-3-031-16983-0_8.

J. I. Pagal (✉) · C. Lane
Jacobs Medical Center, University of California San Diego, La Jolla, CA, USA
e-mail: jipagal@health.ucsd.edu; cbaeza@health.ucsd.edu

C. Dinh
Rehabilitative Services, Scripps Memorial Hospital Encinitas, Encinitas, CA, USA
e-mail: cdinh@yadinneurowellness.com

employee from considering other job opportunities, attract top talent in a competitive workforce, and help maintain the happiness of current employees [1]. Enhancing engagement decreases turnover rate, effectively decreasing the operational cost of the employer. Studies show that replacing an average employee costs 120–200% more than the salary of the position affected [2]. Although multifaceted, resilience is commonly defined as positive adaptation to adversity. Resilience levels are linked in reducing stress, burnout, and work absences. People with high resilience scores demonstrate 10–20% lower rates of depression, absence from work, and have an increased overall productivity [3]. Moreover, it has been shown that work stress causes employees to seek healthcare services, resulting in a 10% reduction in profits for the organization [4]. Seeing as the cost of workplace absenteeism in the USA is $225.8 billion yearly it is of interest to companies to implement mediating interventions [5].

Exercise is one of the best interventions for helping healthcare professionals improve and maintain their overall well-being due to the release of feel-good endorphins in the brain during exercise [6]. Fitness is also an essential component in bolstering resilience [7]. It is proposed that mediating workplace stressors via exercise and fitness modalities would benefit employee satisfaction and employer profits. The deployment of fitness opportunities in the workplace has the ability to address both of these issues by counteracting the effects of stress and engaging the workforce [8].

Regular exercise helps prevent and manage health conditions such as high blood pressure, heart disease, stroke, diabetes, arthritis, and certain types of cancers. Numerous studies have also revealed that these practices are a natural and effective anti-anxiety treatment and have also been proven to treat depression, insomnia, PTSD, and ADHD. Exercise has shown to be a powerful mood booster, improving alertness, memory, concentration, and overall cognitive function. It can also reduce fatigue by helping one sleep better, adding years to their life and ultimately improving one's overall quality of life [7].

Exercise and physical activity have also been linked to an improvement in academic performance. In a review performed by the CDC, 8 of 9 studies found positive associations between classroom-based physical activity and indicators of academic performance [9]. Additionally, 12 of 22 times it was measured, GPA was positively associated with extracurricular physical activity [9]. From these studies, it is suggested that physical activity affects cognitive skills including improved attention, coping, and memory [9]. One study specifically measured acute changes in both executive functioning and attention after just 30 min of resistance training, aerobic training, or rest (control group) [10]. Researchers found that both attention and executive functioning improved after 30 minutes of resistance training, and only executive functioning improved after aerobic training [10]. Meanwhile, the control or "rest" group demonstrated no improvements in either category of cognitive functioning [10]. Another study analyzed the effects of sleep, eating breakfast, and physical activity on psychological distress and anxiety in female medical students (CD 2). It was discovered that the more sleep one received, the less distress and test anxiety these women experienced [11]. Additionally, the study showed decreased likelihood of psychological distress with the introduction of regular physical activity [11]. With the addition of wellness programs promoting exercise in the classroom students are able to perform at a higher level, achieving greater success academically.

Exercise as an intervention to improve engagement and resilience, reduce the prevalence of disease, and enhance academic success has been recognized in organizations paving the way for improved quality of life in the workplace. The American Hospital Association created a roadmap in 2010, a program called Health for Life: Better Healthcare to improve America's Healthcare system. Their Long-range Policy Committee focused on the "Wellness Pillar" creating a culture of health by identifying which emerging and successful practices in the hospital were contributing to the health and wellness of the employees [12].

8.2 Application of Principles into Wellness Practice

The most crucial step is to build a culture of health and wellness among healthcare professionals. One example out of many would be to develop and implement a wellness routine with physical exercises meant to be practiced alone or with other colleagues in the workplace. We formulated a simple, easy-to-follow exercise program for healthcare professionals at any fitness level, listing their physiological benefits. This program is an example of a 10–12-min routine, but if you only have 5 min to spare, a little exercise is always better than none. As a nurse at UC San Diego Health, my clinical advancement project was the creation of a meditation room, where staff members could exercise and meditate. Nurses reported a reduction in stress and burnout levels following use of the meditation room. A project like this cannot be successful without strong support from departmental leadership. We also formed a wellness shared governance committee to continue evolving fitness in the workplace. The team effort of the committee and the support of managers to form the committee helped to enculturate and normalize fitness into the workday. We support and encourage one another to perform fitness activities not just in the meditation room, but also at the nursing station. Interdisciplinary team members such as the respiratory therapists and nurse practitioners are welcome to join any group activity and to use the meditation room.

Consult with your primary care provider prior to practicing any new fitness routine. Listen to your body and stop if exercises cause pain. Focus on what your body and mind are calling for that particular day and time that you are about to exercise. When stressed, choosing exercises and movements that promote calm and peace may be helpful. One example is stretching with slow controlled movements that will ground the mind. However, when feeling sluggish select a more vigorous and stimulating set of exercises. You can exercise indoors or outdoors, alone or with others in small or large groups, play your favorite type of music for motivation or have some silence in a quiet space to calm and refresh the mind. To make it more likely that you will exercise in the workplace, wear comfortable flexible clothing you can move around in easily while on a short break.

The following fitness activities/exercise routines, equipment-free, can be incorporated into breaks, meetings, downtime, and/or team huddles.

1. Waist rotation with swinging arms 10× (Figs. 8.1 and 8.2)
   - Feet shoulder-width apart. Arms hang loose at sides. Rotate waist swinging your arms left then right as opposite heel lifts and you look behind you over one shoulder. Gain momentum, allowing one hand to pat opposite shoulder as the other pats low back. Rotation of waist guides movement of arms.
   - Benefit: A good warm up reducing tension and improving ROM of spine.

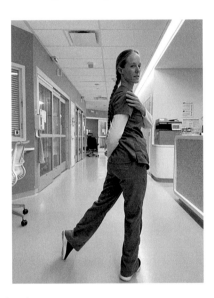

Fig. 8.1 Waist rotation view 1

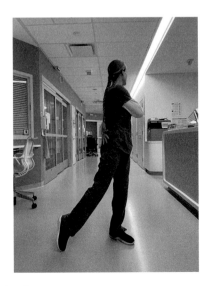

Fig. 8.2 Waist rotation view 2

2. Side stretches 10× (Figs. 8.3 and 8.4)
   - Feet a bit wider than shoulder width apart, bring one arm up and overhead laterally (palm down) tilting spine toward opposite side. The other hand presses into the same leg for support. Switch sides with each breath in a slow, controlled, and fluent motion. Abdomen engaged to support low back.
   - Benefit: Increases blood flow providing lateral stretch to side body. Strengthens abdominal and spinal erector muscles.

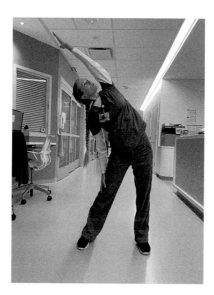

Fig. 8.3 Side stretch view 1

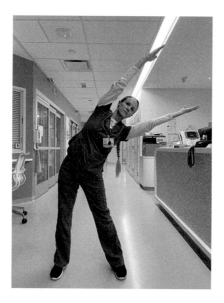

Fig. 8.4 Side stretch view 2

3. Side stretch at a bar or wall 3× breaths each side (Fig. 8.5)
    - Holding a bar (or the edge of a wall/door jamb) with one hand, stand with feet together about one foot away from it leaning hips away reaching outside arm up and over toward the wall, palm down. Repeat on the other side.
    - Benefit: Increases blood flow providing lateral stretch to side body.

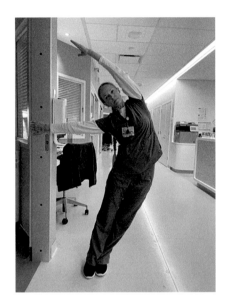

Fig. 8.5 Side stretch view 3

4. Standing backbend holding onto a bar or with arms elevated overhead 3×
   breaths (Fig. 8.6)
   - Placing hands shoulder distance apart behind you on a bar, feet point for-
     ward hip distance apart about 6 in away from wall, lean hips away from wall
     arching back, looking up, open shoulders and chest. Glutes are relaxed,
     allow inner thighs to spiral inward toward space behind you. Inhale to return
     to center.
   - If no bar stand with feet parallel, hip distance apart. Inhale arms up, over-
     head arching back. Palms face one another shoulder distance apart. Look up.
   - Benefits: Releases tension in the neck, back, and shoulders. Stretches
     abdominal muscles. Encourages lung expansion and spine mobility. Lowers
     stress and anxiety.

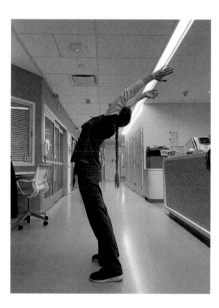

Fig. 8.6 Standing backbend

5. Wall calf stretch 3× breaths each side (Fig. 8.7)
    *   Using a wall if necessary (otherwise place hands on front thigh), step one foot far enough behind you pressing the heel down to feel a stretch in the calf muscle. Front knee stays over ankle. Take 3 breaths then take a little bend in the back knee, bring torso straight up, shoulders over hips, abdominals engaged. Take 3 breaths then switch sides.
    *   Benefit: Increases ROM and flexibility to calves and hip flexors stimulating blood flow.

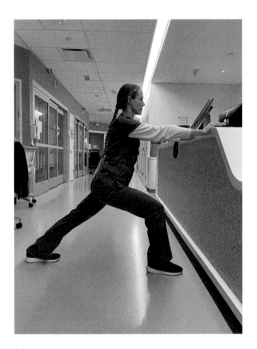

Fig. 8.7 Wall calf stretch

6. Wall sit 30 s× (Fig. 8.8)
   - Find a wall to bring your back against, feet parallel, shoulder distance apart. Walk feet out away from wall so knees stay over ankles (not passed) as you slide your back down the wall achieving a 45–90-degree angle with knees. Knees and toes point straight forward. Hold here for 30–60 s, weight in heels as to be able to lift toes.
   - Benefit: Strengthens quadriceps and stabilize muscles improving balance. Improves endurance.

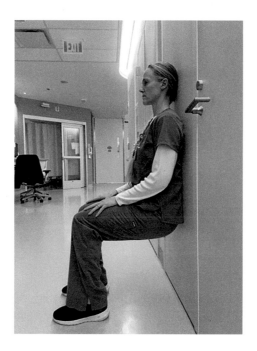

Fig. 8.8   Wall sit

7. One legged bicycles10× each side, then quad Stretch 3× breaths each side (Figs. 8.9 and 8.10)
   - Holding onto a bar or a wall bend one knee up toward chest and slowly extend out at a 90° angle leading with the heel, using the strength of the quad slowly lower toward the floor and repeat making a bicycle pedaling action with one leg 10× then reach behind with same hand taking top of foot drawing heel toward glute muscle. Knee points straight down toward floor bringing it alongside other knee, stretching quad muscle. Hold for 3 breaths.
   - Benefit: Strengthens and promotes quadricep flexibility, lengthening hip flexors as well. Reduces tension and risk of injury.

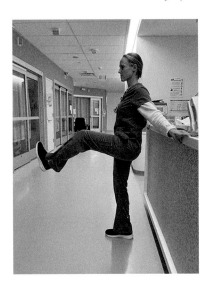

Fig. 8.9 One-legged bicycle

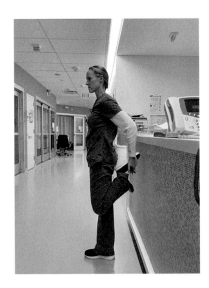

Fig. 8.10 Quad stretch

8. Tricep pushups 20× with hands on a raised surface like a bench, desk, or non-moveable chair (option to finish holding 1/2 way down doing straight leg lifts to the back 10× reps) (Fig. 8.11).

- Find a sturdy raised surface to place hands directly under shoulders, fingers forward. Bend elbows straight back along sides of the body to create a 90-degree angle, upper arms shoulder level. Gaze forward with slight lift in chest. Abdominals engaged to keep body in a straight plank position, hips on same plane as shoulders. After 20 reps hold plank or push up position and lift one leg a few inches straight up behind you while keeping plank position using Abs then the other performing 10 alternating straight leg lifts to the back.
- Benefit: Strengthens triceps, shoulders, chest, glutes, and abdominal muscles. Burns calories.

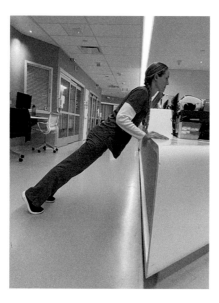

Fig. 8.11 Tricep pushup

9. Modified standing downward dog at wall (option to hold on to a bar or desk) 5×
   breaths (Fig. 8.12)
   • Fold forward halfway grasping same surface or holding a bar while pulling
     hips away from shoulders, biceps come alongside ears lengthening spine as
     feet walk in till a stretch is felt in hamstrings and lumbar spine 5× breaths.
     Release into rag doll (see next pose).
   • Benefit: Improves flexibility of hamstrings and back muscles. Strengthens
     upper body and improves blood flow.

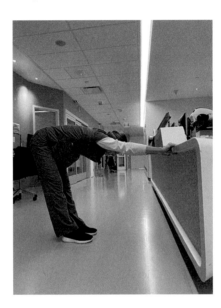

Fig. 8.12 Modified standing downward dog

10. Forward fold into rag doll 3× breaths, then forward fold twist 3× breaths each side (Figs. 8.13 and 8.14).
    - Release torso down toward thighs taking opposite elbows (option to gently sway side to side) 3× breaths.
    - Rotate torso opening shoulder and chest laterally and extend arm straight up toward sky, palm facing out. Soft bend in opposite knee, resting bottom hand on same foot or leg you rotated toward. Look up to hand overhead to challenge balance, opening shoulder. Torso is long. After 3 breaths release arm down and rotate to repeat on other side. Release and keeping a soft bend in the knees roll up to standing one vertebra at a time, head last. Roll shoulders up, down, and back.
    - Benefit: Increases flexibility of the hamstrings. Added rotation of torso stretches muscles of chest and back (Yoga15.com/pose/ragdoll/).

Fig. 8.13   Forward fold rag doll

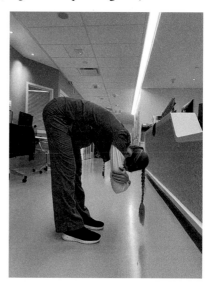

Fig. 8.14   Forward fold twist

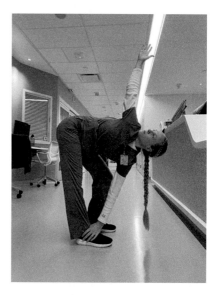

11. Shoulder stretch with hand flat against a wall (option to alternatively clasp hands behind back interlacing fingers to bring palms together if possible, raising arms toward upper back) 3× breaths (Figs. 8.15 and 8.16).
    - Place hand flat on wall chest level. Fingers point outward laterally. Keeping palm anchored slowly turn away from wall opening chest and shoulder. Gaze over opposite shoulder 3× breaths. Switch sides.
    - Benefit: Improves flexibility of chest, shoulders, arms, and wrists.

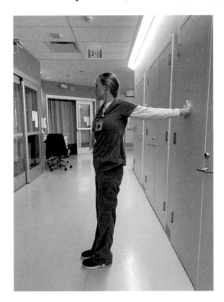

Fig. 8.15 Shoulder stretch

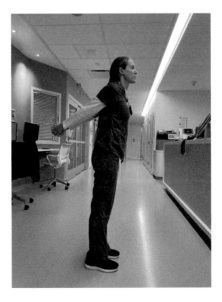

Fig. 8.16 Modified reverse shoulder stretch

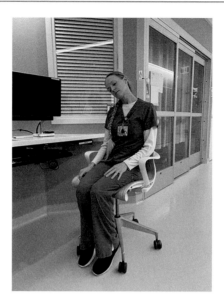

Fig. 8.17 Neck stretch

12. Neck stretch 3× breaths each side (Fig. 8.17)
    - Tilt your head to one side then the other. Ear toward same shoulder as shoulders stay relaxed, down, and back.
    - Benefit: Stretches lateral neck muscles including sternocleidomastoid and scalenes.

8.2.1 Pre-licensure Application in the Academic Environment

Academic institutions for careers in health care would be wise to invest some time into the resilience of the students that graduate from their programs by teaching and encouraging the formation of healthy practices proven to combat burnout healthcare providers often develop. Placing emphasis on physical and mental fitness by detailing examples incorporating time for to practice the strategies outlined above during breaks between courses would help to ensure these practices become habit. Once habituated, physical exercise can be relied upon to persevere through difficult times and help to ensure long-term maintenance of mind and body in an often-stressful environment. Faculty could encourage exercise as a study aide by explaining the evidence-based benefits to cognitive performance. Faculty can promote social events that include physical activities for mental health and team building. The suggestions provided below can also be applied to the academic environment.

8.2.2 Clinical Application Post-licensure

Individual healthcare professionals can set fitness intention into their own practice. Organize an approach to your workday that includes examples such as:

1. Taking the stairs instead of the elevators.
2. Parking farther away.
3. Walking or biking if you live close to work.
4. Conducting meetings/conversations on the go, while walking inside or outside the building instead of sitting in a room.
5. Taking a walking lunch/break with a smoothie.

Volunteer to organize a fitness committee in your own clinic/department. Gather a team of interested colleagues to rotate facilitating opportunities for fitness activities in the workplace. Organize donations for needed equipment or supplies. Publicize and promote fitness activities made available through organizational benefits or human resources.

8.3   Leadership Application

Promoting physical activity for healthcare professionals at the workplace can create a healthy work environment and a healthier workforce, increase productivity, and decrease their risk of developing costly and debilitating chronic diseases as well as improve their physical, psychological, and mental health.

Consider creating safe spaces indoors and outdoors for these professionals for exercise such as during team huddles, breaks, meetings, and conferences, to keep awake, attentive, and energized. Healthcare professionals who are physically active require less sick leave and are more productive and engaged at work. A meditation room, a yoga studio, or an office gym are examples of indoor spaces that can be created for the staff members. Outdoor spaces could include an accessible lawn or garden where staff could safely exercise, practice yoga, or just take a walk. Instructors, be it in person or virtual, are also highly recommended to teach and guide healthcare professionals on a regular basis. The promotion of workplace physical activity should ideally be normalized.

8.4   Opportunities for Future Research

Further investigation would be beneficial to test the best methods of workplace fitness programs.

If organizational leaders in health care would support and implement wellness programs and create infrastructure that encouraged it like rooms dedicated to holding space for one to devote time to their health it would promote a more productive and nurturing work environment.

Research what type of wellness program would be most effective in the workplace for a specific job task and work condition.

Research questions could include:

What effect do fitness programs have on the mental health and overall improvement in wellness of healthcare professionals?

What effect do wellness programs improve patient and job satisfaction or staff retention?

What effect do wellness programs reduce the incidence of work-related injuries?

What is the financial impact of wellness programs for healthcare institutions?

Do fitness programs reduce suicide rates, risky substance use, and mental health issues among healthcare professionals?

Glossary

Anxiety A feeling of worry, nervousness, or unease, typically about an imminent event or something with an uncertain outcome.

Burnout A long-term stress reaction marked by emotional exhaustion, depersonalization, and a lack of sense of personal accomplishment.

Depression It is a constant feeling of sadness and loss of interest, which stops you doing your normal activities.

Physical activity It refers to all movement including during one's leisure time, during transport to get from one place to the next, or as part of a person's work.

Resiliency An ability to recover from or adjust easily to adversity or change.

Stress Any type of change that causes physical, emotional, or psychological strain. Stress is your body's response to anything that requires attention or action.

Turnover rate It refers to the percentage of employees who leave an organization during a certain period of time.

Discussion Questions

1. What are the barriers to implementing these exercises/routines in your daily schedule?
2. How do you think you would feel if you had an allotted time in your day to participate in a set program like this?
3. What would your ideal schedule look like that would allow you to implement these strategies at work—feel free to think "unrealistically."
4. What does a balanced work environment look like to you?
5. What can your employer do to facilitate an environment that reduces stress?

Discussion Guide

1. "If lack of knowledge were the problem to changing a habit, we'd all be billionaires with six pack abs." We know exercise helps stress reduction—so why can't we do it? Particularly, why can't we do it in the workplace?
2. Think specifics:
   (a) Do you think you'd be more productive?
   (b) How do you think your patient care would be?
   (c) How do you think your interactions would be with your colleagues during the day?
   (d) How would your stress levels be?
   (e) How would your job satisfaction be?
   (f) Would you be more/less likely to quit, knowing that the next job lined up may not have this built into its structure/culture?
   (g) Would it be a defining characteristic of whether you would want to stay in a job?
   (h) Would it change whether you would take a job of the same caliber?
3. What if your company/hospital hired someone to run a yoga class for 15 min 2 times per day? Would you go? Encourage people to think about any and every possibility—nothing will change if you never come up with it!
4. We get stuck in these "it will always be like this" mindsets that we forget to think about the possibilities of what "could be." Some of these "wish list" items are not feasible, but I think we will find that some of them are! We just have to remember to implement them.
5. Is there a way to communicate these to leadership roles who can help facilitate even a small introduction to what you need? It helps to deliver a solution management positions.

Discussion Leader Guide

Video for Discussion - Instructional Video: The online version contains supplementary material available at https://doi.org/10.1007/978-3-031-16983-0_8

References

1. Vance. 2006. Employee engagement and commitment. https://www.shrm.org/hr-today/trends-and-forecasting/special-reports-and-expert-views/documents/employee-engagement-commitment.pdf
2. Flash, What is the cost of employee turnover? Compensation & Benefits Review, Sept/Oct 1997: Article #8582, 1998.

3. J Occup Environ Med. 2017;59(2):135–40. Published online 2016 Dec 20. https://doi.org/10.1097/JOM.0000000000000914.   https://www.ncbi.nlm.nih.gov/pmc/articles/PMC5287440/
4. Azagba S, Sharaf MF. Psychosocial working conditions and the utilization of health care services. BMC Public Health. 2011;11:642. https://doi.org/10.1186/1471-2458-11-642.
5. CDC Foundation. Worker Illness and Injury Costs U.S. Employers $225.8 Billion Annually. 2015. https://www.cdcfoundation.org/pr/2015/worker-illness-and-injury-costs-us-employers-225-billion-annually
6. Mayo Clinic. Depression and anxiety: Exercise eases symptoms. 2017. https://www.mayoclinic.org/diseases-conditions/depression/in-depth/depression-and-exercise/art-20046495
7. Robinson, Segal, and Smith. The mental health benefits of exercise. 2021. https://www.helpguide.org/articles/healthy-living/the-mental-health-benefits-of-exercise.htm
8. Johns Hopkins Bloomberg School of Public Health. Physical activity in the workplace: a guide for employers. 2016. https://www.jhsph.edu/research/centers-and-institutes/institute-for-health-and-productivity-studies/_docs/archived-projects/WHRN_PA.pdf
9. Centers for Disease Control and Prevention. The association between school-based physical activity, including physical education, and academic performance. 2010. https://www.cdc.gov/healthyyouth/health_and_academics/pdf/pa-pe_paper.pdf
10. Tsuk S, Netz Y, Dunsky A, Zeev A, Carasso R, Dwolatzky T, Salem R, Behar S, Rotstein A. The acute effect of exercise on executive function and attention: resistance versus aerobic exercise. Adv Cogn Psychol. 2019;15(3):208–15. https://doi.org/10.5709/acp-0269-7.
11. Aziz N. Effect of sleep, breakfast and physical activity on test anxiety and psychological distress. GSC Biol Pharm Sci. 2020;13(2):245–52. https://doi.org/10.30574/gscbps.2020.13.2.0382.
12. American Hospital Association. A call to action: creating a culture of health. 2011. https://www.aha.org/system/files/2018-02/call-to-action-creating-a-culture-of-health-2011.pdf

The Healing Environment: Healthcare Professionals as Leaders in Design

9

Debbie D. Gregory, Terri Zborowsky, and Jaynelle F. Stichler

Abbreviation

EBD   Evidence-based design

Learning Objectives

1. Discover elements of the built environment that impact healthcare professionals, care delivery and well-being.
2. Describe Florence Nightingale's Environmental Adaptive Theory.
3. Discuss evidence-based design research principles and practical application that will enhance the healing environment.
4. Identify the role of healthcare leaders in the design of the caring environment.

D. D. Gregory (✉)
Smith, Seckman, Reid, Inc., Nashville, TN, USA

Nashville, TN, USA
e-mail: dgregory@ssr-inc.com

T. Zborowsky
HGA Architects and Engineers, Minneapolis, MN, USA

St. Paul, MN, USA
e-mail: tzborowsky@hga.com

J. F. Stichler
Castor Nursing Institute, Sharp Healthcare, San Diego, CA, USA

Escondido, CA, USA

© The Author(s), under exclusive license to Springer Nature Switzerland AG 2023
J. E. Davidson, M. Richardson (eds.), *Workplace Wellness: From Resiliency to Suicide Prevention and Grief Management*, https://doi.org/10.1007/978-3-031-16983-0_9

9.1 Presentation of the Science

9.1.1 The Healing Environment: Healthcare Professionals as Leaders in Design

The literature is replete with evidence about the importance of a healthy work environment for healthcare professionals' well-being, retention, focus on the details of complex patient care, and workplace culture [1–3]. Authors cite the importance of inter- and intra-professional relationships, leadership support, shared decision-making, authentic leadership, meaningful recognition, and other attributes [4–8], but there is no mention of the physical environment as an element of a healthy work environment.

9.1.2 The Healthcare Professionals Work Environment

Healthcare leaders are challenged to create a work environment that promotes quality outcomes for patients and supports clinicians in care delivery. The recent pandemic, decompensating aging healthcare facilities, and lack of support have created a crisis for healthcare professionals and our entire healthcare ecosystem. The healthcare workforce, now more than ever before, is challenged to care for their patients at the expense of their own well-being. In a recent systematic review and meta-analysis, Galanis et al. [9] found the overall prevalence of emotional exhaustion was 34.1%, of depersonalization was 12.6%, and the lack of personal accomplishment was 15.2%. Staff are overwhelmed and burned out. The impact of these emotional and physical characteristics of the current healthcare professional's work environment has now been elevated for critical examination and intervention. The American Nurses Association (ANA) recently launched two important initiatives, Healthy Nurse Healthy Nation, and the Well-Being Initiative [10, 11] to support the mental health, well-being, and resilience of all healthcare professionals. While these programs are needed, healthcare leaders must not miss the important discussion of how aspects of the built environment impact healthcare professionals and their well-being. This chapter describes current research related to how the built environment impacts healthcare professionals in all aspects of their well-being. It also discusses how healthcare professionals can leverage research to improve their working life. Florence Nightingale's Environmental Adaptation Theory is introduced because it was her belief that the environment could be altered and improved to allow the laws of nature to influence healing. Her theory emerged from her empirical observation that poor or difficult environments led to poor health and disease, and her theory increases our understanding of how to improve design for healthcare professionals and patients. As healthcare professionals, we need to find ways to tie people, place, and process together, much like Florence Nightingale did years ago to create healing spaces for staff and patients. This chapter provides evidence-based design research principles and practical applications that enhance the healing environment and identify the important role of healthcare leaders in the design of the caring environment for their staff.

9.1.3   Well-Being Defined

According to the American Psychological Association's (APA) *Dictionary of Psychology [12]*, well-being is defined as "a state of happiness and contentment, with low levels of distress, overall good physical and mental health and outlook, or good quality of life" [13]. More specific details regarding the components of well-being or wellness (the terms are often used interchangeably) are offered by the Substance Abuse and Mental Health Services Administration (SAMHSA) at the U.S. Department of Health and Human Services [14–16]. In the SAMHSA framework, well-being (or wellness) is made up of eight dimensions: emotional, environmental, financial, intellectual, occupational, physical, social, and spiritual. A key concept in the wellness framework is recognition of the importance to address and balance all the various dimensions or components in a holistic manner. The environmental dimension of well-being is not often included as a domain in healthcare. While there are current efforts to evaluate well-being and its effect on nurse satisfaction [17, 18], create tools to measure well-being, and identify interventions to promote well-being, healthcare leaders have not taken a lead role in advocating for the built environment as a dimension for workplace wellness. The impact of the environmental domain on healthcare professional's well-being is the focus of this chapter (Fig. 9.1).

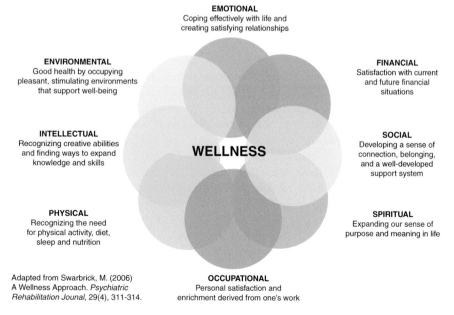

EMOTIONAL
Coping effectively with life and
creating satisfying relationships

ENVIRONMENTAL
Good health by occupying
pleasant, stimulating environments
that support well-being

FINANCIAL
Satisfaction with current
and future financial
situations

INTELLECTUAL
Recognizing creative abilities
and finding ways to expand
knowledge and skills

WELLNESS

SOCIAL
Developing a sense of
connection, belonging,
and a well-developed
support system

PHYSICAL
Recognizing the need
for physical activity, diet,
sleep and nutrition

SPIRITUAL
Expanding our sense of
purpose and meaning in life

Adapted from Swarbrick, M. (2006)
A Wellness Approach. *Psychiatric
Rehabilitation Jounal,* 29(4), 311-314.

OCCUPATIONAL
Personal satisfaction and
enrichment derived from one's work

Fig. 9.1 Substance abuse and mental health services administration well-being. Source: http://www.samhsa.gov/wellness-initiative/eight-dimensions-wellness

9.1.4 Healthcare Professionals' Well-Being

Care and concern over the well-being of clinicians is not a recent discovery. An article in the *Annals of Family Medicine*, entitled "From Triple to Quadruple Aim: Care of the Patient Requires Care of the Provider" [19], became a clarion call to address the well-being needs of healthcare providers and staff. The authors contend that the Triple Aim—to enhance the patient's experience, improve population health, and reduce costs—will be attainable only when high rates of job burnout and dissatisfaction among care providers and staff are mitigated. Provider burnout was a concern before the COVID-19 pandemic began, but now these issues are exacerbated even more, further challenging efforts to achieve and sustain well-being and reduce provider burnout.

9.1.5 Nightingale's Environmental Adaptation Theory

Nightingale was acutely aware of the impact the built environment had on patients— she knew this from direct observation. In fact, all her assertions were from her acute observations of patient or community outcome. Nightingale's environmental theory can be viewed as a systems model that focuses on the "client" in the center, surrounded by aspects of the environment all in balance [20–22]. If one element is out of balance, then the client is stressed, and it is the healthcare professional's role to do what is needed to bring balance back to the client or adapt some aspect of the client's surrounding environment to relieve the stress (Lobo, 2011). If this seems familiar, a similar assertion was used to describe the holistic nature of SAMSHA's Well-being Framework [16]. For Nightingale, it often required the healthcare professional to adapt an aspect of the environment as can be seen in Fig. 9.2.

Through environmental alteration, one can put the patient in the best possible condition for nature to act, thereby facilitating the laws of nature [23]. The environment has internal and external components. Nightingale was as concerned about elements that entered the body—food, water, and medications—as those that directly affected the external being, such as ventilation, light, noise control, stimulation, and room temperature. While Nightingale did not discuss the healthcare professional's well-being in the model, her holistic approach and constructs of interest also affect the healthcare professional.

9.1.6 Healthcare Professionals' Well-Being + the Work Environment

Following the Institute of Medicine's epic report, 'To Err is Human: Building a Safer Health System,' several reports tried to address all aspects of healthcare errors. This was the first time in government reporting that the physical side of the healthcare professionals' work environments began to be addressed [24]. However, it was not until the 2004 report, *Keeping Patients Safe: Transforming the Work Environment*

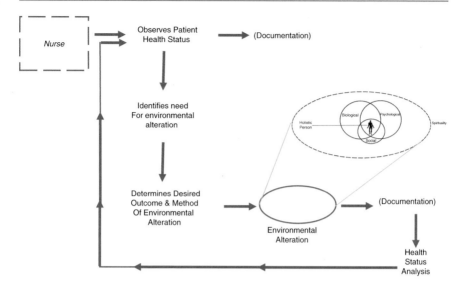

Fig. 9.2 Nightingale's environment alteration theory (modified from Selanders, 1998)

of Healthcare professionals [25] that physical aspects of healthcare professionals' work environment was discussed in depth. The chapter, "Work and Workspace Design to Prevent and Mitigate Errors," dealt specifically with the "evidence on the design of healthcare professionals' work hours, work processes, and workspaces, primarily as they relate to patient safety, but also with respect to efficiency" [25] p. 227. After a thorough review of work issues such as medication errors, fatigue, hand washing, distractions, supply management, acuity adaptable patient rooms among other issues, several recommendations were made, including:

> Nursing leadership should be provided with resources enabling them to design the nursing work environment and care processes to reduce errors, and should concentrate on errors associated with:

- *Surveillance of patient health status*
- *Patient transfers and other patient hand-offs*
- *Complex patient care processes*
- *Non-value-added activities performed by healthcare professionals, such as locating and obtaining supplies, looking for personnel, completing redundant and unnecessary documentation, and compensating for poor communication systems*

Hand washing and medication administration should be addressed [25] (p. 13).

Robert Wood Johnson Foundation (RWJF) published "Ten Years After Keeping Patients Safe: Have Nurses Work Environments Been Transformed?" [26]. The RWJF report revisited the recommendations in the Institute of Medicine's report for averting harm, highlighting both progress and persistent gaps in transforming healthcare professionals' work environments, and showcased research, policies, and tools with the potential to advance the transformation. Given the emotional toll that errors place on the human soul, it can be inferred that the mental health and well-being of the workforce will be improved if the work environment is strategically built to minimize errors. The RWJF document fell short, however, in addressing the role of the built environment in helping to overcome the quality gap. The discussion should focus on people, process and place as interrelated concepts that can improve the healthcare professional's work environment [27]. If environmental alteration were viewed in a holistic manner similar to Nightingale's thinking, staff well-being would be a critical element or domain of the patient healing environment.

9.1.7 Healthcare Professionals' Well-Being + Design of the Work Environment

This field of study is on the rise. Research findings highlighted in the next section address how workplace design elements impact staff well-being. It is important for healthcare leaders to be familiar with this research to connect aspects of the environmental domain to the wellness ecosystem as shown earlier in Fig. 9.1.

9.1.8 Physical Layout that Improves Healthcare Professional Satisfaction and Efficiency

Studies in this section focus on the impact of a hospital unit, or department layout, and the impact on the healthcare professionals' ability to provide care, spend time in non-value-added activities such as searching for supplies, their satisfaction with their job, burn-out symptoms among other aspects of well-being.

9.1.8.1 Nursing Unit Typology, Design, and Assignments

Zborowsky et al. [28] conducted an exploratory study to investigate how nursing station design (i.e., centralized and decentralized nursing station layouts) affected healthcare professionals' use of space, patient visibility, noise levels, and perceptions of the work environment. Using a multi-method approach, the authors found that all nurses were most frequently performing telephone, computer, and administrative duties. However, time spent using telephones, computers, and performing other administrative duties was significantly higher in the centralized nursing stations. Consultations with medical staff and social interactions were significantly less frequent in decentralized nursing stations. There were no indications that either centralized or decentralized nursing station designs resulted in superior visibility. Sound levels measured in all nursing stations exceeded recommended levels during all shifts. No significant differences were identified in healthcare professionals' perceptions of work control, demand, or support in centralized or decentralized nursing station designs. Other researchers reported similar findings comparing centralized and decentralized nursing stations on communication patterns, visibility of the patient and other colleagues, workflow, and steps taken by the nurse [29–31]. Taking all of this into account, the negative impact of decentralization on social interaction [teamwork] needs to be considered when designing for workplace wellness.

To study the effect of nursing unit design on stress and job satisfaction, Parker, Eisen, and Bell [32] administered the Perceived Stress Scale (PSS) and Demand-Control-Support Questionnaire (DCSQ) to 40 nurse participants to evaluate staff stress, job satisfaction, and perceptions of the work environment. In addition, two follow-up focus groups were conducted to expand upon the questionnaire findings. Results suggested that the centralized floor lends itself to better patient access and professional communication. Similar findings were reported by other researchers on nursing unit layout as well [33–38]. Further research is needed regarding healthcare professional burnout and turnover as it relates to nursing unit design.

Copeland and Chambers [34] set out to determine what differences occurred in steps taken and energy expenditure among acute care nurses when their work environment moved from a hospital with centralized nurse stations to a hospital with decentralized nurse stations. Additional goals were to determine design features healthcare professionals perceived as contributing to, or deterring from, their work activities and what changes occurred in reported job satisfaction. They found significant reductions in healthcare professionals' energy expenditure ($p < 0.001$) and steps taken ($p = 0.041$) post-relocation. Overall, healthcare professionals' job satisfaction was high and improved post-relocation, while patient falls decreased by 55%.

9.1.8.2 Design and Staff Productivity

Nazarian et al. [36] found that the arrangement of nursing unit/ward spaces can minimize the distance nurses travel in a shift. Rearrangement of existing space can improve staff productivity. A recommendation was made that architectural planners explore the implications of chosen unit layouts on walking distance and nursing staff productivity. Further, optimizing flow to decrease wasted walking may have an impact on time at the bedside, which would theoretically improve both physical and mental health; further research in this topic of concern is warranted.

9.1.8.3 Unit Typology and Assignments

In a seminal study, the primary goal of Hendrich et al. [35] was to test the hypothesis that healthcare professionals adopt distinct movement strategies based on features of unit topology and nurse assignments. The secondary goal was to identify aspects of unit layout or organization that influenced the amount of time nurses spend in the patient room. Techniques of spatial analysis, borrowed from the architectural theory of spatial syntax, were applied to the Time and Motion data set. Study findings included nurse assignments with greater average centrality to all assigned rooms were associated with a higher number of entries to patient rooms, as well as to the nurse station. Number of entries to patient rooms was negatively correlated with average time per visit, but positively correlated with total time spent in patient rooms. The findngs described two overall strategies of nurse mobility patterns: fewer, longer visits versus more frequent, shorter visits.

9.1.8.4 Single Family Room Layout

Doede et al. [39] conducted a literature review that sought to answer the question: When compared to open bay layout, how does a single-family room layout impact neonatal nurse's work? Many studies reported both positive and negative effects on healthcare professionals—advantages included improved quality of the physical environment; improved quality of patient care; improved parent interaction; and improvements in healthcare professional job satisfaction, stress, and burnout. Disadvantages of the layout included decreased interaction among the NICU patient care team, increased nurse workload, decreased visibility on the unit, and difficult interactions with family. The review suggests that single-family room NICUs introduce a complex situation in which trade-offs occur for healthcare professionals, most prominently the trade-off between visibility and privacy.

9.1.8.5 Pre- and Post-comparison of Burnout and Job Satisfaction on New Versus Existing Psychiatric Wards

In a classical article, Tyson et al. [38] conducted a pre- and post-occupancy comparison of two completely new wards at a rural psychiatric hospital. Measures of the nursing staffs' observed behavior and self-ratings of burnout and job satisfaction were obtained in both the old and the new wards. The results demonstrated that the new wards were associated with largely positive changes in nurse behavior and increased burnout, but there was no change in job satisfaction. However, it was clear that a vital component in the success of any environmental manipulation is an appropriate, corresponding change in the organizational climate.

While these articles are all case studies, they represent important steps in documenting the impact of the built environment on healthcare professionals' well-being. The physical domain of wellness is impacted by the layout of unit as it directly impacts the number of steps or miles that healthcare professionals walk every day. Healthcare professionals today face an increase of wear and tear on their bodies due to time and distance on their feet. Decreasing travel time also increases valuable time at the bedside to perform the care of patients and provides more time for healthcare professionals to have a break or needed respite in their day.

9.1.9 Design Features That Reduce Healthcare Professionals' Stress and Improve Cognitive Functioning

The following section discusses design features that can not only reduce healthcare professional's stress levels but also improve alertness and cognitive functioning. Because patient care is so complex, especially with multiple patient assignments or patients with high acuity levels, cognitive stacking occurs which can contribute to errors of omission or commission [40, 41]. Some design features can address these concerns and facilitate healthcare professional's mental and emotional acuity.

9.1.9.1 Respite Areas

The concept of respite areas has been emerging in the past 5 years and most acutely during the pandemic [42–44]. Some hospitals call the spaces respite rooms, rejuvenation rooms, and even meditation spaces, but they are simply spaces where respite occurs allowing healthcare professionals to restore themselves emotionally, spiritually, and physically [45, 46]. This is especially true in today's pandemic. Break rooms or healthcare professionals' lounges are required space on a patient care unit, but they are often combined with locker and change areas, toilets, eating areas, televisions, and conversations among the healthcare professionals. Nurse lounges are anything other than respite rooms or quiet rooms. Healthcare professionals need immediate access to respite rooms to rest not just their bodies, but to reset from cognitive overload, very common in today's healthcare climate.

9.1.9.2 Access to Nature Views and Daylight

Similar to Pati et al. earlier work demonstrating relationships between nurse alertness and fatigue with views to the outdoors [47], Mihandoust et al. [47, 48] conducted a cross-sectional study that explored the relationship between the subscales (Emotional Exhaustion, Depersonalization, and Personal Accomplishment [EE, DP, and PA]) of the Maslach Burnout Inventory as "outcome variables" and perception of view duration, frequency of exposure to views, view content, and artwork content as "explanatory variables" in a subset regression model. The study model also included organizational stressors, environmental design factors, unit type, workload, and personal factors as control variables. The authors found that the percentage of perceived nature views and organizational stressors were the top two best predictors correlating with EE. Percentage of perceived nature views, organizational stressors, and environmental design were the top three predictors correlating with DP. No significant relationship was found between study variables and PA. The study suggests that a unit and break room design with access to nature views could work as a consistent preventive intervention for burnout.

Gharaveis et al. [49] sought to explore the perceptions of nursing staff regarding the effects of daylighting on various factors including mood, stress, satisfaction, medical error, and efficiency. Despite an extensive body of literature seeking to investigate the impact of daylighting on patients, a limited number of studies have been done for the sake of healthcare professionals' perceptions and behavioral responses. A mixed-methods approach comprised of qualitative explorations (structured interviews) and a validated survey was used. The findings of the study are consistent with the existing evidence that daylighting and view to the outside enhance healthcare professionals' perceptions regarding satisfaction, mood, stress, medical error, and alertness, while reducing fatigue and stress.

9.1.9.3 Exterior View from Healthcare Professional Work Area

A classic article by Pati et al. [47] examined the relationships between acute stress and alertness of nurse, and duration and content of exterior views from nurse work areas. A survey-based method was used to collect data on acute stress, chronic stress, and alertness of healthcare professionals before and after 12-h shifts. Control measures included physical environment stressors (lighting, noise, thermal, and ergonomic), organizational stressors, workload, and personal characteristics (age, experience, and income). Data were collected from 32 healthcare professionals on 19 different units at two hospitals. The association between view duration and alertness and stress is conditional on the exterior view content (nature view vs non-nature view). Of all the healthcare professionals whose alertness level remained the same or improved, almost 60% had exposure to exterior and nature view. In contrast, of all healthcare professionals whose alertness levels deteriorated, 67% were exposed to no view or to only non-nature view. Similarly, of all healthcare professionals whose acute stress condition remained the same or reduced, 64% had exposure to views. Of healthcare professionals whose acute stress levels increased, 56% had no view or only a non-nature view. The authors concluded although long working hours, overtime, and sleep deprivation are problems in healthcare operations, the physical design of units is only now beginning to be considered seriously in evaluating outcomes.

9.1.9.4 Break Rooms

Nejati et al. [50] investigated the main restorative components of staff break areas in healthcare facilities, by assessing usage patterns, verbal/visual preferences, and perceived restorative qualities of specific design features found in break areas for hospital staff. They used a multi-method approach which included a visual ranking of break room spaces. The authors found that staff break areas are more likely to be used if they are near healthcare professionals' work areas, if they have complete privacy from patients and families, and if they provide opportunities for individual privacy as well as socialization with coworkers. Having physical access to private outdoor spaces (e.g., balconies or porches) was shown to have significantly greater perceived restorative potential, in comparison with window views, artwork, or indoor plants.

What these study and others [42–44] have in common is the assertion that access to light, nature or nature-based art in staff break rooms is stress reducing, can enhance healthcare professionals' perceptions regarding satisfaction, mood, stress, medical error, and alertness, while reducing fatigue and stress. Science is mounting and should be leveraged to help support the difficult work environment of today's healthcare professionals.

9.1.10 Technology as Part of the Designed Environment

Technology is changing the world, and nowhere is it more evident than the impact in healthcare settings. Technology is certainly impacting today's work environment and must be considered as a critical component impacting workflow and well-being. Several technologies impacting practice include the electronic health record, mobile devices, tracking devices, and software integration to name a few.

9.1.10.1   Electronic Health Record

Melnick et al. [51] measured nurse-perceived electronic health records (EHR) usability with a standardized metric of technology usability and evaluated its association with professional burnout. In a cross-sectional survey of a random sample of US healthcare professionals EHR usability was measured along with the Maslach Burnout Inventory. Findings concluded the average nurse rated EHR system usability scale (SUS) score was in the bottom 24% of scores across previous studies and categorized with a grade of "F." On multivariable analysis adjusting for age, gender, race, ethnicity, relationship status, children, highest nursing-related degree, mean hours worked per week, years of nursing experience, advanced certification, and practice setting, nurse-rated EHR usability was associated with burnout with each 1 point more favorable SUS score and associated with 2% lower odds of burnout.

9.1.10.2   Mobile Devices

Heponiemi et al. [52] asserted that mobile devices are being used to promote healthcare professionals' workflow, constantly updating of patient information, and improve the communication within the healthcare team; however, little is known about their effect on healthcare professionals' well-being. The authors conducted a cross-sectional population-based survey study to examine healthcare professionals' perceived time pressure, stress related to information systems, and self-rated stress. Healthcare professionals who used the mobile version of their EHR had statistically higher levels of time pressure and stress related to information systems, compared with those who did not use mobile versions. Moreover, the interactions of mobile device use with experience in using EHRs, ease of use, and technical quality were statistically significant for stress related to information systems. Inexperience in using EHRs, low levels of ease of use, and technical quality were associated with higher stress related to information systems and the association was more pronounced among those who used mobile devices. That is, the highest levels of stress related to information systems were perceived among those who used mobile devices as well as among inexperienced EHR users or those who perceived usability problems in their EHRs.

9.1.10.3   Integration and Workflow

According to Wesorick and Doebbeling [53], there is a tension between the use of technology and care delivery (clinical operations). The authors described this tension like a polarity map (see Fig. 9.3). Aligning the technology to support and automate certain behaviors and workflows is an important skill that requires an understanding of the technology and its design intent, the technology integration required for a seamless workflow roadmap, and an understanding of cognitive informatics [54]. The use of cognitive science principles to understand the cognitive part of the healthcare professional's knowledge in problem-solving, decision-making, critical thinking, and clarity on the professional scope of practice is an important aspect of workflow. Usability and competency of technology is a component that must be embedded in this workflow and requires education and

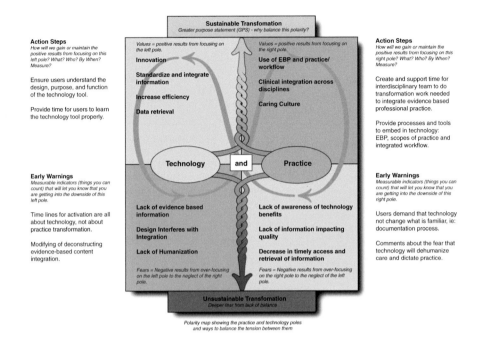

Polarity map showing the practice and technology poles
and ways to balance the tension between them

Fig. 9.3 Polarity map—technology and practice

adoptability. It is important for health systems to provide the proper culture, training, and competency development for their staff. Knowing that your work environment is a safe place for staff and patients improves the outlook on the work environment. It is important as advocates for healthy work environments and healthcare professional resilience to adequately plan and design for the built environment to support healthcare professionals and care delivery. With technology being a large part of the work environment, it is important to include healthcare professionals experienced in technology planning and nurse informaticists to be part of the planning team to align the processes, people, place, and technology.

9.1.11 Evidence-Based Design (EBD)

This snapshot of EBD research reveals how the built environment impacts staff well-being. The research is just a segment of the larger EBD knowledge base that addresses healthcare design elements and their impact on staff and patient outcomes. Nightingale's Environmental Adaptation Theory [23, 55] provides healthcare professionals with the assertion that elements of design are components of the creation of a healing environment. The healing environment is considered a sacred space created when the caregiver and patient come together in a caring relationship. The healthcare professional uses whatever tools they have available to provide healing. The dimensions of wellness are interdependent and holistic and must include the domain of the physical environment to achieve well-being.

9.2   Application of Principles into Wellness Practice

9.2.1   Pre-licensure Application in the Academic Environment

Courses on the application of EBD to enhance healing for patients and healthcare professionals alike should be taught at the entry-level academic programs. Knowledge of the elements of design that impacts outcomes in all healthcare settings, including population health, should be part of the core curriculum and in the graduate education of healthcare leaders. Students should be made aware of professional organizations such as the *Nursing Institute for Healthcare Design* (www.nursingihd.com) which provides education, resources, and advocacy for students.

9.2.2   Student Assignments

Students can learn about the impact of design on the environment through the following exercises and assignments:

- Select and briefly describe a space in your work environment that you would like to transform into a healing environment. Discuss the main aspects of the design you would like to transform and validate with at least one peer-reviewed study.
- Discuss one staff or patient outcome you hope to change based on your design transform and validate with at least one peer-reviewed study.
- Describe a color scheme for your space that will impact your population based on current EBD research and color theory.
- Analyze a staff-only bathroom in your current work environment. Evaluate and discuss the space available, amenities of the bathroom, and materials/colors used. Describe what this tells you about the culture of the healthcare organization.

9.2.3   Clinical Application Post-licensure

Healthcare professionals should be able to use EBD research like their application of evidence-based practice (EBP). Healthcare professionals who select this area of knowledge as a specialty should be encouraged to practice fully in healthcare settings as they can leverage the knowledge to improve the environment for all care providers and patients. Provide feedback to leaders when the design impedes optimal work efficiency, alertness, or aesthetic soothing. Volunteer on committees preparing for re-design or new design during the planning phases.

9.2.4   Leadership Application (Structural and Organizational Considerations)

Healthcare leaders should engage in all aspects of creating healthy work environments that focus on the holistic wellness framework discussed above. Reclaiming the environment as one of the domains in which practicing professionals have input is crucial for closing the gap and assuring that the work environment is supported by the design of the physical space. The physical environment should support healthcare professionals to fully function clinically in providing quality care. Creating and supporting a healthy work environment is the responsibility of all healthcare professionals. Florence Nightingale's Environmental or Adaptive Theory relies on the healthcare professional to give feedback and insight on the physical environment to carry out and support the clinical workflow. Stichler [56] described the healthcare executive competencies necessary to lead in healthcare facility design including communication and relationship building, knowledge of the healthcare environment, business skills, professionalism, and leadership. Support for healthcare leaders that are engaged in optimizing the work environment as a critical domain for healthy work environments can be found at the Nursing Institute for Healthcare Design (NIHD) (www.nursingihd.com).

Leaders have a responsibility to discuss with their employees design features that have not worked as well as anticipated. Typically, what is aesthetically pleasing and features that are successful are published; however, design features that do not work are rarely published. Once a building project is complete, leaders have a responsibility to disseminate information about problematic designs, so they are not replicated in future projects. Healthcare leaders can make an important contribution to the design and function of the caring environment by assessing the environment through a variety of methods. The occupancy assessment can be done internally with an interdisciplinary team or through an external assessment with consultants that can walk through the building to give input. Although, the consultants may not know the mission and vision of those decisions. An internal occupancy assessment can be conducted through an interdisciplinary task force incorporating interviews with staff, patients, and families; interviews with support services; direct observation of operations; and data related to patient safety, patient satisfaction, quality metrics, and facility outcomes. The findings from the task force can then be prioritized and included in the budget or capital improvement plan.

As a healthcare leader, design decisions must be validated and documented. These documents, should explain why specific design elements were included and are ultimately important when trying to value engineer items out of a project. There is a lot to be learned about the built design from what "does not work" after it is built. It is often too late for the organization, but the lessons learned provide useful knowledge to others. There is an opportunity to move past the standard of troubleshooting for the move-in, to also complete a post-occupancy evaluation of what should be done differently next time. This can be performed at iterative intervals, immediate post-occupancy, and then again at 6 months or more to see what problems remain unsolved after staff have had the opportunity to adjust to the new environment.

The healthcare professional's voice needs to be heard after occupancy as well as during design. Often, the nurse's voice determines what they think is best in the design process, but what is built does not often reflect their input. The most common reason is the design feature was taken out during the value engineering process without any feedback from those who work at the front line (e.g., nursing). Nurses are surprised when the features they recommended were not built as anticipated. The value engineering process must be a true interdisciplinary process, otherwise there is no value in value engineering.[57]

9.3   Opportunities for Future Research

Healthcare professionals can lead in research efforts to evaluate the effect of specific design features on best practices, features that impact quality and safety, features that improve efficiency and effectiveness, and features that improve patient outcomes. Healthcare leaders must include clinical healthcare professionals in all phases of the design process and measure the result of their involvement on healthcare professional satisfaction rates, retention rates, professional sensitive indicators, and other operational metrics. Documenting the value of the clinical professional and healthcare leader input during the design process ensures the inclusion of healthcare professionals in future design projects. Since the healthy work environment is a domain of healthcare, the physical design of the work environment must be included and examined for its effect on healthcare professionals' well-being and satisfaction. Publishing the "contrary case" of built designs that fall short of expectations will make it less likely that the value-added design features are not stripped out of plans of future projects. Healthcare professionals can build this "absent" body of literature to inform architectural design.

9.4   Other Resource-Related Healthy Work Environments

Healthcare leaders must be knowledgeable about the evidence related to facility design and patient, provider, and operational outcomes. Sources of evidence are published in the *Health Environments Research & Design Journal (HERD)*. It is an international, interprofessional, peer-reviewed journal that features research and methodology papers, theory articles, case studies, and book reviews focused on the effects of health environments and design on patient, provider, and organizational outcomes. The high impact factor of the scholarly journal indicates its usefulness to healthcare decision makers and the design industry.

Mentioned earlier, the Nursing Institute for Healthcare Design (NIHD) is a non-profit professional association that promotes the engagement and integration of clinical expertise into the planning and design of healthcare environments. NIHD's mission is achieved through education, advocacy, and leadership. NIHD promotes healthcare design standards; fosters inclusion of healthcare professionals and healthcare providers in all phases of the design process; and provides educational programs for members; and disseminates innovations and research evidence for all areas of healthcare design.

The Center for Health Design (CHD) (https://www.healthdesign.org) is an organization with a mission to advance evidence-based design, promote design research, and disseminate knowledge about best practice design examples. An annual conference, Health Care Design Conference + Expo (HCD), also disseminates research and best practice hospital and healthcare facility projects.

Some nursing journals include evidence-based articles and case studies of facility design and outcomes on nursing, patients, and the organization.

9.5   Conclusion

The healthcare profession has come full circle from the knowledge, expertise, and advocacy of Nightingale to current time where healthcare professionals are leading efforts to reinstate the physical design of healthcare environments into the domain of healthy work environments. Nightingale was not only a nurse, but she was a researcher, statistician, and a designer. She used powerful data to persuade decision-makers to improve the design of hospitals, and even influenced people in powerful positions (Queen Victoria and Prince Albert, Johns Hopkins Hospital) to include healthcare professionals' input in the design of new hospitals. Healthcare leaders and clinical healthcare professionals must continue efforts to influence the design of work environments to ensure the "healthy" work environment for all care providers.

Glossary

Design process Includes stages that a building project typically undergoes prior to construction. Pre-design, schematic design, design development and construction drawings must be completed prior to executing the drawings to a contractor.

Design thinking Design thinking is a term used to represent a set of cognitive, strategic, and practical processes by which design concepts are developed.

Empathy Empathy is the capacity to understand or feel what another person is experiencing from within their frame of reference, that is, the capacity to place oneself in another's position.

Environmental design Environmental design is the process of addressing surrounding environmental parameters when devising plans, programs, policies, buildings, or products. It seeks to create spaces that will enhance the natural, social, cultural, and physical environment of particular areas.

Evidence-based facility design Evidence-Based Design (EBD) is a scientific analysis methodology that emphasizes the use of data acquired in order to influence the design process in hospitals. It measures the physical and psychological effects of the built environment on its users. EBD uses formularization of hypothesis, testing/analyzing, and outcome gathering as a framework.

Facility design The business and profession that includes architectural, engineering, and program management to design and construct buildings.

Hospital construction and design The business of designing, building, and activating new healthcare buildings or renovation.

Hospital design The aim of a hospital design is to ensure that their design satisfies the people living and functioning in the space they design. In a hospital this includes the doctors, nurses, staff, and of course the patient. The design of a hospital must meet all their requirements.

Human-centered design Human-centered design is an approach to problem-solving commonly used in design and management frameworks that develops solutions to problems by involving the human perspective in all steps of the problem-solving process.

Interior design Interior design is the art and science of enhancing the interior of a building to achieve a healthier and more aesthetically pleasing environment for the people using the space. An interior designer is someone who plans, researches, coordinates, and manages such enhancement projects.

Discussion Questions

1. Discuss various ways healthcare leaders can advocate for healthcare professionals during a design project.

   Healthcare leaders can lead in healthcare facility design with competencies that include: communication and relationship building, knowledge of the healthcare environment, knowledge of EBD, business skills, professionalism, and leadership.

2. Explain how one healthcare design element might impact the well-being of staff.

   The provision of respite areas that have a window and access to a view to nature might impact the well-being of staff by decreasing their stress level [47]. Those break or respite areas that have access to the outdoors, may impact staff's feelings of restoration [50].

3. What aspects of Nightingale's Environmental Adaptation theory apply to staff as well as patients?

   Nightingale's adaptation theory includes environmental components such as access to daylight, ventilation, light, noise control, stimulation, and room temperature. All impact the staff as well as the patients [23].

References

1. American Nurses' Association. Healthy nurse healthy nation. 2021. https://www.healthynursehealthynation.org/. Accessed 30 Sept 2021.
2. American Nurses' Association. Well-being initiative. 2021. https://www.nursingworld.org/practice-policy/work-environment/health-safety/disaster-preparedness/coronavirus/what-you-need-to-know/the-well-being-initiative/
3. Ritter D. The relationship between healthy work environments and retention of Healthcare professionals in a hospital setting. J Nurs Manag. 2011;19(1):27–32.

4. Shirey MR. Leadership practices for healthy work environments. Nurs Manage. 2017;48(5):42–50.
5. Gillman L, et al. Strategies to promote coping and resilience in oncology and palliative care Healthcare professionals caring for adult patients with malignancy: a comprehensive systematic review. JBI Evid Synth. 2015;13(5):131–204.
6. Connor JA, et al. Interprofessional use and validation of the AACN healthy work environment assessment tool. Am J Crit Care. 2018;27(5):363–71.
7. Monroe M, Morse E, Price JM. The relationship between critical care work environment and professional quality of life. Am J Crit Care. 2020;29(2):145–9.
8. Huddleston P, Gray J. Describing nurse leaders' and direct care Healthcare professionals' perceptions of a healthy work environment in acute care settings, Part 2. J Nurs Adm. 2016;46(9):462–7.
9. Kim LY, et al. Elements of the healthy work environment associated with lower primary care nurse burnout. Nurs Outlook. 2020;68(1):14–25.
10. Sherwood G, et al. Reflective practices: meaningful recognition for healthy work environments. Nurs Manage. 2021;28(3)
11. Galanis P, Vraka I, Fragkou D, Bilali A, Kaitelidou D. Healthcare professionals' burnout and associated risk factors during the COVID-19 pandemic: a systematic review and meta-analysis. J Adv Nurs. 2021;77(8):3286–302.
12. VandenBos GR. APA dictionary of psychology. American Psychological Association; 2007.
13. American Psychological Association. https://dictionary.apa.org/well-being. Accessed 30 Sept 2021.
14. Das, D. Empirical investigation of SAMHSA's (substance abuse and mental health services administration) model of wellness. 2015.
15. Manderscheid RW, et al. Peer reviewed: evolving definitions of mental illness and wellness. Prev Chronic Dis. 2010;7(1):A19.
16. Department of Health and Human Services, Substance Abuse and Mental Health Services Administration. Creating a healthier life: a step-by-step guide to wellness. DHHS publication; 16-4958.
17. Jarden RJ, et al. Intensive care healthcare professionals' well-being: a systematic review. Aust Crit Care. 2020;33(1):106–11.
18. Romppanen J, Häggman-Laitila A. Interventions for Healthcare professionals' well-being at work: a quantitative systematic review. J Adv Nurs. 2017;73(7):1555–69.
19. Bodenheimer T, Sinsky C. From triple to quadruple aim: care of the patient requires care of the provider. Ann Fam Med. 2014;12(6):573–6. https://hsrc.himmelfarb.gwu.edu.
20. Hegge M. Nightingale's environmental theory. Nurs Sci Q. 2013;26(3):211–9.
21. Zborowsky T. The legacy of Florence Nightingale's environmental theory: Nursing research focusing on the impact of healthcare environments. HERD Health Environ Res Des J. 2014;7(4):19–34.
22. Hussian A, Karim K. Enhancing patient's surrounding: application of nightingale's environmental theory into nursing practice. i-Manager's J Nurs. 2020;10(1):45.
23. Selanders LC. The power of environmental adaptation: Florence Nightingale's original theory for nursing practice. J Holist Nurs. 1998;16(2):247–63.
24. Wolfe A. Institute of medicine report: crossing the quality chasm: a new health care system for the 21st century. Policy Polit Nurs Pract. 2001;2(3):233–5.
25. Institute of Medicine, C.o.t.W.E.f.N.a.P.S., ed. Keeping patients safe: transforming the work environment of healthcare professionals. In: Page A, editor. Washington, DC: National Academies Press; 2004.
26. Kurtzman ET, Fauteux N. Ten years after keeping patients safe: have Healthcare professionals' work environments been transformed? 2014.
27. Zborowsky T, Kreitzer MJ. Creating optimal healing environments. In: Kreitzer MJ, Koithan M, editors. Integrative nursing. New York, NY: Oxford University Press; 2019. p. 371–89.

28. Zborowsky T, et al. Centralized vs. decentralized nursing stations: effects on healthcare professionals' functional use of space and work environment. HERD. 2010;3(4):19–42.
29. Fay L, Cai H, Real K. A systematic literature review of empirical studies on decentralized nursing stations. HERD. 2019;12(1):44–68.
30. Freihoefer K, et al. Implications of a decentralized postpartum unit design and clinical operations. HERD. 2019;12(4):39–52.
31. Jimenez FE, et al. Associations of patient and staff outcomes with inpatient unit designs incorporating decentralized caregiver workstations: a systematic review of empirical evidence. HERD. 2019;12(1):26–43.
32. Parker F, Eisen S, Bell J. Comparing centralized vs. decentralized nursing unit design as a determinant of stress and job satisfaction. J Nurs Educ Pract. 2012;2(4):66–76.
33. Rashid, M. Research on nursing unit layouts: an integrative review. Facilities. 2015.
34. Copeland D, Chambers M. Effects of unit design on acute care healthcare professionals' walking distances, energy expenditure, and job satisfaction: a pre–post relocation study. HERD. 2017;10(4):22–36.
35. Hendrich A, et al. Unit-related factors that affect nursing time with patients: spatial analysis of the time and motion study. HERD. 2009;2(2):5–20.
36. Nazarian M, et al. Design lessons from the analysis of nurse journeys in a hospital ward. HERD. 2018;11(4):116–29.
37. Peavey E, Cai H. A systems framework for understanding the environment's relation to clinical teamwork: a systematic literature review of empirical studies. Environ Behav. 2020;52(7):726–60.
38. Tyson GA, Lambert G, Beattie L. The impact of ward design on the behaviour, occupational satisfaction, and well-being of psychiatric Healthcare professionals. Int J Ment Health Nurs. 2002;11(2):94–102.
39. Doede M, Trinkoff AM, Gurses AP. Neonatal intensive care unit layout and healthcare professionals' work. HERD. 2018;11(1):101–18.
40. Sitterding MC, et al. Understanding situation awareness in nursing work: a hybrid concept analysis. Adv Nurs Sci. 2012;35(1):77–92.
41. Jackson J, Anderson JE, Maben J. What is nursing work? A meta-narrative review and integrated framework. Int J Nurs Stud. 2021;122:103944.
42. Stichler JF. Healthy work environments for the ageing nursing workforce. J Nurs Manag. 2013;21(7):956–63.
43. Sullivan CE, et al. Reducing compassion fatigue in inpatient pediatric oncology Healthcare professionals. In: Oncology nursing forum. Oncology Nursing Society; 2019.
44. Stichler JF. Healthy, healthful, and healing environments: a nursing imperative. Crit Care Nurs Q. 2009;32(3):176–88.
45. Keys Y. Mitigating the adverse effects of 12-hour shifts: nursing leaders' perspectives. J Nurs Adm. 2020;50(10):539–45.
46. Gregory D, Lavender C. Designing healthcare spaces to enhance caregiver wellness. Los Angeles, CA: SAGE Publications; 2021.
47. Pati D, Harvey TE, Barach P. Relationships between exterior views and nurse stress: an exploratory examination. HERD. 2008;1(2):27–38.
48. Mihandoust S, et al. Exploring the relationship between perceived visual access to nature and nurse burnout. HERD. 2021;14(3):258–73.
49. Gharaveis A, Yekita H, Shamloo G. The perceptions of healthcare professionals about the behavioral needs for daylighting and view to the outside in inpatient facilities. HERD. 2020;13(1):191–205.
50. Nejati A, et al. Restorative design features for hospital staff break areas: a multi-method study. HERD. 2016;9(2):16–35.
51. Melnick ER, West CP, Nath B, Cipriano PF, Peterson C, Satele DV, Shanafelt T, Dyrbye LN. The association between perceived electronic health record usability and professional burnout among US Healthcare professionals. J Am Med Inform Assoc JAMIA. 2021;28(8):1632–41.

52. TKA H, Gluschkoff K, Saranto K, Nissinen S, Laukka E, Vehko T. The association between using a mobile version of an electronic health record and the well-being of healthcare professionals: cross-sectional survey study. JMIR Med Inform. 2021;9(7):e28729.
53. Wesorick B, Doebbeling B. Lessons from the field: the essential elements for point-of-care transformation. Med Care. 2011;49 Suppl:S49–58.
54. KAMD M. Cognitive informatics: an essential component of nursing technology design. Nurs Outlook. 2008;56(6):332–3.
55. Selanders LC. The power of environmental adaptation:florence nightingale's original theory for nursing practice. J Holist Nurs. 2010;28(1):81–8.
56. Stichler J. Nurse executive leadership competencies for health facility design. J Nurs Adm. 2007;37(3):109–12.
57. Stichler J. Where is the value in value engineering. J Nurs Adm. 2009;39(6):255–9. https://doi.org/10.1097/NNA.0b013e3181a65025.

Developing a Life Safety Plan: Who Will Help You and When?

10

Clare Dickens MBE and Leah Green

Learning Objectives
1. To understand the prevalence of Suicide among Allied Health Professionals.
2. To analyze suicidal thoughts and position them against a continuum of distress.
3. To offer a justification for proactive safety planning for all with some practical steps and guidance for readers to follow.

A report by the English, Office for National Statistics (ONS) in 2017 [1], identified female nurses as having a risk of suicide, 23% above the risk in women in other occupations. Subsequent follow-up exploration conducted by the National Confidential Inquiry found that within this cohort, while clinician-reported adverse life events were common among all the women who lost their life to suicide, 18% of nurses reported problems in the workplace compared with 6% of women in other occupations [2]. A global review of risk factors related to nurse suicide [3] found that collective risk factors leading to such tragedies included knowledge of and access to means, personal and work-related stress, substance abuse, and undertreatment of depression. This should have us reflect further, that while we can chase our tails trying to link cause and effect, gain insight at a population level as to what risk factors may be present at the time of a person's death, a myopic focus on risk factors as a means of being able to categorize and predict risk, may be counter intuitive, and may be ineffective at preventing suicide attempts and completion [4].

C. Dickens MBE (✉)
Academic Lead - Mental Health and Wellbeing, University of Wolverhampton,
Wolverhampton, UK
e-mail: clare.dickens@wlv.ac.uk

L. Green
Priory Group, London, UK

© The Author(s), under exclusive license to Springer Nature
Switzerland AG 2023
J. E. Davidson, M. Richardson (eds.), *Workplace Wellness: From Resiliency to Suicide Prevention and Grief Management*, https://doi.org/10.1007/978-3-031-16983-0_10

By inference, we must consider that there are additional barriers for suicidal individuals to overcome, to include, a preference for self-management, shame, low perceived need, and indeed availability of support [5, 6]. A USA-based study found that compared with other U.S. workers, nurses were at higher risk for suicidal ideation, and nurses with such ideation were more reluctant to seek help than those without it [7]. It could be argued that seeking help from formal services should be easier and they should be more readily available, but this argument should also embrace a consideration that suicidal thoughts and the phenomenon of suicide, is something that requires support via a range of mediums, to include whole community public health provision and self-help.

This argument could go further, in that the default and dominant alignment of psychiatry to suicidality may prove to be detrimental to the aim of suicide prevention [8]. The World Health Organization (WHO) has long highlighted suicide as a complex issue for which no single cause or reason exists. Instead, suggesting it results from a complex interaction of biological, psychological, social, cultural, and environmental factors [9]. Therefore, we need to better understand what suicidal thoughts are, what they are not, and where they appear on a continuum of distress. It is important to recognize that someone's distress triggers may be varied and that it may be disadvantageous to consider that something is "wrong" with them, but instead move toward an acceptance that a lot is happening to them [10]. Some of these issues may not necessarily be bad things, nor should they be viewed through a default deficit-based lens, but concede that they can feel incredibly overwhelming and frightening, nonetheless. Therefore, to offer a summation, there is an acceptance that you do not have to experience mental ill health, nor meet any diagnostic threshold, to experience a thought that your life is not worth living [11], and therefore there is a need for a baseline of understanding of suicidal thoughts and their transdiagnostic span, divorcing them from individual mental disorders [12].

As such, stigma is often cited as a barrier to timely help seeking, and those who perpetuate suicidal stigma perhaps unknowingly, engage in communication and behaviors that include stereotyping, distrust, shunning, and avoidance toward those affected [13]. The United Kingdom, Zero Suicide Alliance promotes a message that we should challenge the inevitability of suicide. This has us delve into a commonly expressed understanding that "if someone is determined to 'do it' there is little we can do to stop them." We must seriously reflect on how attributions such as these may tap into our own perceptions of helplessness, both as helpers, but also as someone who may possibly need help and hope at some point in our life. Instead, we must commence any efforts to create a community of practice and support that can offer an inroad for help-seeking, and which takes care of each other, whereby someone can tip back to a point of safety and a choice to live; with the absolute belief that lives can be saved, that ambivalence does exist [14, 15] and suicidal thoughts are an indication that something in our life needs to change, not that it needs to end.

Suicidal thoughts can occur when someone's prolonged self-perception of burdensomeness, sense of low belongingness, social isolation [16], and feelings of entrapment [17] drive their desire for escape, from what is often intolerable emotional and physiological pain. There is also a proposed shift in thinking which may view suicidal thoughts and attempts representing a "cry for help" (which over the years has been misunderstood to being a "mere" cry for help) to a "cry of pain" where such thoughts, disclosures, and behaviors are a communication of such, of pain [18, 19].

A compassionate approach is reportedly by far the most useful interaction for positive engagement with an individual who is considering that their life is not worth living. Health professionals who are empathetic and compassionate can encourage increased disclosure by individuals about concerns, symptoms, and experiences, and are ultimately more effective at delivering care [20]. They can offer support for individuals to feel validated and heard, and possibly commence a process of co-explored and permitted problem solving, as it has been identified that suicidal and self-harming thoughts can commence from a difficulty or inability to problem solving [21]. This may be because we have never faced such problems before, and therefore have developed limited coping strategies to overcome them.

It should be said that caring and compassion are not offered without consequence, and could come at a price [22]. But what of self-compassion? A UK-based NHS Staff and Learners' Mental Wellbeing Commission set out to discover and review evidence of good practice where the mental health and well-being of staff and learners in NHS organizations has been made an organizational priority. The need for self-care was one of the dominant themes reported, highlighting that if a person is intolerant of their own distress, they may not be able to tolerate the distress of others. A call for action followed in that we need to support a workplace culture which encourages compassion to oneself, where self-care is "normalized" [23].

So, what of shifting the narrative away from characterizing, tallying, and managing risk, to focus instead on compassion, safeguarding, and safety planning **for all**? [24, 25]. Safety planning is the process of thoughtfully laying out a plan of what you could do to seek help or redirect your thoughts if you started having thoughts of self-harm. The plan includes reminders to yourself of what calms you, who you might go for help if you needed it, and where you might seek help. By developing this in advance you will be more likely to call upon the details when needed. If all people had safety plans, a friend or colleague could prompt you through using the safety plan in a time of crisis.

A recent meta-analysis indicated that safety planning has been found to reduce the risk of suicidal ideation by 43% among individuals that have undertaken such an intervention [26]. Similarly, safety planning was associated with improvements in suicidal ideation and behavior, decreases in depression and hopelessness, reductions in hospitalizations, and improvements in treatment attendance [27]. Safety planning is also highlighted as best practice for the management of suicidal ideation and behavior and prevention of the risk of suicide, by the National Institute for Health and Care Excellence (NICE) [28]. However, the quality and specificity of a safety plan can determine its effectiveness [29].

10.1 Application of Principles into Wellness Practice

A safety plan is probably best compared to a plan for what to do if your car breaks down. Most of us who own vehicles have some sense of how it runs, what we need to do in order to keep it running, what might be an indication that it may be breaking down, and what to do if it starts to or does. In summary, we do what we can and that is within our remit to keep it going, and should we find ourselves stranded, most of us would have a pre-considered plan of what to do, and who to call in order to get home safely that day.

How many of us have such a pre-considered, documented, and detailed plan for our own mental health? Emotional pain and suicidal thoughts can happen to any of us at any time, they can commence with no plans or desire to die, with a growing sense of awareness that life is difficult and painful, through to detailed and specific plans, and an ever-growing inability distract ourselves from this distress and to feel hope for the future.

Our own safety plan would include a personalized and individual set of strategies, actions, contacts for support and a commitment to ourselves to enact these principles, underpinned with an absolute belief that we matter, and, that such pain can and will pass.

10.1.1 Components of a Safety Plan

Recognizing Our Warning Signs—Indications that we are becoming overwhelmed are experiencing emotional pain and thoughts that our life may not be worth living. Examples of warning signs might include:

Thinking—"I have no plans to harm myself, but life is so horrible at the moment, if I didn't wake up tomorrow, it wouldn't be a big deal".

Behaving—Coming home from work and having an alcoholic drink before anything else.

Situation—Being unable to perceive solution or hope against the varying things you are experiencing, for example, financial difficulties, relationship breakdown, workplace bullying, burnout.

Mood—Feeling consumed with worry and dark imaginings that at any point, something terrible will happen and disrupt your life which now is going well and is successful.

My own coping strategies—Things we can do, activities we can engage in that don't need us to call up on anyone else. Examples might include:

Thinking—"I matter, this will pass, people love me, and I love them, I have got through this before and I can again, this is temporary, I would not know the value of joy, if I didn't experience sorrow".

Coping—Write a worry list to support cognitive processing and relieve cognitive burden, list the things that are playing on your mind, and consider which of these issues may require support from others, what you can solve on your own, and which may benefit from a differing perspective.

Doing—Relaxation, a bath or shower, distraction and soothing with music, going for a walk, tidying a room, watching TV, drawing, poetry, skimming photographs of people we love and places we want to see.

Reasons for living: Plans to see places and meet new people, career ambitions, those who love me and who I love.

Someone to confide in and somewhere to be—A list of people and places who we can call up on or go to in order to gain social support. Examples might include:

People—Friends, family, colleagues, list who and when—not all our contacts will be available 24/7.

Places—Crisis Café, Safe Haven, Art Gallery, workplace, place of worship.

Making my environment safer—Removing any access to means that we may employ in order to harm ourselves. Examples might include:

Locking medication in a lockable box, placing a photograph of those I love on top of that medication, employing a strategy that means I am not on my own.

Professional services and contacts who i can call up on, and what they can do for me—A list of organizations and services to contact. Examples might include:

talking help lines, professional talking help lines, mental health services, emergency department.

Consider the benefit of saving these contacts in your phone- engage in a practice run of ringing a talking help line before there is an actual need. Contacting these services, or navigating how for the first time, will not be easy during heightened distress.

10.1.2 Clinical Application

An ideal time to engage in safety planning would be during times when we are less overwhelmed [30], to add value and depth to such a safety plan, it is also possibly worth considering engaging in the creation of our safety plan with someone else that we trust being present. It is worth adding that in a clinical situation with patients, it is certainly not best practice to send someone away to complete their safety plan on their own [31]. This way, valuable opportunities for sharing validation, suggestions, and sources of support and hope will be missed. In either situation, whether co-exploring and creating our own safety plan or supporting someone else to co-explore and create theirs, awaiting an invitation for such a plan only once crisis point has been reached, is possibly the equivalent of being stranded with our broken-down car, which we are unaware hasn't been running well for a while, our panic and distress then being heightened as we have had no prior thought of what we need to do, and we have had no prior space to conceive that we can and will get home safely. Safety planning, in the pre-crisis space, affords us and others more capability to explore ways of coping, better reflect on our own emerging signs of distress, and to see our resources more clearly [32].

Safety plans evolve iteratively with us, it is our plan and no one else's, and as we become more familiar with our own internal process, our responses and what helps to remedy our pain, we can add to our plan, highlight those aspects that work incredibly well, and strike off those that haven't, we can add to our own narrative of hope in overcoming such thoughts before, learning from our survival and gaining strength from it. Sticking with the analogy of breakdown cover for our cars, they require a service and refueling at the very least for them to get us from A to B, review your safety plan as life changes. Rory O'Connor offers a compelling vision in his 2021 book *when it is darkest,* in that safety planning does not close the door to suicide, it instead distracts us, prompts us to contact someone else, or do something else, instead of walking through it [33].

A safety plan can scoop us up into an embrace and prevent us from crossing the threshold from suicide being an option, to suicide being the outcome of our pain.

Safety Planning Resources

www.stayingsafe.net

https://papyrus-uk.org/wp-content/uploads/2018/09/Suicide-Safety-Plan-Leaflet.pdf

10.1.3 Leadership Application (Structural and Organizational Considerations)

As leaders, never underestimate how difficult it can be to reflect on our own role and beliefs about suicide prevention. Suicide is a topic that has gone on a journey of being a product of sin, to one of mental illness, and is an issue that has so many layers of complexity, fear, and history wrapped around it. Within the crevices of fear, myth, and misunderstanding, the terror of culpability and the trauma of loss: space can be created for unhelpful attributions to manifest. These casual and unchallenged ascriptions [34] can become more potent and indeed dangerous when they are not viewed as such, but more so as common knowledge and therefore a shared truth.

In their 2005 study, Mackay, Nadine, and Barrowclough [35] applied Weiner's (1980, 1986) attributional model of helping behavior to Accident and Emergency (A&E) staff's care of patients presenting with self-harm. It was hypothesized that where staff attributed precipitants of the act of self-harm to controllable, internal, and stable patient factors, then staff would display greater negative affect, less optimism, and less willingness to help the patient, their findings supported their predictions. Their study concludes that formulating A&E staff's responses to self-harm using a cognitive-emotional model offers the possibility of working with staffs' beliefs, emotions, and behavior to improve the care and treatment of patients who present with self-harm.

In summary, by affording ourselves a time, space and place to explore collective attributions, we can conceive how it may tap into our own perceptions of helplessness. Permission to discuss a topic usually silenced, needs to be offered and shared with others. Here a compassionate community that connects multiple forms of resource, insight, empathy, experience, and hope has a chance to emerge [36]. Health leadership could offer safety planning within workshops on wellness and self-care via professional development and training. A life saved by suicide is no less valuable than any other preventable cause of death, and while updates on CPR and other life-saving interventions are mandatory, there is a call for suicide and self-harm mitigation to be offered the same level of esteem. Starting all employees with a safety plan during orientation would normalize the intervention. The same could be true with students, offering a session regarding the importance of self-care that includes safety planning at the beginning of academic training.

It could be argued that much of the focus of this chapter has rooted suicide prevention firmly at the individual, encouraging us to reach out, consider our own safety planning principles, resources, and early warning signs. This is akin to many public health narratives which encourage the promotion and development of individual resilience. However, this must be met halfway, those in distress must be met halfway, in that when they do seek support, these disclosures are met with empathy and understanding. Beyond this, whatever may be driving their distress, in their workplace context, requires attention at individual, operational, and strategic levels. In addition, in a study on workplace wellness, it was reported that nurses feel cared for when their healthcare leaders recognize them as whole people, acknowledging the issues they might be having personally at home as well as within their work environment [37] There is a for health service and educational settings alike, to conceive their psychological contract with their colleagues providing safe and well-being conscious environments in which staff can work [38].

10.2   Opportunities for Future Research

A 2021 study, having found that in the USA, the risk of suicide completion compared with the general population was significantly greater for nurses, it recommends that further research is needed to assess whether interventions would be associated with benefit in reducing suicide risk among this profession [39]. Research examining the use of safety planning for clinicians and within the workplace is sparse. Interestingly, some research has highlighted that clinicians are somewhat skeptical of the usefulness of safety planning [40], and some require additional training due to poor knowledge and understanding of safety panning and its use, thus, hindering efficacy [41]. This gap in the literature warrants the need for a chapter of this nature, in order to raise awareness and enhance understanding of safety planning among clinicians, to ultimately enhance adoption, improve wellness and mitigate suicide risk within the workplace. There is also an invitation for further exploration of their use and efficacy within the global allied health professional community.

The opening lines of this chapter commenced with a brief summation of an example of tragedies situated within the nursing community in the United Kingdom and the United States of America, and then of an attempt to engage in an exploration of some of the underpinning distress triggers, which may have contributed to our colleagues losing their life to suicide. We must do all we can to continue to learn from any loss of life with the view to inform our understanding, driving our collective commitment to prevent further losses. And yet, while we do this, we must also be receptive to offering space, and affording esteem of living experience expertise to those who have survived. For every story of tragedy, there will be far more stories of hope, we need to hear them. There is a reported protective phenomenon linked to news reports focused on individuals who successfully overcame their suicide crises [42]. Niederkrotenthaler named it the Papageno effect, based on a character from Mozart's opera, The Magic Flute. This character overcame his despair and suicidal crisis after he was reminded of other ways to resolve his problems and distress. Stories of hope and recovery that encourage coping could facilitate the Papageno effect and therefore may prevent loss of life to suicide [43].

Therefore, this chapter also invites a call to action, a plea to all allied health professionals and leaders alike, to not only seek support and help when we are feeling overwhelmed, to recognize the temporality of such distress and the value of their life, to offer a safe space and organizational culture for our colleagues to not only survive but thrive. But to also share our experiences and stories of overcoming darker days, share that we have a safety plan, offer support to our colleagues to explore and create their own, we matter too much not to. We cannot continue to lend on one off anti stigma campaigns at certain points in the calendar year, we must be the agents of change right now through the eloquence of our example, through the sharing of our vulnerability, our humanity, and indeed our strength. Someone who desperately needs to hear it, may well be listening.

Discussion Questions

What suicide prevention strategy specifically for staff, does your organization host?
Should all allied health professionals be equipped with the skills to offer support
and mitigate suicide risk should they find themselves in the role of first responder
to their colleagues and peers?

Should this training also offer a space for them to conceive their own safety planning and wellness needs within a preventative space?
Should we do more to seek out and learn from stories of hope?

References

1. Office for National Statistics. Suicide by occupation, England: 2011 to 2015 Analysis of deaths from suicide in different occupational groups for people aged 20 to 64 years, based on deaths registered in England between 2011 and 2015. 2017.
2. National Confidential Inquiry. Suicide by female nurses: a brief report. 2020. https://www.hqip.org.uk/wp-content/uploads/2020/06/FINAL-nurse-report_20200304.pdf
3. Alderson M, Parent-Rocheleau X, Mishara B. Critical review on suicide among nurses: what about work-related factors? Crisis. 2015;36(2):91–101. https://doi.org/10.1027/0227-5910/a00030.
4. Pokorny AD. Suicide prediction revisited. Suicide Life Threat Behav. 1993;23:1–10. https://doi.org/10.1111/j.1943-278X.1993.tb00273.x.
5. Bruffaerts R, Demyttenaere K, Hwang I, Chui W, Sampson N, Kessler R, Nock M. Treatment of suicidal people around the world. Br J Psychiatry. 2011;199(1):64–70. https://doi.org/10.1192/bjp.bp.110.084129.
6. Andrade LH, Alonso J, Mneimneh Z, Wells JE, Al-Hamzawi A, Borges G, Bromet E, Bruffaerts R, de Girolamo G, de Graaf R, Florescu S, Gureje O, Hinkov HR, Hu C, Huang Y, Hwang I, Jin R, Karam EG, Kovess-Masfety V, Levinson D, Matschinger H, O'Neill S, Posada-Villa J, Sagar R, Sampson NA, Sasu C, Stein DJ, Takeshima T, Viana MC, Xavier M, Kessler RC. Barriers to mental health treatment: results from the WHO World Mental Health surveys. Psychol Med. 2014;44(6):1303–17. https://doi.org/10.1017/S0033291713001943. Epub 2013 Aug 9
7. Kelsey EA, West CP, Cipriano PF, Peterson C, Satele D, Shanafelt T, Dyrbye LN. MHPE original research: suicidal ideation and attitudes toward help seeking in U.S. nurses relative to the general working population. Am J Nurs. 2021;121(11):24–36. https://doi.org/10.1097/01.NAJ.0000798056.73563.fa.
8. Hjelmeland H. 'To prevent suicide, we need to understand (the meanings of) suicidality'—Norwegian University of Science and Technology (NTNU), UK Suicide Prevention Summit Webinar, March 22, 2020.
9. World Health Organization. Figures and facts about suicide (adaptation of the 1999 document). Geneva: WHO; 2020.
10. Dickens C, 2021 Supporting students the role of the NHS in Mallon, S and Smith, J eds. (2021). Preventing and responding to student suicide. London: Jessica Kingsley.
11. Burgess S, Hawton K. Suicide, euthanasia, and the psychiatrist. Philos Psychiatry Psychol. 1998;5:113–26.
12. Glenn JJ, Werntz AJ, Slama SJK, Steinman SA, Teachman BA, Nock MK. Suicide and self-injury-related implicit cognition: a large-scale examination and replication. J Abnorm Psychol. 2017;126:199–211. https://doi.org/10.1037/abn0000230.
13. Cvinar JG. Do suicide survivors suffer social stigma: a review of the literature. Perspect Psychiatr Care. 2005;41(1):14–21. https://doi.org/10.1111/j.0031-5990.2005.00004.x.
14. Hines K, Cole-King A, Blaustein M. Hey kid, are you OK? A story of suicide survived. Adv Psychiatr Treat. 2013;19:292–4. [open access]
15. Dickens C, Guy S. 'Three minutes to save a life': addressing emotional distress in students to mitigate the risk of suicide. Ment Health Pract. 2019; https://doi.org/10.7748/mhp.2019.e1290.
16. Joiner TE. Why people die by suicide. Cambridge, MA: Harvard University Press; 2007.
17. Gilbert P, Allan S. The role of defeat and entrapment (arrested flight) in depression: an exploration of an evolutionary view. Psychol Med. 1998;28(3):585–98.

18. Williams JMG. Cry of pain. Harmondsworth: Penguin; 1997.
19. Niederkrotenthaler T, Voracek M, Herberth A, Till B, Strauss M, Etzersdorfer E, et al. Role of media reports in completed and prevented suicide: Werther v. Papageno effects. Br J Psychiatry. 2010;197(3):234–43.
20. Larson EB, Yao X. Clinical empathy as emotional labor in the patient-physician relationship. JAMA. 2005;293(9):1100–6.
21. Townsend E, Hawton K, Altman DG, Arensman E, Gunnell D, Hazell P, House A, Van Heeringen K. The efficacy of problem-solving treatments after deliberate self-harm: meta-analysis of randomized controlled trials with respect to depression, hopelessness and improvement in problems. Psychol Med. 2001;31(6):979–88.
22. Maslach C. Burnout: the cost of caring. Cambridge, MA: Malor Books; 2003.
23. Cole-King A, Parker V, Williams H, et al. Suicide prevention: are we doing enough? Adv Psychiatr Treat. 2013;19:284–91.
24. Pearson, K. Health Education England—NHS Staff and Learners' Mental Wellbeing Commission available. 2019. https://www.hee.nhs.uk/.../NHS%20%28HEE%29%20%20 Mental%20Wellbeing%20... Accessed Jan 2022.
25. Cole-King A, Platt S. Suicide prevention for physicians: identification, intervention and mitigation of risk. Medicine. 2021;49(3):119–82.
26. Nuij C, Van Ballegooijen W, De Beurs D, Juniar D, Erlangsen A, Portzky G, Riper H. Safety planning-type interventions for suicide prevention: meta-analysis. Br J Psychiatry. 2021;219(2):419–26. https://doi.org/10.1192/bjp.2021.50.
27. Ferguson M, Rhodes K, Loughhead M, McIntyre H, Procter N. The effectiveness of the safety planning intervention for adults experiencing suicide-related distress: a systematic review. Arch Suicide Res. 2021;26(3):1022–45. https://doi.org/10.1080/13811118.2021.1915217.
28. National Institute for Health and Care Excellence. Self-harm in over 8s: long-term management. 2011. https://www.nice.org.uk/guidance/cg133. Accessed 2 Sept 2021.
29. Gamarra JM, Luciano MT, Gradus JL, Wiltsey Stirman S. Assessing variability and implementation fidelity of suicide prevention safety planning in a regional VA healthcare system. Crisis. 2015;36:433–9.
30. Cole-King A, Green G, Gask L, Hines K, Platt S. Suicide mitigation: a compassionate approach to suicide prevention. Adv Psychiatr Treat. 2013;19:276–83. https://doi.org/10.1192/apt.bp.110.008763276.
31. O'Connor R. When it is darkest: why people die by suicide and what we can Do to prevent it. New York: Random House; 2021.
32. Melvin GA, Gresham D. Safety first-not last!: suicide safety planning intervention (SPI). InPsych. 2016;38(1):14.
33. O'Connor R. When it is darkest: why people die by suicide and what we can Do to prevent it. Random House; 2021.
34. Weiner B. An attributional theory of achievement-related emotion and motivation. Psychol Rev. 1985;92(4):548–73.
35. Mackay N, Barrowclough C. Accident and emergency staff's perceptions of deliberate self-harm: attributions, emotions and willingness to help. Br J Clin Psychol. 2005;44(2):255–67.
36. Baggett M, Giambattista L, Lobbestael L, Pfeiffer J, Madani C, Modir R, Zamora-Flyr MM, Davidson JE. Exploring the human emotion of feeling cared for in the workplace. J Nurs Manag. 2016;24(6):816–24. https://doi.org/10.1111/jonm.12388.
37. Dickens C, Guy S. How to support staff to talk safely about suicide. In: Mallon S, Smith J, editors. Preventing and responding to student suicide. London: Jessica Kingsley2021
38. Wilson L, Martin N, Conway J, Turner P. The wellbeing of disability professional in the further and higher education workplace. Report by the National Association of Disability Practitioners. 2020.
39. Davis MA, Cher BAY, Friese CR, Bynum JPW. Association of US nurse and physician occupation with risk of suicide. JAMA Psychiat. 2021;78(6):651–8. https://doi.org/10.1001/jamapsychiatry.2021.0154.

40. Reyes-Portillo JA, McGlinchey EL, Toso-Salman J, Chin EM, Fisher PW, Mufson L. Clinician experience and attitudes toward safety planning with adolescents at risk for suicide. Arch Suicide Res. 2019;2:222–33.
41. Moscardini EH, Hill RM, Dodd CG, Do C, Kaplow JB, Tucker RP. Suicide safety planning: clinician training, comfort, and safety plan utilization. Int J Environ Res Public Health. 2020;17:6444. https://doi.org/10.3390/ijerph17186444.
42. Niederkrotenthaler T, Fu KW, Yip PSF, et al. Changes in suicide rates following media reports on celebrity suicide: a metanalysis. J Epidemiol Community Health. 2012;(66):1037–42.
43. Niederkrotenthaler T, Reidenberg DJ, Till B, Gould MS. Increasing help-seeking and referrals for individuals at risk for suicide by decreasing stigma: the role of mass media. Am J Prev Med. 2014;47(3):S235–S43.

Empathic Communication Part I: Responding to Stress in the Workplace

11

Sharon Tucker and Jacqueline Hoying

Abbreviation

TIC   Trauma informed care

Learning Objectives
1. Review the science of therapeutic and empathic communication that can be adapted for talking with a peer about work-related stress or trauma.
2. Apply key principles to healthy interactions with peers who are exhibiting or expressing stress in the workplace.
3. Develop skills in engaging in healing communication with peers in distress.

This chapter presents concepts, their relationships, and strategies for creating empathic healthy environments.

11.1   Presentation of the Science

11.1.1 Introduction

The healthcare setting is a complex environment with multiple demands and frequent competing priorities. Such demands have grown exponentially over the past few decades with healthcare clinicians and staff faced with more and more

S. Tucker (✉) · J. Hoying
College of Nursing, The Ohio State University, Columbus, OH, USA
e-mail: tucker.701@osu.edu; Hoying.80@osu.edu

J. E. Davidson, M. Richardson (eds.), *Workplace Wellness: From Resiliency to Suicide Prevention and Grief Management*, https://doi.org/10.1007/978-3-031-16983-0_11

technology on multiple fronts, payment incentive plans that require meeting benchmarks and not being paid for conditions considered hospital acquired, an aging population with growing comorbidities, an increasingly informed consumer based on easy access to much information, and unexpected healthcare crises such as infectious disease outbreaks and natural disasters. This is on top of the age-old problem of staffing crises, hierarchical challenges, and ongoing changing practices and education based on new research. The concept of change fatigue has been discussed for decades and yet the degree and pace of change has not slowed down [1, 2]. Moreover, communication has become exponentially challenging based on the numerous venues for sharing information, the reductions in face-to-face communication and with it lost affect and meaning, social connections, and the cognitive overload that leads to distracted attention and a frequent failure to truly listen [3–5]. Finally, clinicians are frequently exposed to situations that can be traumatic for them, given the emotional and psychological impact and triggers from their own past experiences. With all this in mind, it is no surprise that healthcare workers are burning out, struggling with mental health issues and even leaving traditional healthcare settings. In this chapter, we focus on empathic communication as an approach to managing workplace stress including traumatic experiences among clinicians, reducing workplace burnout and incivility, and supporting clinician mental health.

11.1.2 The Impact of Burnout in Healthcare

Burnout has been a growing concern among healthcare professionals for the past two decades. By example, a PubMed search hits for papers on burnout in 1970 were zero, in 2010 hits were 578, and in 2019 hits were 2145 [6]. Burnout is defined as "a work-related stress syndrome resulting from chronic exposure to job stress" (p. 171) [6]. Defined early in the 1970s by psychoanalyst Freudenberger, it has since been widely defined and measured. Maslach et al. [7] developed a definition and instrument to measure burnout and presented three dimensions: emotional exhaustion, cynicism or depersonalization, and reduced personal accomplishment. Burnout matters because of its mental health effects on clinicians and the effects on patients including medical errors [6, 8]. Burnout also results in broken relationships [8], job turnover and loss of productivity, leading to an already shortage of healthcare providers [9], and workplace incivility and aggression [10]. Workplace incivility is defined as "low-intensity deviant behavior with ambiguous intent to harm the target, in violation of workplace norms of mutual respect" (p. 457) [11]. Such behaviors perpetrated by colleagues include raising one's voice, ignoring or excluding a coworker, and doing demeaning things like name calling or humiliating in front of others. Such behaviors undermine a culture of mutual respect and psychological safety and result in many negative effects such as loss of productivity, job dissatisfaction, sleep disturbances, intent to leave the profession, and financial losses [10]. In one study, mental health claims were significantly greater among hospital workers who experienced incivility or bullying [12].

11.1.3 Burnout Mitigation Strategies

Among strategies to help burnout is focusing on relationships and engagement among all healthcare staff. Organizational and individual strategies are necessary [9]. Strategies recommended by Shanafelt and Noseworthy include: acknowledge/ address the problem, engage leadership, develop/implement targeted interventions, cultivate community at work, offer rewards and incentives wisely, align values and strengthen culture, promote flexible work schedules and work-life integration, offer resources for self-care, and fund and conduct science [9]. Inherent in these strategies is increasing empathic communication. A 2017 systematic review examined the relationship between burnout and empathy in healthcare professionals [13]. The review included 10 eligible studies, the majority of which showed a negative relationship between burnout and empathy. Moreover, the studies were cross-cultural demonstrating the universal nature of burnout and what can counter it in healthcare. Thus, as individuals become stressed and burned out, the less empathy they demonstrate, both to patients and colleagues/staff. Whittington et al. suggest that decreasing burnout among healthcare staff might be influenced by increasing empathy. In a similar report, Samra [14] proposed that there is an opportunity to begin training in emotional regulation (empathy and avoiding burnout) during medical school and through residency training. This training would help future physicians and other clinicians understand and manage situational and environmental stress to avoid depleting psychological resources needed for emotion regulation.

11.1.4 Empathy

Empathy is a hallmark of compassionate care as it is about understanding the needs and wants of others. In a 2011 editorial, Dinkins argued that staff who consistently practices empathy in the workplace may find themselves less stressed and more energized—due to the connectedness felt with co-workers [15]. Thinking about our shared humanity brings compassion forward with empathy. Compassion is being able to see and feel the suffering of others. Being empathic and compassionate helps us understand one's suffering and bring support to them. Empathy is considered a vital leadership competency [4]. The Center for Creative Leadership (CCL) stated in an article entitled "The Importance of Empathy in the Workplace" that "Empathetic leadership means having the ability to understand the needs of others, and being of their feelings and thoughts" [16]. Also reported in this article are data from CCL that demonstrates empathy in the workplace is positively associated with job performance.

In addition, empathy emerges more completely when people practice creating a shift in perspective in how they view the world and daily life events. Actively practicing intentional gratitude supports us in our ability to feel empathy and reduce the daily distress with our colleagues, and those we serve [17]. Empathy's transformational powers can be seen in active and reflective listening to understand coworkers' and clients' desires and needs. Empathy necessitates emotional and cognitive awareness on our part to have a deep appreciation of another person's experience, connect with him or her respectfully, and to give voice to what they are feeling, desiring, or needing. When we are empathetic, we recognize the emotion for what it is and are grateful for what it can teach us. Empathy is expressed using specific language that is not hurried, judgmental, or aggressive in nature. This is known as nonviolent communication.

Empathy and honesty are two main components of the Nonviolent Communication Process (see Fig. 11.1) emphasized for centuries among compassion thought and religious leaders, and later integrated into psychotherapies as a part of interpersonal conflict management. The process was further developed and presented in the book *Nonviolent Communication: A Language of Life* by Marshall B. Rosenberg originally in 1999 with a third edition published in 2015. The process is a way of communicating that honors our human shared experience and therefore avoids blame, judgment, and domination. The honesty component highlights that it starts with self and awareness of one's thoughts and feelings in the here and now as we relate to others. It is recognized as a way of communicating as well as a path for healing. The four processes are observation, feeling, needs, and requests. Nonviolent communication begins with being able to look at self as we communicate, understanding, and honoring that all beings have needs, and being able to request what we need in the present moment with clarity and respect for all. Using the process, we pause and select words and meaning that are not violent or hurtful, promoting balance in relationships with intention. The figure provides examples of language that promotes nonviolent communication. For more information, readers are encouraged to visit the Center for Nonviolent Communication at https://www.cnvc.org/.

11.1.5 Trauma Informed Care

Trauma-informed care (TIC) grew out of the 1970s when the physical and mental traumas experienced by Vietnam War vets became apparent [18]. Observations and work with vets evolved to the diagnosis of post-traumatic stress disorders, widely known as PTSD. Clinicians started to learn that PTSD had significant effects on the brain, nervous system, and overall body. As research grew about the experiences of trauma, in 2001 the US Congress and Substance Abuse and Mental health Services Administration (SAMHSA) established the Donald J. Cohen National Child Traumatic Stress Initiative and the National Child Traumatic Stress Network. Concurrently, the landmark study by Anda and Felitti (1997) was published, known as the Adverse Childhood Experiences (ACEs) study. These initiatives led to the need for an approach to working with individuals that recognized they may have experienced trauma in their lives. The approach ensures physical and psychological safety, a partnership with patients/clients, and the understanding and managing of emotions. The approach is now widely recognized with a myriad of settings and individuals trained in a TIC approach to engage with individuals who may have

How You Can Use the NVC Process

Clearly expressing how **I am** without blaming or criticizing	Empathically receiving how **you are** without hearing blame or criticism

OBSERVATIONS

1. What I observe *(see, hear, remember, imagine, free from my evaluations)* that does or does not contribute to my well-being:

   "When I (see, hear) . . . "

1. What you observe *(see, hear, remember, imagine, free from your evaluations)* that does or does not contribute to your well-being:

   "When you see/hear . . . "

   (Sometimes unspoken when offering empathy)

FEELINGS

2. How I feel *(emotion or sensation rather than thought)* in relation to what I observe:

   "I feel . . . "

2. How you feel *(emotion or sensation rather than thought)* in relation to what you observe:

   "You feel . . ."

NEEDS

3. What I need or value *(rather than a preference, or a specific action)* that causes my feelings:

   " . . . because I need/value . . . "

3. What you need or value *(rather than a preference, or a specific action)* that causes your feelings:

   " . . . because you need/value . . ."

Clearly requesting that which would enrich **my** life without demanding	Empathically receiving that which would enrich **your** life without hearing any demand

REQUESTS

4. The concrete actions I would like taken:

   "Would you be willing to . . . ?"

4. The concrete actions you would like taken:

   "Would you like . . . ?"

   (Sometimes unspoken when offering empathy)

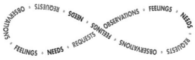

Fig. 11.1 Nonviolent communication process

experienced trauma. Settings include, although are not limited to, child protection services, treatment facilities, criminal justice institutions, healthcare settings, and public schools.

To support TCI, organizational and clinical practices must recognize the complex impact trauma has on both patients and clinicians [19]. Clinicians have been increasingly exposed to the effects of short- and long-term trauma in the lives of clients/patients and communities. The growth has led to attention and advances in the understanding of the potential hazards to clinicians who are regularly exposed to and witnesses to the trauma experiences of persons they serve [19, 20]. An important term recognized in this space is vicarious trauma (VT), originally defined by McCann and Pearlman (1990) as the unique, negative, and accumulative changes that can occur to clinicians who engage in an empathetic relationship with clients [21]. These changes can be profound psychological effects that can be disruptive and painful for the clinician/helper and can persist for months or years after the exposure [21]. A second term that has emerged is secondary traumatic stress, which results from the psychological overwhelm by the desire of clinicians to provide assistance and comfort to individuals observed to be suffering from traumatic experiences [20]. A list of activities to promote empathic communication are provided with a contrary list of actions to be avoided.

11.1.6 Dos of Empathic Communication

11.1.6.1 Individuals
1. Establish rapport with colleagues.
2. Practice active listening without interrupting and reflective listening by paraphrasing.
3. Be objective—make observations not evaluations.
4. Use appropriate non-verbal cues.
5. Validate the other people's perspective (this does not mean agreement, but simply that you understand where they are coming from).
6. Have an attitude of reframing frustrations by taking a different perspective (cognitive reframing).
7. Show concern and support for colleagues in every way possible to help them perform and grow.
8. Look to others for support when stressed for empathy and ideas for coping.
9. Seek training in trauma-informed care.
10. Apply a trauma-informed approach to patient care.
11. Seek training in nonviolent communication as a method for expressing compassion.

11.1.6.2 Organizations

1. Engage leaders in modeling and promoting empathy.
2. Balance empathy in such a way that organizational results are met without burdening employee well-being.
3. Provide education and opportunities for learning about and building one's own empathy, from onboarding to routine operations.
4. Recognize publicly and routinely successful empathy role models.
5. Offer regular sessions on how to remain empathetic even when stressed, and why it matters.
6. Promote employee opportunities for connections.
7. Establish manager rounds with employees focusing on modeling empathy.
8. Use communications, media outlets to elevate the importance of empathy.
9. Provide self-care mechanisms for all employees.
10. Examine patient ratings of empathy of staff.
11. Establish policies for acceptable communication.
12. Hold individuals accountable for empathic communication.
13. Promote team-based work and deliverables.
14. Offer flexible schedules and promote work-life balance.
15. Offer training in trauma-informed care.
16. Build into models of care, trauma-informed care.

11.1.7 Do Nots of Empathic Communication

11.1.7.1 Individuals

1. Make quick judgments.
2. Assume you know how another person feels.
3. Avoid conflict.
4. Use aggressive communication.
5. Blame others for system issues.
6. Personalize conflict.
7. Substitute sympathy for empathy.
8. Make demands instead of requests.

11.1.7.2 Organizations

1. Use punitive-based approaches.
2. Avoid conflict.
3. Overlook employee frustrations and exhaustion.
4. Ignore problems brought forward by employees.
5. Talk about work-life balance yet not show it.

11.2   Application of Principles into Wellness Practice

11.2.1 Pre-licensure Application in the Academic Environment

Students enrolled in healthcare professions programs should be engaged in discussions related to the stress of the healthcare environment, secondary trauma experiences, risks of burnout, nonviolent communication, empathy, and how they can support healthy environments and resilience to manage challenging situations. Helping pre-licensure students appreciate the challenges of the intensive healthcare environment, the potential for stress and conflict, as well as the risks of burnout and how this impacts communication and teamwork is essential. Learning skills to promote healthy, nonviolent communication, respect for all, appreciation for stress, and empathy for patients, families, and colleagues can give students heading into professional roles a realistic plan and strategies for survival and flourishing.

11.2.2 Clinical Application Post-Licensure

Like pre-licensure students, all healthcare clinicians heading into professional roles need onboarding frameworks and strategies that support empathic and nonviolent communication, management of conflict, management of stress, and avoidance of burnout. Being prepared for secondary trauma is important for clinicians so they can recognize when they experience it and know best strategies for managing it. It is common for clinicians to feel unsupported by their leadership and organization, leading to stress, frustration, burnout, and increased likelihood of leaving one's position. This adds to cost, burden for existing clinicians, and fragmented patient care. In contrast, when clinicians work as teams, support each other, challenge each other respectfully using nonviolent communication, and demonstrate appreciation for each other, morale increases, productivity improves, and patient satisfaction improves. Thus, training, resources, and support for healthy, empathic communication are essential for new clinicians as well as for clinicians who may be feeling burn-out.

11.2.3 Leadership Application (Structural and Organizational Considerations)

Healthcare leaders must be committed to promoting healthy environments and empathic communication among clinicians and staff. This should emanate from the mission and strategic plan to be authentically operationalized. Providing resources that allow clinicians and staff to be able to expand their learning about and engage in skills that promote empathic, nonviolent communication is critical. Dedicating key personnel and needed resources, including training and procedures/policies, will promote healthy communication and demonstrate leadership commitment and support. Modeling by leaders in meetings and through rounds can demonstrate standards for nonviolent communication and intolerance for violent communication. Evaluation of empathic environments among staff and clinicians will also be an important strategy to demonstrate change as well as needed refinements in approaches and skills.

11.3 Opportunities for Future Research

Future opportunities for research should focus on organizational mechanisms for promoting and ensuring empathic communication and healthy work environments that can support positive staff, patient, and organizational outcomes. Research can be expanded regarding how students and clinicians can increase their knowledge, skills, and confidence in promoting healthy work environments, nonviolent communication among healthcare professionals, and positive patient care and outcomes. Impact on staff and clinician retention, return on investment, and team functioning are also key opportunities for future research.

Glossary

Empathy Having the ability to understand the needs of others, and being of their feelings and thoughts.

Secondary trauma A term that describes indirect exposure to trauma through a firsthand account or narrative of a traumatic event.

Trauma-informed care A sensitive and empathic approach to working with individuals that recognizes they may have experienced trauma in their lives.

Vicarious trauma The unique, negative, and accumulative changes that can occur to clinicians who engage in an empathetic relationship with clients who have experienced trauma or adverse events.

Workplace incivility Low-intensity deviant behavior with ambiguous intent to harm the target, in violation of workplace norms of mutual respect.

Discussion Questions

1. Why is empathic communication important to clinician settings and practices?
2. What are the risks and stressors currently experienced by healthcare clinicians that impact their ability to engage in empathic communication in the clinical environment?
3. What are strategies for improving work environment communication and healthy communication?
4. How does empathy among healthcare team members promote positive team outcomes, decrease stress and burnout, and promote compassion for patient care?

Discussion Leader Guide

1. Why is empathic communication important to clinician settings and practices?
   (a) It prevents frustration and anger, offers support for all staff, demonstrates caring and compassion, and offers mitigation against burnout.
   (b) It is also a key component of nonviolent communication processes.
2. What are the risks and stressors currently experienced by healthcare clinicians that impact their ability to engage in empathic communication in the clinical environment?
   (a) Work overload, staffing issues, inadequate resources, and new and novel challenges such as COVID-19 all increase risks of burnout and leaving current position. There are also risks for substandard patient care and outcomes.
   (b) Leadership not investing in resources to support staff and clinicians is a major risk and stressor.
3. What are strategies for improving work environment communication and healthy communication?
   (a) Identifying the importance of empathy, its effects on self, colleagues, and patients.
   (b) Using nonviolent communication processes as a way of communicating.
   (c) Appreciating that challenging team dynamics and conflict are inevitable but recognizing them and offering the elements of empathy and nonviolent communication can be highly effective to improving team cohesion and employee self-efficacy and satisfaction with the work environment.
4. How does empathy among healthcare team members promote positive team outcomes, decrease stress and burnout, and promote compassion for patient care?
   (a) Empathy demonstrates that one can understand the needs of others, and awareness of their feelings and thoughts. Empathy includes bringing gratitude in our ability to feel empathy and reduce the daily distress with our colleagues, and those we serve. When we are empathetic, we recognize the emotion for what it is and are grateful for what it can teach us. Empathy is expressed using specific language that is not hurried, judgmental, or aggressive in nature.

References

1. Bernerth JB, Jack Walker H, Harris SG. Change fatigue: development and initial validation of a new measure. Work Stress. 2011;25(4):321–37.
2. Brown R, Way H, Foland K. The relationship among change fatigue, resilience, and job satisfaction of hospital staff nurses. J Nurs Scholarsh. 2017;50(3):306–13.
3. Foronda C, MacWilliams B, McArthur E. Interprofessional communication in healthcare: an integrative review. Nurse Educ Pract. 2016;19:36–40. https://doi.org/10.1016/j.nepr.2016.04.005.
4. Mark S, Seacrest F. The loss of social connectedness as a major contributor to physician burnout: applying organizational and teamwork principles for prevention and recovery. JAMA Psychiatry; 2020.

5. Thomas L, Donohue-Porter P, Fishbein JS. Impact of interruptions, distractions, and cognitive load on procedure failures and medication administration errors. J Nurs Care Q. 2017;32(4):309–17.
6. De Hert S. Burnout in healthcare workers: prevalence, impact and preventive strategies. Local Reg Anesth. 2020;13:171–82.
7. Maslach C, Jackson S. The measurement of experienced burnout. J Organ Behav. 1981;1981(2):99–113. https://doi.org/10.1002/job.4030020205.
8. Reith TP. Burnout in United States healthcare professionals: a narrative review. Cureus. 2018;10(12):e3681. https://doi.org/10.7759/cureus.3681.
9. Shanafelt TD, Noseworthy JH. Executive leadership and physician well-being. Nine organizational strategies to promote engagement and reduce burnout. Mayo Clin Proc. 2017;92:129–46.
10. Viotti S, Guglielmetti C, Gilardi S, Guidetti G. The role of colleague incivility in linking work-related stressors and job burnout. A cross-sectional study in a sample of faculty administrative employees. Med Lav. 2021;112(3):209–18. https://doi.org/10.23749/mdl.v112i3.10732.
11. Andersson LM, Pearson CM. Tit for tat? The spiraling effect of incivility in the workplace. Acad Manag Rev. 1999;24(Suppl 3):452–71.
12. Sabbath EL, Williams J, Boden LI, Tempesti T, Wagner GR, Hopcia K, Hashimoto D, Sorensen G. Mental health expenditures: association with workplace incivility and bullying among hospital patient care workers. J Occup Environ Med. 2018;60(8):737–42. https://doi.org/10.1097/JOM.0000000000001322.
13. Whittington R, Perry L, Eames C. Examining the relationship between burnout and empathy in healthcare professionals: a systematic review. Burnout Res. 2017;6:18–29. https://doi.org/10.1016/j.burn.2017.06.003.
14. Samra R. Empathy and burnout in medicine-acknowledging risks and opportunities. J Gen Intern Med. 2018;33(7):991–3. https://doi.org/10.1007/s11606-018-4443-5.
15. Dinkins CS. Ethics: beyond patient care: practicing empathy in the workplace. Online J Issues Nurs. 2011;16 http://ojin.nursingworld.org/MainMenuCategories/ANAMarketplace/ANAPeriodicals/OJIN/TableofContents/Vol-16-2011/No2-May-2011/Empathy-in-the-Workplace.html.
16. Leading Effectively Staff. The importance of empathy in the workplace. Center for Creative Leadership. November 28, 2020. https://www.ccl.org/articles/leading-effectively-articles/empathy-in-the-workplace-a-tool-for-effective-leadership/
17. Brown B. Daring greatly: how the courage to be vulnerable transforms the way we live, love, parent and lead. New York: Gotham Books; 2012.
18. Gotham. A short history of trauma-informed care. ÎowaWatch: The Iowa Center for Public Affairs Journalism. 2018. https://www.iowawatch.org/2018/06/15/a-short-history-of-trauma-informed-care/
19. Menschner C, Maul A. Key ingredients for successful trauma-informed care implementation. Center for Health Care Strategies, Inc., Robert Wood Johnson Foundation; 2016.
20. Branson DC. Vicarious trauma, themes in research, and terminology: a review of the literature. Traumatology. 2019;25(1):2–10.
21. McCann IL, Pearlman LA. Vicarious traumatization: a framework for understanding the psychological effects of working with victims. J Trauma Stress. 1990;3(1):131–49. https://doi.org/10.1007/BF00975140.

How to Empathically and Honestly Communicate After Harm: Best Practices of Empathic Communication to Support Staff while Mitigating Risk

12

Timothy McDonald and Deanna Tarnow

Learning Objectives

Learners will be able to:

1. Describe the importance of communicating empathically and honestly after harm in healthcare.
2. Utilize a variety of tools that support communicating empathically in the healthcare setting.
3. List the benefits of empathic communication on the well-being of healthcare professionals and the organizations where they work.

T. McDonald (✉)
RLDatix, Chicago, IL, USA

Loyola University School of Law, Chicago, IL, USA
e-mail: TMcDonald@RLDatix.com

D. Tarnow
BETA Healthcare Group, Alamo, CA, USA
e-mail: Deanna.Tarnow@BETAHG.com

© The Author(s), under exclusive license to Springer Nature
Switzerland AG 2023
J. E. Davidson, M. Richardson (eds.), *Workplace Wellness: From Resiliency to Suicide Prevention and Grief Management*, https://doi.org/10.1007/978-3-031-16983-0_12

12.1   Presentation of Science

12.1.1 Harm in Healthcare and the Traditional Wall of Silence Approach

Medical errors are the third leading cause of death in America, at over 250,000 people per year [1]. The financial impact of error and harm is estimated to range from $70 billion and $1 trillion annually in the United States [2]. Beyond the financial impacts are the psychological and emotional costs of medical harm. Delayed and inadequate responses to harm events negatively impact health-seeking behaviors and cause psychological scarring in one-third of patients and produces guilt, distress and feelings of inadequacy in clinicians, while open communication after medical harm has been linked to reduced sadness, depression, and feelings of betrayal by patients and their loved ones [3–6].

In 1905, it was commonplace in medicine to openly discuss and publish mistakes and errors. The famous neurosurgeon, Harvey Cushing, MD, believed the way to attain both clinical judgment and skill in neurosurgery was to learn from one's mistakes. Cushing's experience taught him that it was better to publish mistakes, and warn others while at the same time teaching them how to avoid similar mistakes. He believed this open and honest approach was important for the development of the profession. The Sun printed the names of the patients and the types of medical mistakes they had endured. The Sun later printed when the patients died. Cushing's intent was the pursuit of continuous learning, improvement and perfection through transparency, inviting oversight from professional entities, and creating programs that proffered a transparent approach in education [7].

As it might be expected, his colleagues disagreed with this approach and publicized their disagreements. The public was caught in the crossfire of this public feud among healthcare professionals, but without the foundational knowledge to understand the argument it only generated mistrust and fear. No resolution or publicized appreciation for the pain being caused to patients as a result of these mistakes was offered to the public. As a result, patients and families began to pursue compensation through the legal system perceiving it to be their only option, and malpractice suits began to increase significantly. Transparency and honesty without context were not enough for patients who were harmed, and seeds for an adversarial relationship between healthcare professional and patient were planted. In fact, it was over 100 years ago when the Boston Medical and Surgical Journal published an article entitled, Suits for Alleged Malpractice, where the author recommended physicians stay closed-mouthed and speak to no one about cases with bad outcomes [8]. With this publication we see the first bricks of today's wall of silence being put into place, forcing patients and healthcare professionals to opposing sides of care.

In the following decades, medical malpractice lawsuits continued to increase and in 1934, an article in the *New England Journal of Medicine (NEJM)* entitled, "Malpractice Suits and Their Cause and Prevention," reported that approximately 20,000 suits had been brought in the previous 5 years alone. This article, and suggested way of thinking, became a precursor to the "delay, deny, and defend" litigation strategy now a mainstay employed by the defense bar. The authors offered five rules to safeguard against malpractice suits, and "keeping a cautious tongue" was the first and most prominent of the safeguards. In other words, keep your mouth shut and share little when patient harm occurs [9].

Most all who practice medicine today would agree this shame and blame culture has engendered a fearful, self-preserving environment, the collective "cautious tongue" contributing to the fully constructed wall of silence serving as the premise of Rosemary Gibson's book by the same name [10]. Caring healthcare professionals are regularly prevented by healthcare leadership, more concerned with legal ramifications, from offering an explanation to patients and their families when harm occurs. The knee-jerk reaction to patient harm events today was no doubt defined by the evolution of the healthcare culture over time. It would logically follow, however, that if healthcare professionals have been conditioned to defer accountability to lawyers in these cases, hoping no claim is ever filed or that delay, deny, and defend will cause the patient and family to eventually give up the pursuit of justice or appropriate resolution, we can recondition ourselves to adopt a better way of managing these cases for all involved.

In addition to harming patients, the Wall of Silence culture is destroying good healthcare professionals. Some have offered a firsthand account of the shame and humiliation she felt after a near miss during her training. "It was the shame of realizing I was not who I thought I was, that I was not who I was telling my patient and my colleague I was." She recognized how limiting and self-centered this view is, and shows the depth of emotional intelligence needed to manage the range of complex interpersonal skills required of healthcare professionals; skills that are not covered in depth during training. She writes: "After all, it was the patient who experienced the error. But it is precisely the clinician's emotion—particularly shame—that stands as the major impediment to the full disclosure policies that are increasingly demanded" [11].

In the April 21, 2018 Lancet article, The Art of Medicine: Stories of Shame, the authors discuss the level of distress felt after committing a medical error, and then the guilt and shame that is compounded by a medical-legal system designed to destroy those who enter. "The regulatory body does have the critical task of settings standards for medical practice and protecting the public from doctors whose conduct of performance falls below these values. However, this important goal is currently pursued through what appear to be public shaming rituals aimed at punishment and deterrence, rather than raising the standards of the profession" [12].

As Lucian Leape stated in testimony before congress "the single greatest impediment to error prevention is that we punish people for making mistakes" or just being human [13]. One approach to balancing the need for accountability and a desire to treat people fairly following mistakes is the "Just Culture" concept [14]. Just Culture is a concept that highlights and emphasizes that by and large, mistakes in healthcare are the results of faulty systems rather than incompetent clinicians. However, from the accountability perspective this Just Culture concept also focuses on the behavioral choices of individuals whereby those individuals who commit human errors are supported and not punished while those who engage in reckless behavior are sanctioned or held accountable.

A case that highlights these issues involves a nurse working at the Vanderbilt University Medical Center, RaDonda Vaught, who accidentally administered the wrong medication to a 75-year-old patient, Charlene Murphy, that caused the patient's death [15]. The nurse reported the medication error but the organization's response to the error and death of the patient did not include complete transparency. In fact, consistent with the concerns articulated in the Wall of Silence, Vanderbilt neurologists report Murphey's death to the Davidson County Medical Examiner without mentioning the medication error. Murphey's death was attributed to bleeding in her brain and deemed "natural" [16]. The error was not reported to state or federal agencies, nurse Vaught was fired, and Vanderbilt subsequently negotiated a financial settlement with the family that required the family to not talk publicly about the death or the medication error [16].

Nearly a year later, an anonymous tipster alerted the state and federal agencies of the medication error and subsequent death of the patient. In response, following their investigation, the Centers for Medicare and Medicaid (CMS) threatened to suspend Vanderbilts payments. Shortly thereafter, RaDonda Vaught was arrested and ultimately convicted of criminally negligent homicide and abuse of an impaired adult [16].

Outrage from the nursing and medical community and hospital associations followed the arrest and the conviction of Nurse Vaught. Detailed analyses of Vaught's behavioral choices in the context of the existing systemic issues at Vanderbilt led to the conclusion that a Just Culture approach would not and should not have resulted in the arrest of Nurse Vaught [15]. Furthermore, had Vanderbilt not chosen to hide behind the Wall of Silence and been fully transparent and committed to fixing the systemic issues that led to the error and death, the arrest and conviction of Nurse Vaught, who was left isolated and alone in her defense, would not have occurred. We and many wonder, where is the accountability for an organization that intentionally misled the public following this event and left their employee alone and isolated to defend criminal charges?

Sadly, the collateral damage of this case will undoubtedly cause a chilling effect on the willingness of nurses and other healthcare professionals to feel safe to report and learn from medical errors or mistakes thereby impeding improvements in patient safety, as Lucian Leape warned about in 1997 [13].

12.1.2 Shattering the Wall of Silence

In response to the financial and psychological toll of harm in healthcare and a lack of empathy and compassion well publicized in To Err is Human, organizations have begun to explore a more transparent approach to harm events in healthcare [17]. Early reports provided evidence for the financial viability of a principled approach which included early, open, and honest communication following unexpected harm, coupled with resolution. Some healthcare systems built their patient safety program on the principles of open, honest, and empathic communication. Innovators began to design, launch, and publish their own versions of this approach, none of which to date have reported a negative financial impact [18, 19].

Encouraged by reports of the positive impact of a more principled approach to harm, the U.S. Agency for Healthcare Research and Quality (AHRQ) funded a series of Patient Safety—Medical Liability demonstration and planning grants to learn more about the interface between medicine, law, and tort reform.

Based on data from these grants, AHRQ next funded the creation of a toolkit focused on a comprehensive compassionate response to patient harm. The toolkit was named CANDOR (Communication and Optimal Resolution) and was released in May 2016. The CANDOR approach is based on a comprehensive, principled, and systematic approach to the prevention of patient harm and response to when it occurs. It is especially meaningful to patients and patient advocates, perhaps the most important group of stakeholders, to emphasize CANDOR's potential for learning from failure to prevent future harm. Emotional support for healthcare staff involved in patient safety events has emerged as a powerful motivator for the uptake of CANDOR by healthcare organizations, aligned with increasing interest in organizational strategies to prevent clinician burnout and promote well-being [20].

CANDOR training teaches vital skills and behaviors necessary to increase the perception of compassion—the physical act of empathy. Empathy and open communication are key focus areas of CANDOR. Their application not only has been shown to improve liability outcomes, but also increases patient satisfaction and healthcare compliance leading to improved clinical outcomes and high-quality care. Giving and receiving compassion reduces depression, burnout rates, improves quality of life and well-being. Likewise, robust and patient-centric communication increases positive perceptions of patient–clinician relationships, better recovery from discomfort, decreased diagnostic testing, and reduced healthcare utilization [18].

12.2 Application of Principles into Wellness Practice

12.2.1 Pre-licensure Training

Health science educators have begun to weave the concepts of open, honest, and empathic communication into the undergraduate and graduate education curriculum. Students need to be trained in the techniques of communication to patients once harm has occurred. Attitudes need to be formed early in students that the admission of mistakes and the ability to say "I don't know" are valued, as these attitudes will allow the culture of healthcare to shift away from deny and defend to one of patient safety and continuous learning from mistakes. Students should be introduced to the concept of communication after harm in the undergraduate health science school and allowed to practice this skill with standardized patients using simulated clinical scenarios [21–23].

The Accreditation Council for Graduate Medical Education (ACGME) has responded to the need for a physician workforce capable of providing high quality care grounded in patient safety and professionalism as a part of its Next Accreditation System. The Clinical Learning Environment Review Committee (CLER) Program is designed to provide us teaching hospitals, medical centers, health systems, and other clinical settings affiliated with ACGME-accredited institutions with periodic feedback that addresses key focus areas.

This includes the expectation that the clinical learning environment provides:

1. Residents and fellows with experiential training with their faculty members (e.g., simulated or authentic patient care experience) in the clinical site's process for disclosing patient safety events to patients and families.
2. Ensures that residents and fellows are involved with faculty members in disclosing patient safety events to patients and families at the clinical site [24].

12.2.2 Clinical Application Post-licensure

The goal of empathic communication training for all members of the healthcare team is to effectuate the knowledge and skills transfer to empathically respond to a medical harm event.

The curriculum for this experiential scenario-based empathic communication training begins with a didactic component of defining, describing, and video demonstrations of empathy and the steps in the principled response to harm including planning for the communication with patients and family members. The didactic portion of the communication after harm training is grounded in Karla McLaren's definition of empathy:

"Empathy is a social and emotional skill that helps us feel and understand the emotions, circumstances, intentions, thoughts, and needs of others, such that we can offer sensitive, perceptive, and appropriate communication and support" and focuses on her six essential elements of empathy (Table 12.1) [25].

This empathic communication training approach focuses on not just the ability to recognize, feel, and appreciate the patient or family members predicament and feelings but combine that with appropriate communication of understanding and support back to the persons affected by the harm event that may include acknowledging, validating, normalizing, and encouraging expression of feelings.

These situations are especially unique and challenging as they often involve giving "bad news" but also communicating the bad news may have been the result of errors or mistakes in care. Therefore, the emotional regulation component of the training is especially significant.

Table 12.1 The six essential elements of empathy

Emotional contagion
Empathic accuracy
Emotional regulation
Perspective taking
Concern for others
Perceptive engagement
(from Karla McLaren's The Art of Empathy) [25]

During live, in-person training, learners are given opportunities to practice with actors specifically trained in CANDOR and in ways to respond to harm associated with the medical issues associated with the chosen scenario.

The stepwise approach to the experiential learning process includes:

Facts of a patient harm event case are presented.

Learners are given an opportunity to ponder the approach to communication with the patient/family.

Questions are provided for discussion for 10 minutes prior to the enactment with live actors—**see Huddle Questions**.

Volunteers from the audience of learners are recruited to engage in a conversation with the patient or family.

Enactment of response with live actors takes place with a focus on empathic communication.

Following the communication, the scenario is paused and the debrief takes place. Debriefing is curiosity driven and takes place with the learners sharing

1. A summary of their planning process.
2. Their reflections upon what went well or opportunities to improve.
3. Actors provide their feedback on the quality of the empathic verbal and non-verbal communication and how the conversation "made them feel".

Faculties provide their feedback and open the discussion to other learners in the audience for the reflections.

Opportunities to repeat the scenario with other volunteers or another scenario is introduced [26].

Huddle Questions
1. Are there any special personal or family dynamics, disabilities, language, ethnic, racial, or cultural sensitivities to consider?
2. What are the goals of this conversation?
3. Who should be present for this conversation with the family?
4. What are you going to say to the family? Consider goals above.
5. Would a prop, diagram or X-ray be helpful?
6. Do you need to provide shot[s] across the bow or some warning statement?
   a. Example: what I have to tell you may be very unsettling…
7. After a brief explanation, listen, and deal with feelings first
8. What emotions do you anticipate, how will you name and validate them?
9. What questions do you anticipate getting from family?
   a. Questions may include: who is going to get fired?

10. Who continues to respond to the patient/family as more information is learned?
11. How will you respond to questions of which you may not yet have a definitive answer?
12. Who will support the care team?

12.3 Discussion Leader Guide: Discussion Questions from the HUDDLE

The following "Huddle" questions should be considered prior to entering into a conversation with family members after harm:

- Are there any special personal or family dynamics, disabilities, language, ethnic, racial, or cultural sensitivities to consider?

  In this question, you will want to take into account not only makeup of the family, but any aspects of familial relationships, support systems, any cultural issue that may contribute to particular family dynamics.

  Are there any cultural, ethnic, or racial attributes that need to be considered when identifying the appropriate persons to lead the conversation? Are there any language barriers that might require having an interpreter present?
- What are the goals of this conversation?

  If this is the initial conversation after harm, the goals may be merely to acknowledge that something unanticipated or untoward occurred and to reassure the family that the clinicians and organization are here with them, and will remain present and walk alongside them as they continue to care for their loved one, and seek to understand and learn.

  The goals of subsequent conversations may be to check in with the family, assess how they are doing, provide updates as to the current clinical condition of the patient and ongoing plan of care as well as updates as to what has been learned in regard to what contributed to the event and any performance improvement actions taken.
- Who should be present for this conversation with the family?

  The answer to this question may seem many Medical Staff Bylaws and hospital policies state that it is the role of the attending physician or Licensed Independent Practitioner (LIP) assigned to the patient to "disclose" information related to an adverse outcome of care. However, while the physician assigned to the patient should certainly have a role in these conversations, it is also important to consider other factors such as role within the organization, empathic skills, emotional regulation when delegating responsibility for leading these conversations. In addition, it is important to consider and include organizational leaders and/or others who will be able to respond to operational questions that the physician may not be able to answer.

In some situations, the attending physician, LIP, or other organizational leader may benefit from having another designee, someone who is trained in empathic communication facilitate or participate in the discussion or at a minimum, provide support through coaching the parties in preparation for the discussion. Some questions to consider include:

- Based upon what is currently understood, is the attending physician or LIP in an emotional state to be able to manage their own emotions and empathically carry out the conversation?
- Is there a need to engage a member of a "Communication Consult Team" to provide guidance and support to leading the conversation?
- Who will be responsible for follow-up? This is addressed in a future Huddle question but may also contribute to who should be present for the conversation.

Going through the "Huddle" questions may reveal opportunities to engage others who the family or providers may benefit having present.

What are you going to say to the family? Consider goals above.

This is where practice is critical. The team preparing for the conversation should walk through the facts of what is currently known, the plans are for ongoing monitoring and treatment, how you will support the patient/family throughout the process. How will you, with empathy and in terms the family will understand, relay this information. How will you open the conversation? What specifically do you want to convey? What is the plan for follow-up?

Consider the goals of the conversation and simulate with your team, having the conversation. To the extent possible, it is helpful to have someone portray the role of the family, and help think through and consider questions the family may have. Anticipate and prepare!

- Would a prop, diagram, or X-ray be helpful?

In some situations, a picture or diagram can be very helpful in explaining clinical information. Consider, as you prepare for the conversation, if having a prop, diagram, or other image might help explain facts that will be pertinent to the conversation.

- Do you need to provide shot[s] across the bow or some warning statement?
  - Example: what I have to tell you may be very unsettling…

These are challenging conversations that often include the family hearing information that is difficult to consume. In situations where the information being shared is particularly concerning or perhaps, frightening, it may be helpful to provide a warning statement; a statement that not only provides an early notification that what they are about to hear may be difficult to hear, but also shows that you as the messenger recognize and empathize with how difficult it must be to hear.

- After a brief explanation, listen, and deal with feelings first

Silence is sometimes uncomfortable and challenging. Yet, silence also provides an opportunity for the family to digest what has just been shared and allows an opportunity for them to express their emotions. It is important to acknowledge and validate these emotions.

- What emotions do you anticipate, how will you name and validate them?

    So that you are prepared to deal with feelings and emotions, part of the preparatory huddle should include a process for considering what emotions you might anticipate in response to the information you will share. As you huddle with other members of the team, some who may have different experiences with the family, consider the emotional response the family may have. This is an opportunity for the messenger to exhibit empathy by naming and validating the emotions the family exhibit as a result of what they have just learned.

- What questions do you anticipate getting from family?
    - Questions may include: who is going to get fired? Whose fault is this? Do I need to get an attorney?

    Again, this is a key area of consideration as part of the preparatory process. Questions such as these, while sounding very pointed at an individual, are often based on a family's concern that someone be held accountable. From an organizational standpoint, how will you respond to this type of question. Likewise, questions about getting an attorney may reflect a concern that an organization is not going to be open and honest, or may not openly acknowledge financial aspects of the impact of the event. You will want to consider and be prepared for what a response to questions about the need for an attorney, need to file a lawsuit might sound like.

- Who continues to respond to the patient/family as more information is learned?

    Communicating after harm consists of a series of conversations. It is also about building and maintaining relationships and reinforcing for the family, that they are not alone. With that in mind, it is important to designate a point of contact for the family. This point of contact is an organizational designee, often a patient relations director, patient experience director, clinical leader, or administrator. The designee should develop a rapport with the family and maintain open dialogue throughout the process. It is best to set regular intervals to connect with the family, while remaining available for questions that may come up in between.

- How will you respond to questions of which you may not yet have a definitive answer?

    This is one of the most challenging areas for physician and organizational leaders. As clinicians you are trained to be and often personally expect to be an expert. It is sometimes difficult, when a question is asked to have to respond with "I don't know," or "I do not have the answer to that." Yet, it is very important to not speculate when providing answers. If a question is asked to which the person leading the conversation does not have a definitive answer, it is appropriate to acknowledge this, while also noting you recognize the question as an important one and what you will do to find the answer. It is also important to reinforce for the family that you will share the answer once it is understood.

- Who will support the care team?

    Last, but by no means least, who will support the care team that was involved in or impacted by the event? As noted earlier having a proactive approach to providing emotional support for members of the care team is critical to addressing the impact patient harm has on clinicians, building resilience and decreasing burnout among the healthcare team. It is important to have a proactive process for identifying and reaching out to members of the team early. Regardless of whether members of the team exhibit the need for support, it is the proactive approach to offering peer support that will help decrease the emotional burden of these events.

12.3.1 Impact of Virtual Training

Virtual training takes place with the use of previously recorded video scenarios created from deidentified, real events and selected based on organizational needs. All videos utilize professional actors; some videos taken from live training where healthcare workforce members roleplayed as the persons providing empathic communication support to patients, family members, or loved ones. Following viewing of the videotaped scenario, breakout sessions take place lasting approximately 7 min were utilized to stimulate discussion in small groups. Debrief and sharing of breakout discussions are conducted with all participants.

This approach to empathic communication has been studied and demonstrates that learner participants demonstrated statistically significant improvements in interpersonal communication during complex scenarios, developed better understanding and confidence in conducting empathic conversations with peers, patients and their families. Self-reported empathy scores improved significantly. Improvements in compassionate communication behaviors occurred in a variety of healthcare disciplines [26, 27].

12.3.2 Case Example of Applying the "Huddle" Approach: Experiential Learning

The following is a scenario in which parents of a 27-week critically ill, premature infant meet with the physician to learn about certain events related to their baby's care, current clinical condition, and plans for ongoing monitoring and treatment. As you watch the video, consider the Huddle questions and empathic behaviors presented in earlier chapters pertinent to this type of situation:

Facts of the Scenario
- A 27-week gestation infant is born and is extremely critical, requiring chest compressions and advanced airway intervention at birth. At a few hours of age intravenous fluids were started.
- Practitioner #1 ordered dextrose 15% with 5000 units of heparin in 500 cc of IV fluid.
- 15% dextrose seemed to be a usual concentration, because of this, the pharmacist considered the heparin amount to be intentional and did not question the 5000 units per 500 cc.

- The bedside nurse scanned the fluid and began infusing in a peripheral vein. Forty (40) min later it was determined that the fluid should be infused through the umbilical line instead of peripherally. The fluid needed to be re-ordered for the different site.
- During the process of re-ordering, practitioner # 2 noted that the concentration of heparin was 10× more than what should have been ordered. The fluid infusion was stopped. The new order indicated the heparin concentration was changed from 5000 units to 500 units per 500 cc of fluid.
- The following day, the infant was noted to have grade III and grade IV bleeding on a cranial ultrasound. This is the first ultrasound since birth and the team considers the cause to be related to extreme prematurity and complications at the time of delivery.
- It is subsequently determined that the Heparin may have played some, yet uncertain role in the bleeding.

Setting
- The day after the parents have been told about the bleeding noted in the ultrasound.
- A quiet room near the NICU. Parents have been told there is a need for a "meeting" and they are seated in the room waiting for the meeting to start.

Scene: In the scenario you are about to see, the volunteer is portraying the role of the physician who is meeting with the parents of a 27-week newborn.

Debrief:
It is easy to understand how the volunteer prepared for the conversation and how using the huddle questions, he was able to engage in a well-planned, patient/family centric conversation. The following are examples of how he prepared for the interaction:

Huddle Questions that were clearly considered include:

- Considered family dynamics: The volunteer inquired as to other family being able to be geographically present to be with and provide support to the parents.
- The volunteer considered the goals of the conversation—which he shared with the parents at the beginning of the interaction so that they knew what to expect.
- Prior to telling the parents about the medication error, he provided a shout across the bow—"I need to share with you an event from yesterday that may have complicated care…".
- He anticipated questions and stopped the conversation, letting the family know that he wanted to provide time to allow them to ask questions.
- He allowed for silence.
- He planned for next steps.

More specifically, you may have noticed how, through considering the huddle questions, the volunteer embraced the family and provided very difficult and frightening information in an empathic manner:

Preparation:

You may have noticed that in preparing for the conversation, the volunteer identified some key points he wanted to be sure he addressed and in doing so, prepared and kept with him, a few notes that he could refer to if needed. These notes served as reminders about both emotions to consider and points that he wanted to convey.

12.3.3 Setting the Stage, Beginning the Conversation.

In this scenario, when the volunteer walked into the room, he immediately sat down, placing himself at the same level as the parents. He also leaned in, both physically and emotionally, providing a kind introduction, speaking slowly and calmly and acknowledging how difficult this must be for the family. These actions help to build rapport and trust and ease fear.

- Early in the conversation the volunteer acknowledges the difficult situation, the fact that the clinical course is not what anyone had anticipated or planned and how difficult this is for the family.

Next, he set the agenda for the conversation—goals of which were:

- To hear from parents as to how they are doing.
- Provide an update as to current treatment and care.
- Make parents aware of some specific concerns.
- Share a specific event that occurred the day prior.
- Answer questions.
- Reaffirm commitment to being present for the family.

The volunteer did an excellent job of displaying empathy and reassurance for the family. His "emotional contagion" for what the parents were going through was palpable. He showed deep concern for them and took the opportunity to validate for them that often times when infants are born prematurely, parents think/wonder if it is due to something they did. He then confirms for them, that their baby's current condition is not related to anything they did or did not do, and that this is not their fault. In doing so, he relieves them of any perception that they may be accountable and removes any potential feelings of personal guilt they may have felt.

12.3.4 Anticipating and Responding to Questions (Huddle)

The volunteer allows time for questions—having thought through and anticipated what questions the parents may have in response to what they have just heard, as well as what they have observed through the course of their baby's care, the physician is able to a provide thoughtful response.

Is our baby going to die? The volunteer again takes this opportunity to acknowledge how frightening and overwhelming it must be to see all of the medical equipment/devices and the fragility of their baby's condition. Having anticipated the question, he is able to provide his honest clinical opinion that while their baby is critically ill, he does not anticipate that he is in immediate risk of death. He then proceeds to provide additional information as to the baby's clinical condition and what the clinicians are doing to monitor him and provide ongoing treatment and support. He also opens the conversation as to what the team is watching for going forward, who the parents might see at the bedside and their roles and the plan for responding to any complications.

These details reassure the family of what to expect and that they are with them through the process.

Introduces and explains the complication; in this case the error in the baby's care.

The volunteer provides a clearly stated statement of the facts, in this case, noting that the event is in fact an error "the baby, for at least an hour, was receiving a dose of Heparin that was higher than what it should have been and that this error may have contributed to the bleeding."

The volunteer then stops allowing time for the information provided to settle in and the family to come to closing the conversation.

The volunteer announced when he had come to the end of what he had to share, noting that he wanted to provide an opportunity for the parents to sit with what they had just heard, and ask any questions they may have. This was an explicit pause, allowing for silence and time for the parents to reflect on the significant amount of information that has been provided.

12.3.5 Role and Importance of Leadership

Successful implementation of a principled, open, and honest approach to harm grounded in empathic communication necessarily depends upon leadership support and role modeling. Leaders must demonstrate to the healthcare team that they should feel safe and protected from retribution when they empathically share sensitive information to patients, family members, or loved ones after unexpected harm in healthcare.

Leadership needs to ensure collaboration between all of the critical stakeholders in this approach including the Departments of Nursing, Pharmacy, Social Work, Patient Safety, Risk Management, Legal Affairs, and the Medical Staff [28].

In addition, appropriate resources must be devoted to the necessary training and supportive clinical and administrative infrastructure to sustain such an approach [29].

12.4 Opportunities for Future Research

There is an abundance of research opportunities related to empathic and honest communication after harm in healthcare. Such opportunities extend from the effectiveness of various education methodologies for the transfer of empathic communication knowledge and skills transfer at all levels of the educational spectrum—pre-licensure and post-licensure for all healthcare professions and disciplines.

As argued earlier, patient safety experts have advocated for greater transparency following harm as a condition predicate for improving quality and safety outcomes and, with the expansion of empathic communication programs, linking the improvement in empathic communication to a broad set of patient safety outcomes remains an important opportunity. We have learned giving and receiving compassion reduces depression, burnout rates, improves quality of life and well-being but future research could answer the question of whether the implementation of empathic communication programs can effectively reduce burnout during unique circumstances such as a global pandemic.

Finally, most of the published improvement of liability outcomes associated with open and honest communication arise from major academic medical centers and future research focused on such outcomes in the non-academic and non-acute care setting are clearly warranted.

12.5   Conclusion

Preventable harm in healthcare remains a significant problem that negatively impacts the well-being of patients, families, loved ones, and healthcare professionals. Unfortunately, healthcare organizations too often respond to these harm events with a delay, deny, and defend approach that involves erecting a "wall of silence." The wall of silence can be shattered with a comprehensive, principled, and systematic approach to harm that is grounded in empathic and honest communication. Organizations that reliably approach harm events in healthcare with a holistic, empathic, and honest approach experience improvements in patient safety learning, patient experience, healthcare professional wellness, reductions in serious safety events, and mitigation of risk. Leaders and their organizations must commit to eliminating the shame and blame response to harm and, instead, vigorously support and defend a psychologically safe culture of transparency that fosters learning, improving, and emotional well-being for all healthcare professionals. Leaders in education and the delivery of clinical care must also commit the necessary resources to support the training and infrastructure needs for sustaining this approach. Empathy can be taught and best practices are emerging related to ways of reliably implementing this approach in any healthcare setting.

References

1. Makary MA, Daniel M. Medical error-the third leading cause of death in the US. BMJ. 2016;353:i2139.
2. Andel C, Davidow SL, Hollander M, Moreno DA. The economics of health care quality and medical errors. J Health Care Finance. 2012;39(1):39–50.

3. Ottosen MJ, Sedlock EW, Aigbe AO, Bell SK, Gallagher TH, Thomas EJ. Long-term impacts faced by patients and families after harmful healthcare events. J Patient Saf. 2018. PMC ahead of print 17 Jan 2018. https://doi.org/10.1097/PTS.0000000000000451.
4. Prentice JC, Bell SK, Thomas EJ, Schneider EC, Weingart SN, Weissman JS, et al. Association of open communication and the emotional and behavioural impact of medical error on patients and families: state-wide cross-sectional survey. BMJ Qual Saf. 2020;29(11):883–94.
5. Seys D, Wu AW, Van Gerven E, Vleugels A, Euwema M, Panella M, et al. Health care professionals as second victims after adverse events: a systematic review. Eval Health Prof. 2013;36(2):135–62.
6. Ullstrom S, Andreen Sachs M, Hansson J, Ovretveit J, Brommels M. Suffering in silence: a qualitative study of second victims of adverse events. BMJ Qual Saf. 2014;23(4):325–31.
7. Pinkus RL. Mistakes as a social construct: an historical construct. Kennedy Inst Ethics J. 2001;11(2):117–33.
8. Gay GW. Suits for alleged malpractice. Boston Med Surg J. 1911;165:406–11.
9. Stetson HG, Moran JE. Malpractice suits and their cause and prevention. N Engl J Med. 1934;210:1381–5.
10. Gibson R, Singh JP. Wall of silence: the untold story of the medical mistakes that kill and injure millions of Americans. Washington, DC: LifeLine Press; 2003.
11. Ofri D. What doctors feel: how emotions affect the practice of medicine. Boston: Beacon Press; 2013. p. 129.
12. Lyons B, Gibson M, Dolezal L. The art of medicine: stories of shame. Lancet. 2018;391(10130):1568–9.
13. Testimony, United States Congress, House Committee on Veterans' Affairs, Dr. Lucian L Leape, MD, October 12. 1997.
14. Marx DA. Patient safety and the "just culture": a primer for health care executives. New York, NY: Trustees of Columbia University; 2001.
15. Marx D. Reckless homicide at vanderbilt: a just culture analysis. http://bit.ly/2TflzBbVanderbilt
16. https://www.tennessean.com/story/news/health/2020/03/03/vanderbilt-nurse-radonda-vaught-arrested-reckless-homicide-vecuronium-error/4826562002/
17. Institute of Medicine. To err is human: building a safer health system. Washington, DC: The National Academies Press; 2000. https://doi.org/10.17226/9728
18. Lambert BL, Centomani NM, Smith KM, Helmchen LA, Bhaumik DK, Jalundhwala YJ, TB MD. The "seven pillars" response to patient safety incidents: effects on medical liability processes and outcomes. Health Serv Res. 2016;51(Suppl 3):2491–515.
19. Kachalia A, Kaufman SR, Boothman R, Anderson S, Welch K, Saint S, Rogers MA. Liability claims and costs before and after implementation of a medical error disclosure program. Ann Intern Med. 2010;153(4):213–21.
20. Communication and Optimal Resolution [CANDOR] Toolkit. Content last reviewed October 2020. Agency for Healthcare Research and Quality. Rockville, MD. https://www.ahrq.gov/patient-safety/capacity/candor/modules.html
21. Mayer D, Klamen D, Gunderson A, Barach P. Designing a patient safety undergraduate medical curriculum: the telluride interdisciplinary roundtable experience. Teach Learn Med. 2009;21(1):52–8.
22. Gunderson AJ, Smith KM, Mayer DB, McDonald T, Centomani N. Teaching medical students the art of medical error full disclosure: evaluation of a new curriculum. Teach Learn Med. 2009;21(3):229–32.
23. Cantor M, Barach P, Derse A, Maklan C, Woody G, Fox E. Disclosing adverse events to patients. Jt Comm J Qual Saf. 2005;31:5–12.
24. CLER Evaluation Committee. CLER pathways to excellence: expectations for an optimal clinical learning environment to achieve safe and high-quality patient care, version 2.0. Chicago, IL: Accreditation Council for Graduate Medical Education; 2019.
25. McClaren, K. The art of empathy: a complete guide to Life's Most essential skill. Sounds True; 10/16/13 edition (October 1, 2013).

26. Samuels A, Broome ME, McDonald TB, Peterson C-H, Thompson JA. Improving self-reported empathy and communication skills through harm in healthcare response training. J Patient Saf Risk Manage. 2021;26(6):251–60.
27. Pehrson C, Banerjee SC, Manna R, Shen MJ, Hammonds S, Coyle N, Krueger CA, Maloney E, Zaider T, Bylund CL. Responding empathically to patients: development, implementation, and evaluation of a communication skills training module for oncology nurses. Patient Educ Couns. 2016 Apr;99(4):610–6.
28. McDonald T, Van Niel M, Gocke H, Tarnow D, et al. Implementing communication and resolution programs: lessons learned from the first 200 hospitals. J Patient Safety Risk Manage. 2018;23:73–8.
29. Gallagher TH, Boothman RC, Schweitzer L, Benjamin E. Making communication and resolution programmes mission critical in healthcare organisations. BMJ Qual Saf. 2020;29(11):875–8.

Using Improvisation Skills to Improve Communication for Workplace Wellness

13

Jeffrey Katzman

Learning Objectives
1. Become knowledgeable about the forces and impact of burnout among health-care clinicians and how improvisation might help to address this.
2. Learn specific improvisation techniques that might help clinicians to communicate better with patients.
3. Appreciate how specific improvisation experiences might promote cooperation and wellness within a healthcare team.

13.1 The Science of Burnout, Resilience, and Improvisation

Recall the best doctor you've ever known. Who comes to mind and why? Was it their skill in documentation? Was it their success in meeting quality metrics established by insurance companies? Was it their use of jargon and medical terminology outside of your understanding? Likely not. While life-saving sophisticated technologies and automated medical records have brought tremendous advances, the sense of connection between providers and patients and between teams of clinicians has often waned [1]. When any of us find ourselves in the role of patient, we experience at least a bit of anxiety and are hopeful that we can interact with a person who

J. Katzman (✉)
Department of Psychiatry, University of New Mexico School of Medicine, Albuquerque, NM, USA

Silver Hill Hospital, New Canaan, CT, USA

Department of Psychiatry, Yale University, New Haven, CT, USA
e-mail: JeKatzman@salud.unm.edu

can attune to and understand our situation, respond empathically, and spend some time with us in the present moment, particularly if this involves an experience of receiving difficult news.

There is growing evidence that the application of improvisation skills training is quite helpful both for individuals and for teams in the workplace. In the challenging arena of providing healthcare, clinicians can likely buffer against the experience of burnout and enhance their ability to provide medical treatment by improving their capacity for communication, learning to respond quickly to changing situations, decreasing the consequences of microaggressions and harassment, and learning to communicate spontaneously and authentically [2].

Improvisational theater is creating something onstage in the moment. It is unscripted theater that emerges instantaneously. Imagine two actors on stage. They ask the audience only for a single suggestion of a relationship, and perhaps a location. From there, they create an entire show knowing nothing about where they are going. They create characters together, a story, and moments of meaningful engagement that often move the audience. They may venture toward great comedy, or perhaps take a moving dramatic turn unexpectedly. What they know is that by trusting each other and relying on a set of well-practiced skills, they will create something on a stage for all to see without a script [3].

Actually, experiences in healthcare are not so different. We don't know what will happen when a patient and clinician meet—they will form a relationship and begin to tell a story together. This may be highly scripted by checklists, or it may involve some spontaneous wonders and curiosities as they get to understand the context of their meeting and how they can best work together. Similarly, medical teams do not know from moment to moment how they will function or what will come their way, but by knowing that members can rely upon one another to work flexibly with a situation and to face any particular evolving narrative coming their way, a sense of trust and engagement in work transpires.

13.1.1 Burnout in Healthcare

Unfortunately, many of our healthcare providers suffer psychologically through the many burdens placed upon them. Over the past decade, the healthcare industry has paid greater attention to issues of wellness in the workplace, burnout prevention, and the development of resilience in healthcare workers. Burnout has been defined as the state of mental and physical exhaustion related to the work or caregiving activities [4] and has commonly included symptoms of emotional exhaustion, depersonalization, and low personal accomplishment [5]. It is a psychological syndrome characterized by energy depletion, increased mental distance from one's work (i.e., cynicism or negativism), and reduced professional efficacy [6]. Burnout in the healthcare system is often associated with excessive workload, family/work conflicts, clerical issues and inefficient systems of care [7]. Burnout has dire and lasting consequences for the healthcare system and the communities they serve. Economically, the American Medical Association has estimated that physician burnout can cost an organization $500,000 to $1 million per provider, with costs related to lost billing, recruitment, and sign-on and onboarding costs [8]. The experience of burnout is widespread for healthcare clinicians across the world, effecting, for example, an estimated 40% of physicians in the United Kingdom [9].

Burnout for healthcare providers has only become a greater problem since the COVID-19 pandemic. A recent study conducted at the center of the outbreak in China reported that more than 70% of frontline health workers had psychological distress after caring for patients with COVID-19 [10]. While workplaces in almost all industries have fallen victim to "the great resignation" of 2021, healthcare has been particularly vulnerable. Healthcare providers have worked tirelessly, facing grief and stress beyond what had been imaginable in the past. Many clinicians have also experienced detachment from a sense of meaning in the workplace, and alienation from one another, as many meetings and patient visits have moved from in-person to telehealth platforms [11].

13.1.2 Resilience in the Healthcare Workplace

There are several models and best practices focused on reducing burnout, and they generally focus on creating a greater sense of resilience among providers. Resilience is a complex process that "concretely manifests itself at specific moments in order to face certain circumstances" [12]. The development of resilience is complex, and often involves psychoeducation about mental health disorders, training in response to traumatic experiences such as Psychological First Aid, training in stigma and implicit bias, education about communication, as well as specific practices of mindfulness, relaxation skills, and the development of networks of personal connections. Resilience also requires attention from employers to develop programs within their organizations committed to the wellness of its employees, a lesson learned acutely through the experience of clinicians in the recent pandemic [13–15].

It is interesting to consider the development of a workplace focused on the development of resilience. While many hold wellness workshops, provide education, and even offer experiences such as yoga or noon-time exercise, the call for wellness is often experienced by clinicians as yet another administrative demand. Few healthcare organizations actually focus on the network of social relationships so important to the health of any organization. In healthcare in particular, one would imagine that the existence of social networks and the experience of a sense of belonging would buffer the individual employee from burnout and other psychological experiences during times of stress. The Gallup organization has identified this for decades in its consultations to the workplace. It has long identified that "having a best friend at work" is a critical predictor of employee engagement and retention, and one could imagine that the mechanism of this would be a buffering against the experience of burnout.

The evolution of quality relationships is very normal and an important part of a healthy workplace. In the best workplaces, employers recognize that people want to forge quality relationships with their co-workers, and that company allegiance can be built from such relationships [16].

When we spend most of our days in the workplace, one can imagine the importance of feeling connected with our work groups. To foster this, teams need actual experiences of connecting, perhaps even more than they do instructions about how to take care of themselves to stay well. When we feel connected to one another at work—we wake up with an attitude of excitement about getting there. The University of Minnesota School of Medicine has recognized the importance of interpersonal connection in the prevention of burnout among its employees. In borrowing from a longstanding idea in the military, the Battle Buddies program developed as a check in experience, in which pairs of healthcare employees checked in with one another daily [17]. Much like the Gallup idea of a best friend at work, this program underscores the potential impact of being known in the workplace and the importance of relationships in buffering against burnout.

Traditionally, wellness activities focus on activities that an individual must undertake to take care of themselves—exercise, eating right, sleep, meditation, getting to nature. Though something else may be critical in building a successful workplace wellness program—connecting through fun. The FISH leadership program demonstrates this to us as they teach leadership by throwing a fish wildly from person to person on the Seattle docks, truly enjoying being with one another. Their mottos: Be There... Play... Make Their Day... Choose Your Attitude [18]. Of tremendous interest, there appears to be a direct connection between healthcare employees' satisfaction and customer satisfaction—mediated through multiple variables. One of these: fun at work [19].

Unfortunately, adults are not necessarily skilled at the experience of having fun. While children are expected to engage in play-dates and to have fun at school and afterward, adults make little time for this. This is particularly true for healthcare providers, many of whom have spent a lifetime working long hours studying to get to where they are. Improvisational theater legend Keith Johnstone writes about a sense of dullness that can come upon as we age.

As I grew up, everything started getting gray and dull. I could still remember the amazing intensity of the world I'd live in as a child, but I thought the dulling of perception was an inevitable consequence of age—just as a lens of the eye is bound gradually to dim. I didn't understand that clarity is in the mind [20].

Might the experience of play and fun at work buffer against the dullness that might come with aging, stress, and predictable work experiences? Might burnout itself be a result of a lack of play?

The author's experience in providing improvisational theater workshops for healthcare providers has been quite inspiring [21]. Participants begin to bring themselves to their role of physician, with an ability to play and embrace their humanity. Interdisciplinary teams of providers, who may not even know each other or cared about each other, come to respect and understand one another in a new way. Improvisation provides a playground where people can actually engage with others—the thing that most healthcare providers yearn for over the course of the day. At its core, healthcare is a series of relationships, and if we get good at relationships, there is a greater chance that providers and patients can align in treatment goals, and that healthcare teams can effectively work together.

Improvisational theater has at its heart the relationship between people. The rules of this art form guide us to build and collaborate together, to become curious about our partners, to develop our sense of empathy, and to begin to imagine new possibilities. What if these became the very pillars of a medical system? Why shouldn't they be?

Medical systems are beginning to realize the value of improvisation in training clinicians and in enhancing teamwork [22–27]. Of course, scripting is critical in medicine. Healthcare providers need safe protocols to accomplish their tasks, and discovering the best evidence-based ways of doing this is important. But such an emphasis on quality has led us all astray from a critical aspect of healthy medicine—the relationship between providers of care and those who receive it. We need human beings to take care of us, and we need to be able to be human and vulnerable when seeking help.

13.1.3 Communication

The importance of communication in the healthcare system cannot be overstated. It is critical that clinicians gather information from patients relevant to the context of their presentation. This is most often done when a patient has a sense of trust for the provider collecting the information. When a provider is asking questions off a checklist, it can be more off-putting than if the same questions were asked amidst a connected, trusting relationship, even if that happens in just the first few moments of engagement. Though the electronic medical record has afforded greater communication within healthcare organizations in many ways, providers often find themselves looking at computer terminals while meeting with patients, greatly impacting the critical interpersonal relationship.

When healthcare professionals and patients can communicate well with each other, they engage in the story of the presenting symptoms, and the details of the story can come alive. Resilience programs emphasizing the importance of communication, both formally and socially, make a good impact for frontline healthcare workers [28]. An immersion in the experience of improvisational theater allows an individual clinician to focus on the relationship with fellow participants, and the emerging story, as they collaborate back and forth, much like a clinician and patient would in the actual medical setting. This is not a theoretical idea—research demonstrates that students who participate in such a program develop enhanced communication skills [29]. Another program demonstrated that patients rated their medical student physicians as better able to listen to them after an experience of improvisational theater [30].

Even basic improvisational theater warm-up games can provide healthcare students and professionals with an experience of enhanced focus, deliberate communication, and listening. Consider the classic improv warm-up game of zip, zap, zop. In this game, participants in a circle pass around a sequence of sounds—zip, zap, zop—repeating this over again as they pass the sound with a clap of the hand, pointing specifically at someone else in the circle. The game emphasizes specific, clear, and deliberate communication—otherwise a mistake will be made and the game starts over again. It is also energetic, fast-paced, and can lead to a sense of raucous fun and engagement for a team [31, 32].

The Alan Alda Center for Communicating Science has used improvisation to enhance the ability of scientists to tell the stories of their science. Through improvisation exercises, scientists learn how to best communicate with a particular audience and how to create relevance while bringing a particular piece of research to life. Similarly, this group has shown the impact on medical student communication through an ongoing course of applied improvisation [22].

Additionally, communication can be hampered by issues of status—consider a student learning that a patient had a drug allergy, yet not sharing this information with the team due to fear generated by a low status position, inaction leading to potentially life-threatening situations. When teams participate in improvisation theater training, they learn to play together—from check-in clerk to physician. They develop an experience of familiarity with one another, and come to see each other as people. After even a brief experience of playing zip or other improvisation games, communication is likely fostered in the real-world medical situation. Lives saved and suffering diminished.

13.1.4 Changing Situations

As given in healthcare is that situations change—sometimes quite suddenly and without sufficient information. A patient in the emergency room or on the medical floors can suddenly develop new symptoms or unstable vitals, and the clinician must adapt to the situation. If the healthcare industry has learned anything from the recent pandemic, it is that the context of delivering healthcare continues to change in the presence of a mutating, dangerous, contagious virus. Clinicians who can adapt to change are better prepared for such experiences. Hospitals that have developed ongoing strategies of communication such as daily reports and town halls have likely fared better.

Improvisational theater training actually provides an experience in which individuals can develop greater ease at coping with the unknown [33]. In particular, the enhanced comfort with the unknown comes through a decreased sense of paralysis and inhibition to act. One can imagine that participating in improvisation, building something with little information and advancing the narrative despite this may provide a direct model for acting in the face of the unknown and build an individual's confidence in doing this. Such a development would likely advance the flexibility and adaptability of a healthcare provider, allowing for adjusting to ongoing shifts in practice such as those as created by the recent pandemic. One might anticipate that this would decrease provider burnout as well, as clinicians feel more comfortable changing with circumstances and acting in the face of less than optimal information.

Improvisation has at its core adapting to change. When two actors are working together, one will offer something unexpected…. "That's an alarming cough you've got, Uncle Willie." Such an endowment from one actor to another invites an adaptation to change—one actor is suddenly a coughing Uncle Willie, though when the scene started he thought he was 9 years old Billy Jones, sad about a broken bicycle. As the scene develops and endowments such as this continue from one actor to another, those in the scene must continually adapt to what is "offered" and give up the notions they had carried just seconds prior.

13.1.5 Trust, Perspective Taking, and Microaggressions

In the world today, it has become imperative for individuals to have experiences in which they can understand perspectives that might be different than theirs. Medical providers must enter the world of many other cultures and backgrounds in the delivery of healthcare, and experiences emphasizing the skills of curiosity of another person's background are quite helpful. Improvisation allows for the development of curiosity into the experience, ideas, and background of others.

Consider the following wonderful improvisation game: I'm playing you in a movie [34]. Participants break into pairs and are given 5 min each before switching roles. Person A is instructed that they are going to play Person B in a movie. They need to get information about their background to do a good job. They are instructed to ask questions about Person B's growing up, focused on a particular age. The questions are guided by Person A's curiosity in response to each answer. The trick is in the pronoun shift—Person A, who will be playing B in the movie, says, "What was I like when I was eight?" Person B responds, "You were a kind little girl… you liked to make presents for others in the class for no particular reason." Person A: "What was one present I made?" "You painted a rock for another little boy who was having a hard time on the playground." In this way, participants really experience the background of the other, through their own reality. People describe this exercise as really teaching them about curiosity, and some describe wanting to spend much more time getting to know more details. It is also easily adapted as an online exercise.

Other improvisation games help to build a sense of trust among team mates, while teaching participants to closely follow the lead of another person to feel a sense of connection. The classic mirror game is one frequently used to warm up by improvisation ensembles. A and B face each other, and person A moves his hands, face, etc. slowly so that B can copy in near-real time what he is doing, as though they are gazing in a mirror. The result of this, as they close in on the timing of their movements, is to feel extremely connected with an emergent experience of trust between the two. The implications of this are clear: this is what ideally can develop between a healthcare professional and a patient, and a sense that can permeate a healthcare team generally.

One can imagine that in a healthcare workforce lacking an experience of trust and facility in perspective taking, projections, and misunderstandings arise. Without the experience of getting to know each other, individuals are more apt to talk badly about one another or to verbally harm each other, intentionally or not, with the potential formation of in-groups and out-groups. Evidence shows, however, that when individuals work together toward a common goal, greater friendships and interactions across gender and race occur [35]. The Irondale Theater in Brooklyn has employed this strategy successfully for years. Improvisation games played together by police officers and civilians followed by a dinner appear to break down previously held ideas by allowing individuals to interact with one another and to learn about each other's perspectives [36].

As mentioned, improvisation exercises also often involve the idea of status. Status is part of many stories, and many improvisational exercises bring awareness to this. One such game involves a status shift, in which a low status person and a high-status person gradually shift status over the course of the narrative. Exploring and playing games with status leads participants to wonder about the role of status in their lives, how it works, how it impacts relationships, and how it can be addressed.

Finally, improv facilitates an experience of moving a scene forward by committing to an idea [37]. For many, this is an experience in leadership development. If a group, for example, is doing an improvised fable, and the story is going nowhere, someone will need to make a bold move against the inaction of the scene. They need to break the inaction, or "waffling" as it is called in improv. Perhaps they discover a magical tulip, or call out to a secret visitor landing in the meadow, or transform themselves from a tree into a wish granting elf. The point is, scenes often "waffle" because no one is daring to move them forward. When improvisers learn about the idea of "waffling," they often see how they fail to take a stance in their lives. This can certainly involve the need to speak out against hate comments or microaggressions in the workplace, rather than "waffling" as a bystander. Individuals participating in improv in this way often have an experience of discovering their voice and using it in their real lives.

13.1.6 Spontaneity and Authenticity

Ultimately, improvisation affords us the opportunity to look inside ourselves and discover what's there. In spontaneous moments, we are greeted by our own ideas and feelings and are taught to honor and embrace them. In this way, improvisation gives an individual an experience of their own authentic and spontaneous connection to themselves through the experience of honoring their ideas, which are in turn built upon by fellow improvisers. As mentioned, when patients work with clinicians who they experience as humans, they are more likely to share their story and the associated important information that might guide treatment. Patients are more likely to take their medications, to follow a treatment plan, and to honor the advice of their clinician if there is a sense of an alliance between them. It is the alliance between provider and patient that ultimately most robustly connects treatment outcomes [38].

Warm-up exercises common in improvisational theater ensembles invite the participant to check in with their imagination and their feeling state to add something to the ensemble. This experience facilitates familiarity with spontaneity and authenticity, both so important in being a real person in the therapeutic relationship, and in being a part of a medical team.

The games are not complex, and the list of examples is lengthy. Imagine a group in a circle, and the leader starts with a blob of clay. It is passed to the person on the right, who is asked to receive it, play with it a bit, and see what it becomes. It is now a rubber four-square ball. Then next a poky cactus. Then a kitten… each participant experiences the transformation authentically. Or the leader presents a wooden cane to the group, with the description of a detail of the cane: It is extremely smooth. The next person adds a detail: it smells like old oak. Then the next: There are initials carved on the bottom: LR. The cane is passed around the circle picking up details. Then the leader receives the cane back and adds a detail to the back story of the cane: it was found in the back of the auditorium. Then the next: It was used in a murder (the group laughs!) The next, laughing, adds, it had been in the Sterling family for 100 years. No one had planned this developing story, but each participant honors what comes to them as they are immersed in the story of the cane. We have similar experiences in healthcare, wondering about details of patients as we engage with them in the narrative of their health presentation. Such experiences from improvisation connect participants to their authentic and spontaneous selves so they might be better participants in the collaborative history taking with their patients.

13.2   Applications of Improvisation into Wellness Practice

13.2.1 Pre-licensure Application in the Academic Environment

Famously, many medical schools have a play at the end of the first year, in which feelings can be expressed through songs and skits and impersonations. It would be no stretch to imagine that pre-licensure students would benefit from the experience of improvisational theater as a component of the curriculum. In fact, they do.

To date, most improvisation occurring at the pre-licensure level has involved a focus on communication skills. Many improvisers and improvisation companies have brought the application of improvisation to enhance communication. One particular article [39] summarizes the potential applications of improvisation in pre-licensure health professionals generally and medical student training specifically. The point is made that improvisation skills represent a potential vehicle to teach communication skills and to bring traditional medical competencies to life. They represent a transition from the pre-clinical to the clinical years by providing an experience of interaction. The point is also made that medical improvisation at this level of training also potentially enhances wellness and professionalism. Most all published articles of improvisation courses in pre-licensure programs describe a positive experience as rated by trainee participants. Research at Northwestern and Stonybrook demonstrates the consistency of this over multiple years. One study of pharmacy students demonstrates an enhanced performance on clinical simulation following the improvisational skills program [40].

Critically, the level of burnout and depression is significant in medical school. This grows more significant over the course of medical training, with higher levels of emotional exhaustion and depersonalization and lower levels of personal accomplishment seen in third year compared to first year students. Improvisation courses may well help alleviate this experience as discussed earlier [41].

13.2.2 Clinical Application Post-licensure

The use of improvisational theater has been less implemented in post-licensure training programs. Yet the need could be considered even stronger. The level of burnout in residency training programs is quite high—far greater than the general public, often exceeding the level of medical students [42]. Few improvisation applications have been made to general residency programs in any field of medicine. Though it has certainly been applied and described in the literature in various post-licensure training contexts including psychiatry, OB/GYN, and pediatrics [21, 43]. One surgical program describes the use of a "stretch circle" described as similar to medical improvisation in which one person stretches and talks spontaneously, followed by another, prior to every surgery [44]. It has been used specifically to work with healthcare trainees at various levels to learn to break bad news to patients [45]. Improvisation skills have also been used to teach respect for members of other professions within healthcare teams as trainees from different post-licensure programs work together learning to improvise [26].

13.2.3 Leadership Application (Structural and Organizational Considerations)

Professional improvisation consultation to leadership of organizations has almost become standard practice. Fortune 500 companies often turn to improvisers to conduct retreats and to interact with their leadership teams. Leadership in healthcare has been slower to incorporate this. Generally, healthcare teams participating in teamwork development programs describe some specific themes that influence the utility of such interventions. In one review of this literature, the following ideas emerged as important to consider: These included "the context that the program was delivered in, the diversity of healthcare teams, starting points of individual learners, the type of tools utilized in education programs, the levels of confidence and motivation of learners post training and the opportunity to transfer into practice new learning" [46]. This author's experience of delivering improvisation workshops to leadership teams, interdisciplinary healthcare teams, and department faculty at the University of New Mexico has been quite eye-opening. In most all cases, participants describe wanting more—they describe often seeing others in a new light, craving the experience of play at work, dropping past projections of one another, and being able to do actual work much more expeditiously and in a more focused manner following an experience of improvisational theater games. Given these potential positive impacts, it would be the responsibility of leaders to fiscally support improvisation programs to enhance communication between faculty, students, and staff as part of a holistic wellness program and to optimize patient experience.

13.3 Opportunities for Future Research

As the role of applied improvisation expands into the healthcare arena, many interesting and important questions arise. As these programs develop, it will be important to collect data to understand some of the following questions:

- Can a short course in improvisational theater promote resilience and prevent burnout in the healthcare arena? Must it be ongoing to have sustaining impacts?
- Are the improvisational theater skills such as communication introduced in the medical student curriculum and other predoctoral training programs long lasting? Do they translate into better communicators among physicians years later?
- How does the participation of a clinician in an improvisational theater course impact the experience of their patients and patient ratings of the therapeutic alliance?
- Do some disciplines within healthcare respond better to the introduction of improvisational theater applications?
- Are variables such as comfort with the unknown sustained long after participation in an improvisation course?
- How does participation in improvisation impact the leadership of a healthcare organization?
- What would an improvisational theater curriculum look like as a best practice at various levels of participant's experience in healthcare?

13.4 Conclusion

To really shift our healthcare systems, we need to be able to engage with each other in all levels of this system. It is critical that we become present and learn to respond to each other in collaborative ways if we want to truly shift our delivery system and prevent burnout in providers. This will involve developing tools to facilitate engagement for patients, trainees, healthcare providers, and all of those who touch our healthcare system. To that end, the ability to improvise is a critical skill. We do it most every day in one way or another. And to do it successfully, we can turn to the experts in this area—professional improvisational theater artists. They spend years perfecting the art of spontaneity and adapting to evolving characters and stories. By learning about improvisational theater and the guidelines it offers us, we can all learn to collaborate better, to wake up to spontaneous moments, and to access our imagination. These are critical skills that can help us to learn to engage in a new way and can re-establish our healthcare system as one centered on acknowledging each other and on healing.

Glossary

Burnout The state of mental and physical exhaustion related to the work or caregiving activities.

Improvisational theater Creating something onstage in the moment; unscripted theater that emerges instantaneously.

Microaggression A statement, action, or incident regarded as an instance of indirect, subtle, or unintentional discrimination against members of a marginalized group such as a racial or ethnic minority.

Resilience A complex process that allows an individual, team, or organization to face certain difficult circumstances.

Residency training Graduate medical education programs following medical school that lead to licensure after the first year, and specialized training often connected to board certification in a specific field of medicine.

Waffling Postponing by lack of ideas and failing to take a stance to add to an improve scene.

Wimping Accepting the offer of another player but not building upon it.

Discussion Questions

What are forces leading to clinician burnout and what are ways to address this?

How are current forces in healthcare impacting the clinician–patient relationship?

How might an experience of improvisation impact the sense of burnout for a healthcare team?

How might improvisation help teach or remind a clinician how to engage with patients or with other members of their healthcare team?

How might improvisation impact the sense of trust and reduce microaggressions in the healthcare system?

What can be gained by healthcare providers participating in an improvisational theater course?

What evidence is there that improvisation might help with changing healthcare forces?

Discussion Leader Guide

Improvisational theater applications have the potential to assist with the burnout that has come to healthcare providers. By reinvigorating the clinician patient relationship and healthcare teams, experiences with improvisation have the potential to enhance the wellness of all those who touch the healthcare system. They offer the potential to enhance communication, spontaneity, flexibility, a sense of trust, an experience of authenticity. The literature describes the use of improvisation in multiple contexts of the healthcare system, from pre-licensure to leadership roles.

What experience do healthcare providers recall about improvising within their roles? These are often remembered with a bit of joy as problems were addressed in new and creative ways. Through the impact of the COVID-19 pandemic, healthcare providers need to find new ways to engage in work, and to find fun and spontaneous ways to connect with one another. Perhaps an introduction to improvisation could facilitate this.

References

1. Ceriani Cernadas JM. Is it possible to revert doctor-patient relationship deterioration? Arch Argent Pediatr. 2016;114(4):290–1. https://doi.org/10.5546/aap.2016.eng.290. Epub 2016 July 4
2. Hanley MA, Fenton MV. Improvisation and the art of holistic nursing. Beginnings. 2013;33(5):4–5, 20–2.
3. Katzman J, O'Connor D. Life unscripted: using improv principles to get unstuck, boost confidence, and transform your life. Berkeley: North Atlantic Books; 2018.
4. Ishak W, Nikravesh R, Lederer S, Perry R, Ogunyemi D, Bernstein C. Burnout in medical students: a systematic review. Clin Teach. 2013;10(4):242–5. https://doi.org/10.1111/tct.12014.
5. Romani M, Ashkar K. Burnout among physicians. Libyan J Med. 2014;9:23556. https://doi.org/10.3402/ljm.v9.23556.
6. Raudenská J, Steinerová V, Javůrková A, Urits I, Kaye AD, Viswanath O, Varrassi G. Occupational burnout syndrome and post-traumatic stress among healthcare professionals during the novel coronavirus disease 2019 (COVID-19) pandemic. Best Pract Res Clin Anaesthesiol. 2020;34(3):553–60. https://doi.org/10.1016/j.bpa.2020.07.008.
7. West CP, Dyrbye LN, Shanafelt TD. Physician burnout: contributors, consequences and solutions. J Intern Med. 2018;283(6):516–29. https://doi.org/10.1111/joim.12752. Epub 2018 Mar 24
8. Berg S. How much physician burnout is costing your organization. Am Med Assoc 2018. https://www.ama-assn.org/practice-management/physician-health/how-much-physician-burnout-costing-your-organization. Accessed 21 Aug 2021.
9. Khan A, Teoh KR, Islam S, Hassard J. Psychosocial work characteristics, burnout, psychological morbidity symptoms and early retirement intentions: a cross-sectional study of NHS consultants in the UK. BMJ Open. 2018;8(7):1–11.
10. Lai J, Ma S, Wang Y, et al. Factors associated with mental health outcomes among health care workers exposed to coronavirus disease 2019. JAMA Netw Open. 2020;3:e203976. https://doi.org/10.1001/jamanetworkopen.2020.3976.
11. Shachak A, Alkureishi MA. Virtual care: a 'Zoombie' apocalypse? J Am Med Inform Assoc. 2020;27(11):1813–5. https://doi.org/10.1093/jamia/ocaa185.
12. Trockel M, Bohman B, Lesure E, Hamidi MS, Welle D, Roberts L, Shanafelt T. A brief instrument to assess both burnout and professional fulfillment in physicians: reliability and validity, including correlation with self-reported medical errors, in a sample of resident and practicing physicians. Acad Psychiatry. 2018 Feb;42(1):11–24.
13. Adibe B. COVID-19 and clinician wellbeing: challenges and opportunities. Lancet Public Health. 2021 Mar;6(3):e141–2. https://doi.org/10.1016/S2468-2667(21)00028-1.
14. Klatt MD, Bawa R, Gabram O, Blake A, Steinberg B, Westrick A, Holliday S. Embracing change: a mindful medical center meets COVID-19. Glob Adv Health Med. 2020 Dec;11(9):2164956120975369. https://doi.org/10.1177/2164956120975369.
15. Kiser SB, Bernacki RE. When the dust settles: preventing a mental health crisis in COVID-19 clinicians. Ann Intern Med. 2020;173(7):578–9. https://doi.org/10.7326/M20-3738. Epub 2020 June 9

16. Gallup, Workforce. https://www.gallup.com/workplace/237530/item-best-friend-work.aspx. Accessed 26 May 1999.
17. Albott CS, Wozniak JR, McGlinch BP, Wall MH, Gold BS, Vinogradov S. Battle buddies: rapid deployment of a psychological resilience intervention for health care workers during the COVID-19 pandemic. Anesth Analg. 2020 Jul;131(1):43–54. https://doi.org/10.1213/ANE.0000000000004912.
18. Fish philosophy website. https://www.fishphilosophy.com/
19. Jackson T, Wood BD. Employee and customer satisfaction in healthcare. Radiol Manage. 2010;32(2):20–5; quiz 26–7
20. Keith J. Impro: improvisation and the theatre. New York: Routledge; 2015. p. 13.
21. Fidler D, Trumbull D, Ballon B, Peterkin A, Averbuch R, Katzman J. Vignettes for teaching psychiatry with the arts. Acad Psychiatry. 2011;35(5):293–7. https://doi.org/10.1176/appi.ap.35.5.293.
22. Fessell D, McKean E, Wagenschutz H, Cole M, Santen SA, Cermak R, Zurales K, Kukora S, Lantz-Gefroh V, Kaplan-Liss E, Alda A. Medical improvisation training for all medical students: 3-year experience. Med Sci Educ. 2019;30(1):87–90. https://doi.org/10.1007/s40670-019-00885-0.
23. Kaplan-Liss E, Lantz-Gefroh V, Bass E, Killebrew D, Ponzio NM, Savi C, O'Connell C. Teaching medical students to communicate with empathy and clarity using improvisation. Acad Med. 2018;93(3):440–3. https://doi.org/10.1097/ACM.0000000000002031.
24. Sawyer T, Fu B, Gray M, Umoren R. Medical improvisation training to enhance the antenatal counseling skills of neonatologists and neonatal fellows: a pilot study. J Matern Fetal Neonatal Med. 2017;30(15):1865–9. https://doi.org/10.1080/14767058.2016.1228059. Epub 2016 Sept 5
25. Watson K, Fu B. Medical Improv: a novel approach to teaching communication and professionalism skills. Ann Intern Med. 2016;165(8):591–2. https://doi.org/10.7326/M15-2239. Epub 2016 July 26
26. Zelenski AB, Saldivar N, Park LS, Schoenleber V, Osman F, Kraemer S. Interprofessional Improv: using theater techniques to teach health professions students empathy in teams. Acad Med. 2020 Aug;95(8):1210–4. https://doi.org/10.1097/ACM.0000000000003420.
27. Leonard K, Libera A. Improvised caregiving or how a famous comedy theatre found itself in health care. AMA J Ethics. 2020;22(7):E619–23. https://doi.org/10.1001/amajethics.2020.619.
28. Pollock A, Campbell P, Cheyne J, Cowie J, Davis B, McCallum J, McGill K, Elders A, Hagen S, McClurg D, Torrens C, Maxwell M. Interventions to support the resilience and mental health of frontline health and social care professionals during and after a disease outbreak, epidemic or pandemic: a mixed methods systematic review. Cochrane Database Syst Rev. 2020;11(11):CD013779. https://doi.org/10.1002/14651858.
29. Phelps M, White C, Xiang L, Swanson HI. Improvisation as a teaching tool for improving oral communication skills in premedical and pre-biomedical graduate students. J Med Educ Curric Dev. 2021;8:23821205211006411. https://doi.org/10.1177/23821205211006411.
30. Grossman CE, Lemay M, Kang L, Byland E, Anderson AD, Nestler JE, Santen SA. Improv to improve medical student communication. Clin Teach. 2021;18(3):301–6. https://doi.org/10.1111/tct.13336. Epub 2021 Mar 8
31. "Zip, Zap, Zop" Drama-Based Instruction (DBI) Network: activating learning through the arts. https://dbp.theatredance.utexas.edu/node/29. Accessed 3 Nov 2021.
32. "Zip, Zap, Zop" Laughter for a Change. https://www.youtube.com/watch?v=lyWKVGoXKak. Accessed 3 Nov 2021.
33. Felsman P, Gunawardena S, Seifert C. Improv experience promotes divergent thinking, uncertainty tolerance, and affective well-being. Think Skills Creat. 2020;36
34. Katzman J, O'Connor D. Ensemble! Using the power of Improv and play to forge connections in a lonely world. Berkeley: North Atlantic Books; 2021.
35. DeVries DL, Edwards KJ. Student teams and learning games: their effects on cross-race *and cross-sex interaction.* J Educ Psychol. 1974;66(5):741–9. https://doi.org/10.1037/h0037479.

36. Irondale Theater. To protect, serve, and understand. https://irondale.org/to-protect-serve-and-understand/
37. "Waffling", Improv Encyclopedia. http://improvencyclopedia.org/glossary/Waffling.html. Accessed 3 Nov 2021.
38. Katzman J, Coughlin P. The role of therapist activity in psychodynamic psychotherapy. Psychodyn Psychiatry. 2013 Mar;41(1):75–89. https://doi.org/10.1521/pdps.2013.41.1.75.
39. Fu B. Common ground: frameworks for teaching improvisational ability in medical education. Teach Learn Med. 2019;31(3):342–55. https://doi.org/10.1080/10401334.2018.153788 0. Epub 2018 Dec 31
40. Boesen KP, Herrier RN, Apgar DA, Jackowski RM. Improvisational exercises to improve pharmacy students' professional communication skills. Am J Pharm Educ. 2009;73(2):35. https://doi.org/10.5688/aj730235.
41. Elkins C, Plante KP, Germain LJ, Morley CP. Burnout and depression in MS1 and MS3 Years: a comparison of cohorts at one medical school. Fam Med. 2017;49(6):456–9.
42. Dyrbye LN, et al. Burnout among U.S. medical students, residents, and early career physicians relative to the general U.S. population. Acad Med. 2014;89(3):443–51. https://doi.org/10.1097/ACM.0000000000000134.
43. Cai F, Ruhotina M, Bowler M, Howard E, Has P, Frishman GN, Wohlrab K. Can I get a suggestion? Medical improv as a tool for empathy training in obstetrics and gynecology residents. J Grad Med Educ. 2019;11(5):597–600. https://doi.org/10.4300/JGME-D-19-00185.1.
44. Shahawy S, Watson K, Milad MP. The stretch circle: a preoperative surgical team improvisation exercise. Acad Med. 2019;94(12):1846. https://doi.org/10.1097/ACM.0000000000002981.
45. Kukora SK, Batell B, Umoren R, Gray MM, Ravi N, Thompson C, Zikmund-Fisher BJ. Hilariously bad news: medical Improv as a novel approach to teach communication skills for bad news disclosure. Acad Pediatr. 2020;20(6):879–81. https://doi.org/10.1016/j.acap.2020.05.003. Epub 7 May 2020
46. Eddy K, Jordan Z, Stephenson M. Health professionals' experience of teamwork education in acute hospital settings: a systematic review of qualitative literature. JBI Database Syst Rev Implement Rep. 2016 Apr;14(4):96–137. https://doi.org/10.11124/JBISRIR-2016-1843.

The Power of Microaffirmations

14

Desiree N. Shapiro

Learning Objectives
1. Identify microaggressions and their impact
2. Understand microaffirmations and their impact
3. Learn practical strategies aimed to improve workplace wellness

---

14.1 Presentation of the Science

In healthcare settings, teamwork is essential in delivering quality and empathic care. Each member on the team plays an important and valued role. Teams include patients, families, nurses, physicians, social workers, case managers, therapists, technicians, custodial staff, and many more. Among these valued individuals, there are endless interpersonal interactions that many do not think twice about, given the chaos in a day. However, small interactions add up and have the power to contribute to positive, affirming, and encouraging workplace cultures. We spend most of our days at work; intentionally finding ways to make the experience positive, meaningful, and enjoyable is important for personal well-being and the well-being of those we are trying to help. Encouraging authenticity and safety in the workplace can sustain our healthcare workforce.

Supplementary Information The online version contains supplementary material available at https://doi.org/10.1007/978-3-031-16983-0_14.

D. N. Shapiro (✉)
University of California, San Diego, La Jolla, CA, USA
e-mail: dlshapiro@health.ucsd.edu

Waking up in the morning on a workday, many of us have routines that lead us to the clinic, hospital, or academic institution. When we walk into those doors or start a meeting virtually, we are collectively contributing to workplace culture whether we are speaking or not. There are expectations, roles, and structures that we learn about explicitly and implicitly. With many dynamics circulating, there are clear moments that engage us or throw us off course. We easily may become stuck, knowingly or unknowingly, on how an interaction made us feel. At the end of the day or on the drive home from a shift, we may recall, remember, and hold onto those feelings of discomfort and possibly pass them on to loved ones or others in our lives. Perhaps your idea was ignored, you were left off a meeting invite, a colleague was cut off, or you did not receive the credit or acknowledgement you felt was appropriate for your effort. Just because these are *micro* in duration does not mean they are not *macro* in impact. The experience we have at work and the environment we work in can lead to fulfilment, acceptance, agency, and mastery; however, it can also be associated with feelings of dread, self-doubt, and perseverative thinking. Staying stuck prevents full presence at home, outside of work, which has the capacity to buffer us against burnout. The good news is that with intention, organizational culture can be molded into one that is inclusive, positive, and safe. No workplace is without conflict or disagreement or stress, but as safe and trusting spaces are cultivated, conversations and encounters become enriched with personal and organizational growth.

Dr. Derald Wing Sue describes microaggressions as the "everyday verbal, nonverbal, and environmental slights, snubs, or insults, whether intentional or unintentional, which communicate hostile, derogatory, or negative messages to target persons based solely upon their marginalized group membership" [1]. Microaggressions may involve any marginalized group including race, ethnicity, language, country of origin, gender, sexuality, ability status, and religious or spiritual identification [2]. Microaggressions may be verbal or nonverbal. A colleague may have used a derogatory term when discussing a case or a situation. Someone may physically distance themselves from another with side glances. Oftentimes, there is not an awareness that these are offensive or even occurring. Microinequities involve a similar concept of small and subtle events that are unintentional, unrecognized, in addition to covert messages that involve people who are outside of the dominant group [3]. These are often demonstrated through gestures, vocabulary, tone, or eye or facial expressions. These occurrences may lead to employees doubting themselves or preventing those who witnessed the event from contributing in an optimal way. The more frequent these microinequities and microaggressions occur, the deeper they become a part of organizational culture. Without creating space for healthcare professionals to be authentic and share ideas to improve systems, we are discouraging growth and innovation; we are holding ourselves back. Embracing and celebrating differences with diverse leadership team increase performance and problem solving [4]. Individuals with different knowledge, processing, and perspectives enhance solutions. Diversity in all settings drives us forward.

Identifying the problem and awakening ourselves to the microinteractions with macroimpact on those around us can lead to greater workplace well-being. When individuals witness these microinsults, microaggressions, or microinequities, it is important to challenge them no matter one's role. Identifying these as barriers to workplace wellness begins the process of change. Teams can identify ways to openly discuss and explain their experience of interactions and comments made. Interrupting or talking over individuals is a common occurrence in the workplace, especially given the sensation of feeling rushed. Encouraging processing of all input may add some time to a meeting but also may add a unique approach to a patient care situation or even a quality improvement opportunity. Discussing meeting dynamics and tendencies along with offering agreed upon norms are ways to use structure to change culture. These conversations may occur in groups, meetings, or individually after an event has occurred or to set norms. Teams can also collect general and specific feedback as a group or anonymously. Aligning everyone with the truth that others want the best for them and the health of the workplace environment welcomes honesty and invites investment towards positive change.

When thinking about assigning tasks or delegating work, it is important to pay attention to any tendencies for individuals to be stereotyped or looked over. Perhaps a leadership role has always been assumed by a vocal and outgoing individual, placing value on these characteristics; however, the organization may benefit from considering opening the position up to someone with a different style or approach without assuming one is better than the other. Other examples include assuming a young professional, also a parent, would not be able to serve in a leadership role because of their home life, or a search committee discounting someone because of known struggles in an applicant's personal life. We must challenge ourselves and our systems to prevent the limitations that we fall into out of routine and the hierarchies we were raised in, noting that individuals from these examples might be outstanding in these roles.

Creating cultures that allow for voices to be heard and individuals to be valued in healthcare leads to excellent patient care and better systems. Environments where individuals treat one another with dignity and honor strengths allow team members to be their best. Microaffirmations are acts that promote the success of others, small and inclusive acts that involve listening and generously crediting others [3]. Microaffirmations may improve workplace wellness, productivity, and overall satisfaction. In the same way, small glances, comments, or dismissals can have negative impact on someone's work productivity and ability to enjoy their free time; microaffirmations are ways to welcome all members of the team into discussions and dialogues while also move agendas forward and get the work done. These microaffirmations can buffer and build teams to become fuller and more whole. In these occurrences, individuals are affirmed and there are clearer opportunities for success.

14.2 Application of Principles into Wellness Practice

How does a practice or team build in microaffirmations, especially if the current culture does not have the foundation for this setup?

14.2.1 Meaningful Listening

Many times, in meetings or discussions, we are distracted by our lists of things to do or internal dialogue about how we may contribute or be perceived. Rarely do we listen mindfully and with intention, leading to colleagues feeling devalued or ignored. In workplace settings where there are many hidden or not so hidden rules about who speaks when, it can require courage to verbalize an idea. When someone does speak up and an idea is ignored, belittled, or glossed over for any number of reasons, confidence can be affected, and an individual may feel less engaged or invested in sharing ideas in the future. Not everyone's idea will work or be the winning one; however, being sure to listen and reflect upon an idea may make the difference in inspiring creativity and creating an encouraging environment long term. To achieve meaningful listening, groups can practice the skills of active listening. How teams communicate is often modeled by the leader of the group so team leaders and individuals with named privilege and power may aim to share that power with the group invite people in. Being transparent about decisions being made and how input will be factored is one way to allow team members to trust the process, especially processes of change. Using good eye contact, encouraging tones, and reflecting what was heard are good strategies to employ. Asking follow-up questions that seek understanding and clarity is another way to encourage comments. Group leaders may rotate who leads meetings to experience different styles and strengths. Group leaders may also call on individuals or ask, "what voices have I not heard from regarding the disposition of this patient?" Those who are not group leaders may also model microaffirming statements of praise when witnessing inclusive practices. When we mindfully listen, we hear and discover more. Sometimes the greatest gift we can give someone is the entirety of our attention. Set aside the multitasking, which is unproductive in and of itself, to be fully present. When healthcare professionals come to work feeling unseen or invisible, the gift of presence is powerful.

14.2.2 See and Acknowledge Othersing

In healthcare settings, we are paid to do work and that part is transactional. However, in healthcare there is an opportunity for transformation. When individuals are allowed and encouraged to be their best, they have the power to transform systems, situations, and futures. In childhood, there is always someone to impress or please and the amount of feedback seems never-ending. There are grades, progress reports, input from coaches, choir leads, art, and music instructors, and more. As we advance in our careers, there are less structured opportunities for receiving microdoses of feedback; and feedback is usually batched into a semiannual or annual performance review or faculty review. If there is an adverse event, complaint, or error, there is timely feedback for the safety of others. Adding acknowledgement and validation of hard work done is a positive strategy to increase engagement in the workplace.

Many workplaces have a system in which to honor peers who have gone above and beyond. This may be an anonymous submission on computer desktops or an email address that collects positive praise. These instances are usually ones that capture a healthcare professional helping a colleague, taking another shift, staying late, or saving the day in some way. Routine and meaningful work that gets done every single day can and should also be seen and acknowledged. Some teams might build positive microaffirmations into the meeting. Starting off a meeting asking if anyone would like to shout out appreciation to a colleague can set the tone to one that is uplifting and collaborative. Mixing in fun examples also lightens the mood and reminds us that in addition to the workplace, we have lives outside of the office or clinic and blending them in small doses can increase community. For example, someone might complement a colleague for bringing in a baked good to share or motivating them to run a race on the weekend. There is also the opportunity to integrate these acknowledgements into the meetings themselves. Identifying individuals' strengths can remind the group of how strong the collective is; for example, when reviewing the patient list in the morning someone might acknowledge the way a nurse spoke with a patient and their family and how the family mentioned it on the discharge.

Healthcare professionals are raised in competitive environments. Competition can only bring us so far; if we exchange competition for compassion and collaboration individual success will spread to others and elevate the group. Whatever someone brings to an idea, acknowledge them for it. While it may be easier to focus on the product or outcome, the process and the journey are also important. It is rarely one person who thinks of and completes tasks or projects. Credit the roles people played in getting something launched or done. Publicly and privately, we can identify the contributions of others. Certain environments are inherently competitive. If you are sitting in one of these situations, consider if the healthcare professionals in your organization feel like they can trust one another.

When microaffirmations become consistent and routine, they are more likely to be adopted and spread to other spaces. Increasing morale, productivity, and enjoyment at work is well worth the effort.

14.2.3 Calm Conversations

In any healthcare setting, we will face conversations that are challenging and emotionally charged. Some people instinctively avoid the emotional response and target the action items and solutions. While effective in some situations, when we create space for emotions and feelings to be affirmed and appreciated, we are able to better understand our coworkers and our patients. In having difficult conversations, labeling affect and emotion for ourselves and inviting others to identity their feelings can be empowering. When a frustrating patient encounter has taken place, identifying those feelings may allow the conversation to productively illuminate how the team of individuals can grow and learn. When we are emotionally charged, leading with questions and curiosity yields better results than assuming statements. If a colleague is experiencing stress related to a clinical encounter, help them label their emotions and offer to discuss it with them in a calm and quiet setting. Calming down and self-soothing will always save us time and minimize harm.

14.2.4 Intentional Inclusion

In all healthcare situations, there are things that can be done to create welcoming environments. One important approach is to allow all members of the team to be seen for who they are. When meeting someone for the first time, ensure that you are saying their name correctly and ask what they prefer to be called in the workplace. Behavioral gestures may include intentionally keeping open body language and using expressions that are neutral or encouraging. Being curious, asking questions, and being genuinely present and interested may create dialogue that would not have occurred without intentional effort. Intentionally scanning one's environment for positive work being done or kindness being shared is one way to maintain gratitude for others. Including others and welcoming their authentic identity may seem daunting to some and beyond the scope of the workplace; however, checking in briefly about a meaningful event, trip, or hobby may deepen relationships and build trust. Through small acts of listening, acknowledgment, caring, and inclusion, our well-being increases.

14.2.5 Examples

Learn to properly say team members' names
Respect and share pronouns
Acknowledge the wholeness of your colleagues and their lives/identities outside of medicine
Use positive praise when starting meetings and when delegating tasks
Give your presence and mindfully listen
Routinely invite all voices and perspectives
Build space for validating experiences
Challenge workplace norms that are not inclusive
Identify microaggressions, microinsults, and microinequities openly
Provide platforms for colleagues and patients to identify positive experiences
Build trust and safety by welcoming difficult conversations
Be mindful of facial expressions
Give credit and recognition to others generously
Avoid generalizations about personal lives or practices
Invite sharing about cultural practices, interests, hobbies
See the good in others
Notice your own patterns and assumptions

| Keep an open mind and be willing to learn |
| Embrace different styles and appreciate unique strengths |
| Prioritize collaboration over competition |
| Ask about what make workdays meaningful |
| Offer safe opportunities for sharing experiences and feedback |
| Have productive and empathic conversations to move teams forward |

14.2.6 Pre-licensure Application in the Academic Environment

In medical/clinical training, there are opportunities to increase self-awareness and leadership skills in coursework and discussion. Learning how to provide care is core to one's training; however, adding time to reflect on how to best work on an interdisciplinary team and realize the importance of interpersonal interactions can benefit the larger learning environment. Including and prioritizing well-being and emotional awareness and regulation into curriculum across all disciplines may improve present and future learning and workplace cultures. Faculty might consider implementing strategies in their in-person or virtual classrooms and on the wards. Starting classes off with an optional arrival practice such as one deep breath or a grounding mindfulness exercise may improve cohesion. During classes or learning settings where there is more time available, trainees or students can pre-submit anonymous comments or words that describe their colleagues. Starting a meeting or class off with an appreciation coming from peers builds a safe and welcoming environment. Gathering these affirmations prior to a class can be relatively easy to do with the positive impact on well-being. Academic settings often involve closely working with one another and opportunities to praise and celebrate peers can be done at the beginning or end of any gathering. Microaffirmations and appreciation can be tailored to the time and setting. Including trainee champions to lead and organize efforts is one way to engage groups and empower change.

14.2.7 Clinical Application Postlicensure

In established clinical positions, focus on compassion and empathy during patient interactions is emphasized. However, all members of the clinical team benefit when microinteractions between physicians, nurses, and other healthcare professionals are positive and affirming. As clinicians travel throughout their day, finding opportunities to encourage all members of the team will impact clinic flow and in turn, patient care. Completing tasks in a supportive setting can remind hard working clinicians of the meaning and purpose in work done each day.

14.2.8 Leadership Application (Structural and Organizational Considerations)

Leaders have a platform to integrate microaffirmations frequently throughout one's day in conversations, meetings, presentations, emails, and reports. Allowing leaders to build a culture that is welcoming and validating requires time. Assigning value to creating a healthy workplace culture allows the entire organization to witness and appreciate efforts. Leaders can model and they can also learn from their teams about what might be working well and what might be working less well, being receptive to adaptations and suggestions. Consider this exemplar:

Sarah is a nursing manager on a busy pediatric service. She interacts daily with many healthcare professionals and frequently responds to problems and complaints.

In her desk, she has a drawer of cards with beautiful and soothing images. After creatively solving or responding to a challenging clinical scenario, she routinely stops by her office to take a moment to reflect. In this brief, grounding moment she writes a message of appreciation on a card to team members she worked alongside. Perhaps her colleague endured a tragedy or selflessly managed a crisis; the card allows Sarah to reflect on her gratitude for her team and allows her team to shine despite inevitable hardship. She makes it a point to write cards after challenging and emotionally draining situations. Sarah has seen her physical cards displayed on workstations and desks years later, an enduring reminder of the impact of being recognized. Similar messages can be verbalized or emailed. Setting an intention to recognize three colleagues a week is a way for healthcare leaders to build this into their routine of recognition, leading teams away from fear in crisis but rather towards acceptance and acknowledgement.

14.3 Opportunities for Future Research

Creating affirming workplace environments may add to the well-being and enjoyment of healthcare professionals, connecting us all to the deeper meaning of serving patients and families. There are small but powerful, research-based strategies to cultivate more affirming workplace environments. However, more research is needed to assess content, mode of delivery, dose, frequency, and impact. We need to explore outcome metrics and distinguish how to best teach and implement these interventions. How might certain populations benefit more, less, or differently? Are there settings or times in which microaffirmations are best delivered? What may be unknown consequences or impacts? Because individual personalities and preferences vary widely, more research is needed to explore whether these strategies impact individual or community emotional well-being or workplace satisfaction in the short and long term. Hearing from healthcare professionals on their perception of these strategies is essential in determining feasibility. Future research may uncover how to teach the practice of microaffirmations efficiently and effectively, for clinical leaders to adopt for their teams. In searching for the most impactful ways to implement microaffirming practices, research might also determine what implementation and evaluation model has the most success.

Glossary

Microaffirmations Microaffirmations are actions and comments that celebrate the strengths and successes of individuals working together.
Microaggressions Verbal or nonverbal communications that are hurtful, harmful, or offensive.

Discussion Questions

Compared to microaggressions, how do microaffirmations add to workplace wellness?
What are examples of microaffirmative practices in the workplace setting?
How might microaffirmations be integrated into busy clinical settings?

Discussion Leader Guide

Video for Discussion - Instructional Video: The online version contains supplementary material available at https://doi.org/10.1007/978-3-031-16983-0_14

References

1. Sue DW, Capodilupo CM, Torino GC, Bucceri JM, Holder AMB, Nadal KL, Esquilin M. Racial microaggressions in everyday life: implications for clinical practice. Am Psychol. 2007;62(4):271–86.
2. Sue DW. Microaggressions in everyday life: race gender and sexual orientation. Hoboken: John Wiley & Sons; 2010.
3. Rowe M. Micro-affirmations and micro-inequities. J Int Ombudsman Assoc. 2008;1:45–8.
4. Hong L, Page S. Groups of diverse problem solvers can outperform groups of high-ability problem solvers. Proc Natl Acad Sci U S A. 2004;101(46):16385–9.

Authentically Restructuring the Workplace to Promote Diversity, Equity, and Inclusion: Building Capacity for a More Just Healthcare Future

15

Chloe O. R. Littzen, Jessica Dillard-Wright, Shena Gazaway, and Patrick McMurray

Learning Outcomes
1. Define the key concepts related to diversity, equity, and inclusion in healthcare.
2. Identify the significance of diversity in their healthcare role.
3. Recognize, understand, and analyze their own privileges that impact their healthcare role.
4. Apply and evaluate strategies to enhance diversity in their healthcare role.

15.1 Introduction

When we think about leadership in healthcare, we wish to recognize the immediacy and urgency of healthcare workers on health outcomes, health systems, the provision of healthcare, and broader implications for global humankind. To this end, as scholars

---

Authors' Disclosure: The authors consider their work here fully coequal.

Supplementary Information The online version contains supplementary material available at https://doi.org/10.1007/978-3-031-16983-0_15.

C. O. R. Littzen (✉)
Biobehavioral Health Sciences Division, The University of Arizona College of Nursing, Tucson, AZ, USA
e-mail: clittzen@email.arizona.edu

J. Dillard-Wright
Department of Physiological and Technological Nursing, Augusta University College of Nursing, Augusta, GA, USA

S. Gazaway
School of Nursing, University of Alabama Birmingham, Birmingham, AL, USA

P. McMurray
University of North Carolina Medical Center, Chapel Hill, NC, USA

© The Author(s), under exclusive license to Springer Nature Switzerland AG 2023
J. E. Davidson, M. Richardson (eds.), *Workplace Wellness: From Resiliency to Suicide Prevention and Grief Management*, https://doi.org/10.1007/978-3-031-16983-0_15

209

of nursing, health equity, systems, and leadership, we recognize diversity as a foundational prerequisite for healthcare, as a point of entry for establishing values like equity, inclusion, justice, and human dignity [1]. This means that considerations of diversity, equity, and inclusion must be central to substantive and meaningful healthcare leadership, rather than an afterthought. We adopt a definition derived from the American Association of Colleges of Nursing, and understand diversity to "encompass a broad range of individual, population, and social characteristics, including but not limited to age; sex; race; ethnicity; sexual orientation; gender identity; family structures; geographic locations; national origin; immigrants and refugees; language; physical, functional, and learning abilities; religious beliefs; and socioeconomic status" [2]. As this definition suggests, diversity itself is complex and robust, but is ultimately descriptive. Because of this, diversity is a starting place rather than a final destination. We understand diversity in concert with inclusion, equity, and justice as fundamental for building a more just, equitable future for healthcare, for the strength of our workforce, and for the communities for whom we care.

As we navigate through our discussion of diversity and its significance for healthcare workers, we wish to acknowledge the complexity of considerations of diversity, equity, and inclusion. In considering diversity, equity, and inclusion in healthcare, we explicitly attend to the intersections inhabited by all healthcare workers. We therefore implicitly include considerations related to the communities and systems for whom healthcare workers care because of the nature of their work. Additionally, there are important workforce considerations related to diversity, equity, and inclusion that healthcare leaders need to be comfortable with to lead fellow colleagues to thrive. Leadership by healthcare workers is critical to creating safe environments for their colleagues from diverse backgrounds to work, grow, and develop. Without this essential leadership, both formal and informal, individual healthcare workers from disparate backgrounds may feel singled out or marginalized, experience increased stress and anxiety related to job performance, and ultimately suboptimal well-being; this may eventually lead to these healthcare workers leaving their jobs and even healthcare at large [3–6]. To this end, healthcare leaders must understand the role they play in creating safe environments for healthcare workers as well as the people and families, communities, and systems for whom they care. Given all of this, healthcare leaders must come to their praxis with a strong foundation in diversity, equity, inclusion, and justice in order to create a work environment that supports their staff, their patients, and overall system functioning.

15.2   Thinking About Diversity in Healthcare

As we unpack ideas around diversity, equity, and inclusion in healthcare, it is important to recognize that science plays a central role in how healthcare understands itself and what it values [7]. Science enforces normative values in healthcare that are not always apparent to those most deeply invested, a function of the privilege of inhabiting a normative positionality [8]. Healthcare disciplines have entangled histories of reifying white supremacist heteropatriarchy, in both subtle and not so subtle ways. These disciplines frequently mobilize the vernacular of care work as a strategy for deflecting scrutiny of problematic ideas [8]. In other words, healthcare professionals use the excuse that, because they care, they are somehow exempt from being oppressors [9]. We sometimes see healthcare workers avoiding difficult conversations around race and racism, gender and sexism, sexuality and heteronormativity, ability and ableism, and class and elitism [9–12]. These issues are framed as political and somehow outside healthcare. Many approaches to diversity, equity, and inclusion-related issues in healthcare (including "cultural competence") devolve into stereotypes, centering the individual healthcare worker who is either leading or providing care rather than the individual on the receiving end.

Moreover, as many healthcare disciplines, including nursing, medicine, pharmacy, physical therapy, and more, fashion themselves as primarily scientifically based, health disciplines reify white-male coded philosophy of empiricism as the dominant way of knowing in healthcare [13, 14]. This reinforces encoded whiteness in these disciplines and practices, that may, at first glance, appear invisible to *some*. For example, as nursing increasingly sought professionalization and legitimacy as a scientific discipline in the middle of the twentieth century, we leaned into an existing structure for scientific community and funding [7]. This effort meant adopting a trope of success in academic nursing that looked very much like existing tropes of white masculine-defined status, complete with the trappings of federal funding, bench science, and academe. Along with this turn, nursing also embraced empiricism and later evidence-based practice as a primary way of knowing in nursing. But this turn was incomplete and challenged by the inherently interdisciplinary and gendered aspects of the discipline [7].

Furthermore, nursing has historically been constructed as an extension of the feminine role of caring. Because of this essentialized biological assumption, the labor, skill, and sophistication of nursing as care work is minimized. The profession has retained an overwhelming majority white female composition. And while nursing has struggled to retain autonomy in the masculine-coded medical field, the discipline of nursing is itself grappling with issues of racism, colonialism, ableism, sexism, cisnormativity, and more. This struggle, all too often, prioritized (and prioritizes) the white feminine sensibilities that underpin much of nursing work at the expense of people who do not embody nursing's white cisgender feminine norms [15]. Of course, nurses are not alone in this snarl: healthcare is dynamic, complex, and interdisciplinary, rife with intersecting oppressions and power dynamics. With this in mind, we implore healthcare workers, especially healthcare leaders, to challenge the status quo that limits what is possible, embracing equity and justice as guiding aspirations in the delivery of healthcare. First stop, diversity.

15.3   Diversity: A Prerequisite

Diversity is a buzzword, all too often a placeholder for more challenging ideas. A euphemism, we often use diversity without a clear understanding of its meaning. Critically, "diverse" is a word that describes a group of individuals rather than an attribute of any single person. Diversity is connected to many things—the visible and invisible attributes that make us who we are. And while the concept is broad, diversity is not an end in and of itself. Instead, it is a point of departure, the earliest kernel of beginning. Workforce diversity in healthcare is a prerequisite for excellence and health equity, but it is a reality not yet manifest as disciplines such as nursing remains overwhelmingly white and female [2]. This has far-reaching implications including reinforcing the conditions of white supremacy that structures sociocultural conditions beyond healthcare in the United States, which creates a hostile environment for workers and people receiving care alike. A qualitative study examining the ways in which racism-related stress affects the well-being and career trajectories of Black nurses and certified nursing assistants found that 78% reported experiencing both subtle and explicit racism in the workplace from patients, peers, and their supervisors [6]. Moreover, participants described a stark absence of People of Color from supervisory roles in their organizations, suggesting that these folks were often passed up for these positions, frequently to those who were less qualified and white [6].

As an aspiring or established healthcare leader, we encourage you to examine your understanding of diversity—and the related concepts of equity, inclusion, and justice—and its significance in your approach to leadership and provision of care. Take the time to recognize how dimensions of diversity, including your own privilege, impact every facet of healthcare. Recognize the interconnections between power and identity, asking yourself how that shapes healthcare and communities. Your engagement with diversity is not complete when you finish this chapter, either. That is when your work *starts*. That is when it is time that you put one foot in front of the other and *do* the work. That means learning and practicing every day; being open to making mistakes and to redirection. That means recognizing corrective feedback as the gift that it is, particularly when someone takes time out of their life to give it. That means choosing to not let hegemonic norms rule what you do or say. We construct our spaces, realities, and institutions. Being able to construct our reality is powerful because it means that we can build a present and a future as we imagine it, not simply how it has always been. Choose to continuously develop your understanding of how diversity, and the many concepts you will learn about in this chapter, impact you, your colleagues, patients, communities, and systems.

15.4   Our Critical Assumptions

We, as nurses from a variety of different nursing backgrounds including research, practice, policy, and education, are allied in our understanding that healthcare workers must engage together to dismantle oppression and embrace diversity, equity, inclusion, and justice in holistic fashion (Table 15.1). Therefore, our vision for this

Table 15.1 Positionality table

Author	Pronouns	Key identities	Salient assumptions and biases
Chloé Littzen-Brown	She/her/hers	White-cis-hetero-woman Chronically abled, immigrant Settler-colonizer, educator, scientist Theorist, activist	Intermodernist; all nurses have epistemic authority and nursing Can be an act of justice. Committed to the personal, daily, lifelong consciousness-raising Required to enable justice and equity for those who have been Historically and/or contemporarily marginalized and Oppressed.
Jess Dillard-Wright	She/they, her/their, hers/theirs	Fat, white, queer and gender queer parent-nurse-activist-educator-writer-crafter who struggles with major depression	Learning and unlearning all the time. Justice is a worthy end in itself. Planetary survival is contingent on collaboration. The same tools, techniques, and tactics that got us here will not take us anywhere new. Nursing can be about liberation, if we choose it.
Shena Gazaway	She/her/hers	Black-cis-hetero-woman, chronically abled, mother, wife, scientist, educator	Nurses have a duty to be lifelong learners, engaged in providing quality, compassionate, bias-free care to diverse patients, families, and communities.
Patrick McMurray	He/him/his	Black, cis-hetero-man, educator, Jehovah's witness, chronically abled, scientist	Nursing should be an act of justice, and it is in a perpetual state of metamorphosis. Learning to live up to the principle of "doing right by folks," which means not only treating others as you wish to be treated, but treating them as THEY wish to be treated.

chapter is to provide a critical space to promote healthcare leaders' understanding of these complex but foundational issues as an entry point for fostering equity within healthcare, and provide tools for success to help lead *all* healthcare workers to thrive. It is our hope that healthcare leaders themselves become champions of diversity, equity, and inclusion, embrace their role as change agents in work environments, and lead healthcare to become more diverse, equitable, inclusive, and just discipline than ever before.

15.5 Our Critical Assumptions

- Diversity is a prerequisite, not an end point.
- Diversity without equity is performative.
- Diversity is sometimes a way that people sanitize more difficult concepts, like racism, sexism, homophobia, and transphobia.
- Fostering a diverse, equitable, and inclusive workforce and work environments requires resources, commitment, intentionality, and attention from leaders and stakeholders.
- Diversity influences every aspect of healthcare.

- Healthcare professionals from diverse backgrounds must be seen, heard, and respected in their work environments.
- Healthcare has a historical and contemporary lack of diversity, inclusion, equity, and justice.
- Historical and contemporary healthcare normalizes the ideals of ableism, elitism, sexism, classism, cis-heteronormativity, and ethnocentric whiteness.

15.6   Theoretical Guidance

As we work toward modes of leadership that encourage individual healthcare workers to creatively, competently, and compassionately care for people, communities, and systems, we recognize a complex constellation of individual attributes and systemic factors that interact to create the world around us. To this end, as we think about leading to foster a more diverse, inclusive, equitable, and just future for healthcare, we draw our theoretical guidance from two key frameworks. The first, developed by Black feminist legal scholar Kimberle Crenshaw, is *intersectionality* [16]. The second, a collaborative effort led by physician Johnathan Metzl drawing on earlier works by folks as disparate as Black Panther Stokely Carmichael and nurse Patricia Butterfield and in collaboration with legal scholar Dorothy Roberts, is *structural competency* [17–20]. Together, these schema account for individual experiences as well as the larger forces that shape our lives, providing an organizing framework that we, as leaders, can use to enable us to think about how we can effectively lead while attending to the unique challenges faced by the nurses, staff, and patients with whom we work.

Intersectionality first appeared in the literature in 1989 in a legal essay entitled "Demarginalizing the Intersection of Race and Sex: A Black Feminist Critique of Antidiscrimination Doctrine, Feminist Theory and Antiracist Politics." In it, Crenshaw developed the concept of intersectionality to account for the differential intersections of oppressive forces, attending to the limits of both Black masculine-coded civil rights politics and white liberal feminism in adequately accounting for the experiences of Black women [16]. This creates interlocking and irreducible matrices of domination that shape the lived experience of women of color, specifically Black women [16, 21]. Intersectionality makes space for a broad array of possibility and analyses, not foreclosing any possible combination of identities as invalid or unimportant. This is because intersectionality implores us to recognize that complexities of identity and oppression are not reducible or equivalent from individual to individual and across groups, a product of the manner in which hegemony is manufactured through legal, social, cultural, and political systems. In healthcare, intersectionality demands that we, for example, recognize the normative whiteness of our disciplines, what that means for Black, Indigenous, and healthcare professionals of Color, and what that means for the patients in our care.

If intersectionality attends to the ways individual experiences are shaped by intersecting identities, *structural competency* is a strategy useful for understanding the ways that broad systemic forces structure our individual choices, possibilities, and realities. In a 1968 address to a community of psychiatrists, organizer and Black Panther Stokley Carmichael declared that dealing in individuals when it came to power was inadequate—a cop-out—because of the institutional and structural powers that create individual conditions [19]. Building from Carmichael's work, physicians Johnathan Metzl and Helena Hansen advanced structural competency as an approach to medical education that accounts for the downstream manifestations of upstream inequities [17, 20]. The model for structural competency is predicated on an understanding of the structural factors that individuals have little or no control over by virtue of the institutions, systems, and governmental factors that shape individuals' daily lives, including things that determine health [17]. So that means thinking about things outside the caregiver/care-receiver dyad is required for meaningful care. Health is not possible, for example, in the absence of clean water, making the community campaign for clean drinking water in Flint, Michigan, a relevant and necessary structural intervention for the health, well-being, and thriving of the community and the people in it.

15.7 The Words We Choose: Why Diversity Isn't Enough.

Words can inspire. And words can destroy. Choose yours well.
Robin Sharma

Now we need to unpack important background knowledge for healthcare leaders to consider regarding diversity, equity, inclusion, and justice. This part of our conversation leaves the more comfortable terrain of diversity and inclusion, and moves us into uncomfortable but necessary considerations regarding power, oppression, equity, and privilege. We will then discuss some of the glaring statistics that characterize health inequities in our communities, linking them to considerations for healthcare leadership. That foundation thus secured, we will address some common misconceptions about diversity and inclusion and their more substantive complements, justice and equity.

15.8 Uncomfortable Terrain

Diversity is a concept that sometimes is used to deflect more difficult conversations. If we are talking about diversity and inclusion, we are likely not talking about racism and injustice. Some assert, as feminist astrophysicist Chanda Prescod-Weinstein has, that diversity and inclusion initiatives, as they presently exist, are a diversion designed to engineer good feelings in white, usually male, allies [22]. This kind of performative allyship prioritizes *looking* the right way instead of engaging in the substantive, hard, and uncomfortable work of *being* an ally [23]. Relying on "diversity" as a shorthand, placeholder, or euphemism for every socio-political-cultural-historical issue at hand reifies the true systemic problems linked to inequality, inequity, injustice, power imbalance, and oppression.

Healthcare leaders need to get comfortable in the dis-ease of working on topics like racism, sexism, oppression, and heteronormativity to challenge the worldviews that make these inequities possible in order to truly lead all healthcare workers to thrive. Resisting this disease prolongs the underlying problems, delaying fairness, equity, and justice—which has implications for the healthcare workforce and for the people we serve. As a healthcare leader, you have the power and privilege to educate yourself. Use that power and privilege to proactively create a more just and equitable future for healthcare, and dismantle the structural inequalities that exist in the world. The following are foundational concepts you can add to your lexicon as you build your inclusive leadership vocabulary.

15.9 Key Terms and Definitions

- **Equality:** is "treating everyone the same and giving everyone access to the same opportunities" [24]. In order for equality to actually work, everyone has to *start* from the same place and *need* the same things—which is not reality [24].
- **Equity:** "the ability to recognize the differences in the resources, or knowledge needed, to allow individuals to fully participate in society, including access to higher education, with the goal of overcoming obstacles to ensure fairness" [2, 25]. Equity is often used interchangeably with the concept of equality, but these concepts are distinct. In contrast with equality, equity accounts for the differential advantages and disadvantages that individuals and groups are placed at in society, and promotes the fair distribution of needed resources in order to promote high-quality care for individuals, communities, and systems.
- **Oppression:** dehumanization of individuals of a particular group identity [26]. According to Eliason and Chinn, oppression results from the combination of power and prejudice of a dominant group [27]. This dominant group creates and imposes standards for society, called hegemony. These standards enforce imposed inequity for the marginalized other, dehumanizing them [28]. Examples of oppressed group behavior within healthcare include silencing of whistleblowers and persistent lateral violence [29].
- **Politics:** a topic healthcare seems to shy away from, politics are simply power-structured relationships [30]. Politics, then, are something we all engage in every day. This is as true for healthcare workers as for any other group of individuals. We ignore this at our own peril, abdicating our chance to define our own perspectives. Because of this, we recognize that healthcare is political.
- **Power:** drawing from French poststructuralist Michel Foucault, we understand power as a practice, a negotiation that takes place at each interface, relational and exercised within disciplines and between interlocutors [31]. This practice is intimately connected with knowledge and the authority to construct truth.
- **Privilege:** the "unearned benefits and advantages" that have been handed to a group of individuals as a result of systemic norms and standardizations, the system structures, policies, and practices pave the road for this one group of indi-

viduals while creating obstacles for other groups [32, 33]. If you've never been uncomfortable, or felt unsafe about some aspect of your identity, you have experienced privilege. Learning about something that you have never experienced similarly is a privilege. Having privilege means you are actively benefiting from the oppression of others, and therefore contributing to the structural inequalities, such as white supremacy, that exists. If you are not aware of the barriers others face, you will not see them, be much less be motivated to remove them, especially if they are an advantage to which you feel entitled [8].

15.10 Promoting Meaningful Diversity

To make the term diversity meaningful, the healthcare leader must possess a clear and accurate understanding of what diversity exists, and how to maintain and establish this diversity as a pillar of their leadership and organization. Diversity also extends beyond external and internal optics for the leader or the organization in which they function. Diversity, equity, and inclusion must be more than an optical illusion for those the organization serves and those who are a part of the organization. There are circumstances where cultivating diversity within a system is little more than political correctness, a box to be checked, a one-off. Healthcare leaders must strive to practice diversity in a more intentional and meaningful way. To make the practice of diversity meaningful, it will require the healthcare leader to have a willingness to navigate uncomfortable conversations and topics within their sphere of influence and beyond. In addition to the desire to navigate discomfort, impactful healthcare leaders must become proficient in how to respond to and handle issues involving diversity. Addressing issues within diversity often requires the healthcare leader to demonstrate qualities of humility and include others who may be more experienced and qualified in a particular aspect of diversity. Leaders who practice diversity in a meaningful way will seek to be informed on how various decisions or changes could impact those who work with them and those whom their team(s) serves. Diversity should enhance the quality of decisions and better facilitate change, even in situations where that means change requires more planning and time. Lastly, the healthcare leader must demonstrate that diversity is not a barrier to progress, rather it is the key for opening the door to potential, creativity, and value in their institutions.

15.11 Your Privilege as a Healthcare Leader

Understanding and acknowledging your privilege as a healthcare leader enable you to recognize where your limitations might be and to identify things that you might fail to see without seeking to do so. Privilege as a healthcare leader influences those you lead, the patients they care for, and the function of systems at large. Privilege is the "invisible package of unearned assets" [34] afforded a group of individuals as a result of systemic norms and standardizations. The system structures, policies, and practices pave the road for some to enjoy power while creating obstacles for others. We must realize the privilege that some healthcare professionals inherently possess by nature of being in the demographic majority: white. The disproportionate make-up of our professions can be seen at the point of entry to healthcare, such as in schools of nursing and medicine [35]. Our goal here is to present this section as a gateway to understanding and acknowledging privilege when you see it and recognize when you are benefiting from it as well as seeing when others are disadvantaged. In that way, the section is designed for active engagement through application and reflection. These activities were mindfully selected to challenge the reader as you journey with us to identify the areas in which personal growth needs to begin so that professional growth can occur.

Discussions of privilege can be emotionally charged. We acknowledge that and ask that the reader make space in yourself for grace as you grapple with and acknowledge your feelings when they occur. You will not benefit from this reading if you elect not to engage and opt not to get comfortable in the discomfort of interrogating your own deeply held beliefs, their origins, and what privilege may be informing this. We ask you to recognize the emotional response you may be feeling in talking about some of these issues. Sit with it for a while. Then recognize that your emotional reaction may be a deflection, a denial of the lived realities of people who experience the world differently from you. This kind of response ultimately shores up ideologies of injustice. Seek to understand your own response so that you may begin to understand where others are coming from.

Privilege is a marker of a system or structure that is inherently inequitable. And we all have privileges and disadvantages, depending on our personal identities, families of origin, life experiences, chosen families, and more. Acknowledging privilege is not a denial of your hard work. No doubt *you* accomplished what you needed to be successful, but depending on who you are, your relative advantages and disadvantages may be quite different from those of us writing this chapter. Your struggles may not include struggles around racialization, gender identity, sexuality, disability, and so forth. And that is fine. What is not fine is failing to recognize that privilege exists, creates an uneven footing for people from go, and has a pernicious influence on even what we may perceive as neutral interactions and exchanges.

Unchecked privilege contributes to ongoing inequity. Inequity has no place in healthcare and privilege assigned because of skin color, perceived absence of disability, gender identity, and/or sexual orientation has no place within the ethos of healthcare leadership. Dismantling unchecked privilege requires conscious and thoughtful reflection and subsequent action. As authors we humbly request that you come along with us and explore your privileges. Do not skip this section because it raises feelings of unease, this is expected and welcomed, what we ask is that you examine those feelings and leave this section better prepared to identify privilege in yourself and others.

15.12 Consciousness Raising: Part 1

To begin your journey in exploring your own privilege we ask you to be honest and not read ahead. The following activity, based on an activity developed by the School Reform Initiative called "Paseo or Identity Circles," the result of collaborative work by Debbi Laidley, Debbie Bambino, Debbie McIntyre, Stevi Quate, and Julie Quinn at the winter 2001 meeting [36]. This can be conceptualized as a *consciousness raising exercise*, a means for you to gain an understanding of what your privileges are, how those privileges may be different from those you lead, and how those privileges influence your work environments.

Consciousness Raising Instructions:
1. Take out a pen and a piece of paper.
2. Draw a circle in the middle of your paper.
3. Draw four to five additional circles surrounding the center circle with a line connecting each circle to the center circle.
4. Write your name in the central circle.
5. In each of the surrounding circles, write down a word or phrase that represents **your** identity. For example, one of the authors grew up in Canada, so she wrote "Canadian." Don't spend too much time on this.
6. After you have filled out each circle, put the pen and paper aside. We will revisit what you wrote for this consciousness raising activity later.

15.13 The Impact of Privilege

Our privileges impact our everyday lives. As a healthcare leader, your individual privileges impact what you see as a problem, and similarly, prevents you from seeing what others may see as a problem. Moreover, your privileges project false expectations and limitations on others. As a healthcare leader, unless you take the time and examine your individual privileges, and how others without those privileges have been disadvantaged, you will never truly be able to lead authentically. To be an effective leader you have to know where you are, which will enable you to meet people where they are.

Knowing yourself links up with foundational thinking in nursing by way of Carper's "Fundamental Patterns of Knowing in Nursing," where one of our professional obligations in nursing practice is to recognize what we bring with us to our practice and thus leadership [37]. This takes practice and time and may be an uncomfortable process, if your efforts at self-knowing challenge your previously held assumptions about yourself. Making excuses, saying you "didn't know," is unacceptable. This excuse-oriented, exculpatory mindset perpetuates the systemic problems that exist today, creating a false truth that inhibits healthcare from becoming a more equitable, inclusive, and just discipline. We must be accountable for our actions—both the ones we take and the ones we do not. The story that follows was developed by Andrea Dalzell, BS, RN, known on Instagram and Twitter as the Seated Nurse. Andrea uses a wheelchair and wrote the following narrative for this chapter with the aim of illustrating how privilege operates, in part through the failure of imagination by those who occupy spaces of privilege. Having likely never confronted the world from a perspective like Andrea's means not having Andrea's perspective on the work of nursing and healthcare. This lack of imagination leads to problematic and harmful assumptions, as Andrea narrates below.

15.14 Vignette: Ability and Privilege in Nursing

I am the first person in a wheelchair to graduate from a nursing program in New York City. I graduated with my associates degree in nursing in January of 2018. I applied to over one thousand nursing positions, and got a call back to over 100 interviews in a 7-month span. Out of the 100+ interviews, I interviewed for 76 acute care bedside positions. I would get asked questions about what I would do if a patient fell on the floor and I was the only nurse on the floor. I was asked how I would be able to do CPR, or how I could hang an IV bag even though I proved my abilities in nursing school. I interviewed with one facility over 4 times and the Human Resources manager actually made me walk through my techniques to caring for patients and then was told that the nurse manager decided to move onto another candidate.

Nursing with a physical disability is perceived to be a hindrance versus an asset. Disability is considered to be a death sentence. Living an active life with a disability let alone being a nurse with a disability is like finding a "needle in a haystack". Nursing leaders have to understand that: (1) Nursing is not one size fits all. The multiple different facets of nursing must be taught and accessible to students so that the profession can open to anyone who wants to be a nurse. (2) Understanding that disability may seem limiting; however, those with disabilities have figured out their way through life and their innovation is key to progression. (3) The perspective that nurses with disabilities give to those we treat impacts the communities we are in.

15.15 Consciousness Raising: Part 2

The above vignette highlights two critical concepts. First, healthcare providers can and do have bias about folks who may appear different from the white, cisgender, able, heteropatriarchal norms that characterize healthcare—in this case regarding physical ability, though these forms of bias take any number of shapes. Second, it accentuates privilege experienced by those who have never faced the kind of extrinsic limitations imposed by ableism. Folks who do not live with disability may not have ever had to think about it. Andrea was (and is) able to safely and effectively complete the jobs she was interviewing for. She demonstrated it during their interviews. She graduated nursing school and successfully completed the NCLEX-RN, our disciplinary threshold for safe practice and licensure. The assumptions projected onto Andrea delayed the start of her career in nursing. This has financial, mental, and emotional implications, from the time spent to experiences of harm. This experience is not unique and happens in all the places we work, consciously and unconsciously. It speaks to the necessity of reflecting on our own positions and privileges and especially the limitations and biases this may build into our worldviews.

Now that we have spent some time looking at what privilege is, how it impacts leadership, and read some examples of privilege, you now need to acknowledge your personal privileges as a leader. Knowledge of self is critical to mindful, belonging-oriented leadership. To begin, take out your piece of paper and pen that you put aside from earlier, be open to learning something new, and embrace being uncomfortable.

Consciousness Raising Reflections:
1. Looking at your piece of paper, take a moment to read what you wrote in each circle.
2. Draw a checkmark next to any circle that if you wrote any of the following identifiers down:
   - Age
   - Generational Membership
   - Citizenship or residency status
   - Education level
   - Ethnicity
   - Gender
   - Health status or ability
   - Job status or profession
   - Marital status
   - Sexual orientation
   - Socioeconomic status
   - Race
   - Religion

1. From the above list, on the side of the paper write down the words that you did not have a checkmark for in any circle.
2. Take a moment to reflect. Does the omission of these dimensions mean anything? It is possible that it does not: perhaps you are simply not a religious person and omitted that dimension. But perhaps the absence is significant: have you ever had to navigate the immigration system? Have you ever worried that you would not be able to access a space due to physical limitations? Consider what this could signify in terms of privilege for you.

The words that you do not list are often aspects of yourself you do not have to think about. When you as an individual do not have to think about something—say, choosing a shirt that hides your cleavage or gritting your teeth and smiling when a stranger tells you to—you have a privilege. You do not have to navigate being Black in a white-normative space or being feminine in a masculine-coded environment. White people may not write the word "white" in one of their "identity" circles because they do not have to think about their race, an unearned privilege of being part of a given structure. The same goes for cisgender men, who may not write the word "man" because they often do not have to think about gender. Moving forward as a healthcare leader, educate yourself on the topics you wrote down. Think about what you did not write and, more importantly, why. Use this consciousness raising activity as a chance to interrogate your privileges. For some this may seem daunting, but if you approach this challenge humbly, accept that you will make mistakes, you will create a thriving work environment for all whom you lead, and the individuals they care for. In order to facilitate you in this journey, please see our personal and professional growth resources section at the end of this chapter.

15.16 What Is a "Diversity Issue?"

When we think about the phrase "diversity issue," it sets our teeth on edge. "Diversity issues" are one of those times where we substitute palatable, euphemistic language to do the heavy-lifting for what we really mean. Framing a behavior, conflict, or problem as a "diversity issue" reinforces the dominant group—white, cisgender, heterosexual, able, masculine, etc.—by suggesting that conflicts related to gender, to sexuality, to ability, to age, and so on are the result of folks not adhering to normative expectations. It is important to recognize that these ideologies are at play everywhere, including in communities, in healthcare systems, and beyond. As we navigate through the remainder of this chapter, we encourage you to reflect on what is being implied by the term "Diversity Issue." Consider adopting more specific language that clearly names a problem and the underlying considerations that culminated with the "diversity issue."

As a group, healthcare disciplines have a track record of exculpating themselves from these kinds of difficult topics. It is important to both acknowledge and interrogate this historical legacy and to use what we can learn from this legacy to create a future for healthcare that is founded in meaningful equity and justice [12]. Even more, a future founded in equity and justice that is meaningful to the communities with which we partner. Healthcare disciplines use the discourse of "care" as a strategy to avoid deep reflection, difficult conversations, and substantive transformation. Deflection. You can absolutely be homophobic, racist, patriarchal, ableist, sexist, fatphobic, problematic in any number of ways *and still be a healthcare worker*. These things are not mutually exclusive, as much as we might like to think they are.

Moreover, healthcare is frequently complicit in regimes of oppression, actively propagating reinforcing and constructing racism. Take, for instance, the so-called "race correction" of glomerular filtration rates, which afforded different lab thresholds for normal kidney function for Black people versus other people. The impact of this specious science is twofold: first, it reinforces faulty assumptions about race as biological; second, it delays transplant eligibility for Black people with kidney disease, prolonged courses of dialysis as well as increased burden of morbidity and mortality [38]. Even more immediately, the crises that have characterized the racialized disparities in health outcomes during the COVID-19 pandemic to the simultaneous uprising against police brutality, state-sanctioned violence, and inequities at large - has resulted in any number of healthcare workers interrogating their own biases for the first time, some by choice and some as a consequence of sharing racist, xenophobic, or otherwise-problematic content on social media.

The right time to develop your understanding of diversity, equity, inclusion, and justice and their implications for healthcare is now. Envision a culture of belonging, where people are valued for the full complement of the skills, insights, attributes, and strengths they bring with them, as desirable and possible. Achieving such a vision will require ongoing work and effort and will require co-ownership of the vision with those who must operate within it. Resources abound, in more formats than we can imagine. Let this chapter serve as a launch pad for renewed personal responsibility and accountability for building the knowledge and skills necessary to create a more diverse, equitable, and inclusive world. As you do this, it is vital that you recognize that this is *your* journey.

This means that *you* need to do the work. As authors, we come from a wide array of backgrounds. We voluntarily come together to share our insights; we are happy to do so and share what we have learned and experienced. But what we cannot do is speak for everyone. We cannot and do not represent all perspectives. We cannot and do not speak for all members of the groups to which we belong. We respectfully ask that you recognize that it is no one's job to educate you about their experience, irrespective of your intent or burning desire to know. Think about it: people experience considerable trauma from their experiences of racism; they experience trauma linked to their sexual identity; they experience trauma related to classist assumptions. If someone walked up to you and demanded that you explain your experiences of trauma, how would that make you feel? What if it was asked by someone who had harmed you in the past? What if the real answer to the question put you in danger?

Real learning is necessary. Starting from a place of good faith—one that we assume you are coming from simply by getting this far in our chapter—is essential. But it is only the very first step in what will ultimately be a lifetime of learning. Seek to understand. Do not make it anyone else's job to help you understand, unless they offer. Recognize that you will slip. If you are lucky, someone will graciously (or not) point it out to you. Instead of becoming defensive in those moments, recognize it for the gift it is—receive the correct, reflect, and change your course accordingly. Apologize, change your behavior, and seek deeper understanding. The following are examples of harms and biased behaviors you may face in healthcare. This is not an exhaustive list, but captures some of the common problems that may arise within the practice environment:

- **Gaslighting:** Gaslighting is an abusive strategy in which an individual is made to feel as if their concerns are irrational, disproportionate, unreasonable, or misinterpretation in an effort to undermine the confidence of the person being gaslighted, to the point on occasion of question their own sanity [39]. Gaslighting is related to tone-policing and the two are often used in tandem. For example, after voicing a concern about perceived bias, a leader responds to a colleague, "I wish you'd calm down, it's not that big of a deal." Instead of diminishing people's lived experience when they share something with you, believe them. Acknowledge the problem and seek to understand their perspective as you work to resolve the conflict. This is difficult and gaslighting can be, by its very nature, subtle.

- **Microaggressions**: Coined by the Black Harvard psychiatrist and professor Dr. Chester Pierce in studying the persistent presence of stigmatizing representations of Black people in television, Pierce defined microaggressions as "subtle, stunning, often automatic and nonverbal exchanges which are 'put-downs' of Black people" (p. x) [40]. Sue, Bucceri, Lin, Nadal, and Torino further expanded that definition to include, "brief and commonplace daily verbal, behavioral, and environmental indignities that communicate hostile, derogatory, or negative slights and insults to marginalized individuals or groups" [41]. Whether intentional or not, microaggressions are a form of discrimination that have many focuses such as race, gender, sexual orientation, religious affiliation, physical capability, age, generational affiliation, social status, and their intersections. Do not allow the prefix "micro" cause you to underestimate the impact of microaggressions. While some believe that microaggressions are harmless, research has repeatedly revealed that microaggressions have significant negative impacts on people's mental and physical health [42]. Moreover, microaggressions by healthcare providers against patients are harmful to patient's health and lead to negative healthcare outcomes [43]. Leaders should be explicitly aware that their personal perceptions may not allow them to understand the microaggressions that others experience and report. Sue et al. further identified three subtypes of microaggressions, including microassaults, microinsults, and microinvalidations [41].
  - **Microassaults**: "verbal or nonverbal attacks meant to hurt the intended victim through name-calling, avoidant behavior, or purposeful discriminatory actions" (p. 274) [41].
    Example: Making a stereotypical joke about someone's age (e.g., older nurse) or generational membership (e.g., millennial nurse) and saying you were "just joking."
  - **Microinsults**: "communications that convey rudeness and insensitivity and demean a person's racial heritage or identity" (p. 274) [41].
    Example: A healthcare administrator telling a native English speaking Asian American that they "speak good English" during an interview.
  - **Microinvalidations**: "communications that exclude, negate or nullify the psychological thoughts, feelings, or experiential reality of a person of color" (p. 274) [41].
    Example: A white physician telling a BIPOC physician that racism does not exist.
    What can you do about Microaggressions? First and foremost, in facing microaggressions it is important for the healthcare leader to examine their own biases first. You can think of this as some deeper "consciousness raising" that enables you as the leader to potentially understand where your

biases and prejudices may limit your ability to face microaggressions in the workplace, and in yourself. A great place to begin this work is with Project Implicit, a non-profit organization and international collaboration of researchers who are interested in social cognition, or more specifically, "thoughts and feelings outside of conscious awareness and control" [44]. With Project Implicit, you can take individual tests on different areas where you may hold implicit biases. For more information, please see the section below, *Assignment #2: Creating a Culture of Belonging: Implicit Bias.* Second, you must educate yourself on how to recognize, respond, intervene, and prevent microaggressions in the work environment. Lastly, if you commit a microaggression it is important to be accountable for it. According to Nadal et al. (2014), as people *we all make mistakes*, but it is our duty as nursing leaders to admit when we are at fault, learn from our own wrong doings, and apologize.

- **Tokenism:** is defined by *Encyclopedia of Race and Racism* as the "policy of admitting an extremely small number of minorities to work, educational, or social activities to give the impression of being inclusive, when in actuality these groups are not welcome" [45]. Tokenism has been in place since the Civil Rights Act of 1964 so that predominantly white institutions could present as if they were meeting the federally mandated desegregation of the workforce and schools to adequately include African Americans. While this practice did benefit some, research has supported that tokenism is harmful to the identity of African Americans and leads to a sense of isolation and an increased need to prove oneself under more severe scrutiny.
  - *What can you do about Tokenism?* As healthcare leaders it is important that you are mindful to not draw constant comparisons between your groups of people, especially those who are historically oppressed and if they are few in numbers. To be singled out, as the pristine example of all things that are supposed to be good about a culture or identification group places that individual in an uncomfortable situation. The goal is to give praise and acknowledgement where it is due and to do so in ways that are distinctly different for healthcare workers from diverse backgrounds actually serves to alienate them from their peer group and can lead to negative feelings associated with inadequacy and imposter syndrome.
  - Additionally, make sure to have a comprehensive program for promotion and acknowledgement. Ensure that all employees are getting the praise they deserve and highlight complex and different things about how each individual contributes to the workings of the unit. Refrain from highlighting the same individual(s) performance above others solely because you feel that is now time for a "diverse: member of the team to be acknowledged" because this kind of recognition negates the hard work and dedication the diverse nurse has given to have excelled to this point in their career. When you are seeking thoughts about diverse matters or concerns, do not fall victim to tokenism and stay aware and reflective of who you include and exclude as you make decisions and seek advice.

- **Tone-policing:** Tone-policing is a strategy used to set the terms of a conversation by a person in power, often dictating the terms of engagement through an appeal to civility or rationality. Tone-policing diminishes the concerns of the person raising an issue while centering the needs of the person or entity doing the policing [46] (Hugs, 2015). Appeals to professionalism and civility are common in healthcare and are sometimes used to stymie dissent or objections. Tone-policing can be subtle and seem well-meaning: "People would be able to hear you better if you just contain your anger." Do not seek to control how people express themselves, instead prioritize understanding over your own emotional reaction.
- **Whataboutism:** is a term that has been revived in the modern vernacular of personal and professional communications. Merriam-Webster describes the term "whataboutism" as going beyond a simple deflection or changing of subject. Instead, whataboutism reverse engineer a topic or argument, constructing an accusation out of the original statement [47] for selective application [48]. Whataboutsims are social tools that healthcare leaders wishing to meaningfully practice diversity will need to avoid, as they often create divisive and dismissive discourses and also center defensiveness during critical conversations and moments. The repartee of "All Lives Matter" in the face of the "Black Lives Matter" Movement provides a propitious moment to further examine the inherent harm in whataboutisms. The whataboutism in this case makes the assumption that an accusation by a collective stating "Black Lives Matter" somehow indicates that other lives are not equitably important. This selective application harms in that it aims to silence, delegitimize, and misframe the statements or efforts of the opposing side. The error in this thinking may be most easily demonstrated when we consider other applications: We do not see people showing up at breast cancer events shouting, "All Cancers Matter."

15.17 Creating a Culture of Belonging: Examining Implicit Bias

When we are faced with issues that challenge our worldview, we often react and become defensive rather than take the time to step back, reflect, and ask ourselves *why* we responded the way we did. This assignment is a chance to unpack this "why," and perhaps lend insight into the way you interact with others. As described above, Project Implicit is a non-profit, international collaboration of researchers who are interested in social cognition, or more specifically, "thoughts and feelings outside of conscious awareness and control" (para. 1) [44]. This is commonly referred to as implicit bias. Hosted by Harvard University, Project Implicit provides an online Implicit Association Test (IAT), where you can learn about your attitudes and beliefs about race, gender, age, disability, religion, sexual orientation, and many different important and diverse topics that impact your ability to lead nurses to thrive. Your assignment is to **pick at least three** different IATs—choose ones that you think can provide you with the most insight. After you complete those IATs, take a moment to browse the resource list at the back of the chapter. Use the IATs results, which may help you identify your biases, and pick at least one resource to actively challenge those biases and enhance your ability to lead ALL to thrive.

Copy this link for Project Implicit's IATs: https://implicit.harvard.edu/implicit/takeatest.html

15.18 Leading Healthcare to Thrive with Plans for Action: Application of Principles

One of the key takeaways we hope you leave this chapter with is the **imperative for action**. Not just any action, either, but **intentional, contemplative action informed by critical self-reflection, and accountability for the future of healthcare** *and* **the world**. Not taking action, which includes not doing the personal work and not speaking out against the status quo, is complicity with a status quo that continues to inscribe inequality, injustice, inequity. As a leader, it is your responsibility to face challenges head on, and that includes issues that face healthcare today related to a lack of diversity, equity, inclusion, and justice. It is now your time as a leader to step up and challenge yourself, and the status quo, and do what is right for your patients, your colleagues, your communities, and the systems in which you lead. It's time for you as a healthcare leader to lead healthcare professionals, and healthcare, to thrive.

But, *where do I start?* This is a great question—and we have some suggestions. The first order of business is deep learning where you as a healthcare worker take the time to figure out your own strengths and weaknesses, taking time to remediate your knowledge deficits. We have suggestions for you but we also have ideas for collaborative strategies to help you build a network for collective action and developing a culture of belonging in your organization. We've outlined our suggestions below.

1. **You as the Leader**
   (a) *Assess yourself:*
       Starting this work starts with you. It doesn't matter if you are in academia or the clinical environment. First and foremost, it is first important *for you* to understand where your beliefs, assumptions, and biases exist as it relates to the key concepts we have covered in this chapter such as diversity, equity, inclusion, and justice. With this personal work, you will be able to see where your blinders are as it relates to issues related to these concepts. Assessing yourself may seem like an insurmountable task at first, but if you make the choice to do this work in tiny bite size pieces every day, you will see positive change over time.
       1. Start with the *Consciousness Raising* assignment.
       2. After you complete the Consciousness Raising assignment, complete the *Creating a Culture of Belonging: Examining Implicit Bias* assignment.
       3. From the Creating a Culture of Belonging: Examining Implicit Bias assignment, identify your personal biases. Seek out specific resources

that educate you on those biases. Take an active role in seeking out resources that don't support your current biases, and allow yourself to engage in intentional, critical, and informed self-reflection.

(b) *Diversity Mentorship*:

We all have knowledge gaps, and mentors can help us identify and refine those gaps—especially when it comes to areas such as diversity, equity, inclusion and justice. Mentors possesses patience, enthusiasm, knowledge, a sense of humor, and respect [49, 50]. Along with these characteristics and skills, mentors should be knowledgeable about the field and have the ability to support novice professionals [51, 52]. Mentorship can take place in multiple settings and in a variety of ways. Mentors provide guidance, support, and encouragement throughout many of life's challenges. Most are familiar with mentors in the sense of professional growth and development, but many seek guidance and have called individuals mentors to aid in life's transitions.

Professional mentorship can occur formally, if assigned by management, or informally, as an organically developed relationship between a novice and an expert nurse [53]. These relationships can be time consuming, but if done correctly they can provide multiple benefits for both parties in the relationship. Mentees benefit from the relationship by improving leadership abilities and professional engagement and the mentor benefits by experiencing joy and satisfaction in nurturing a newer professional [54]. Mentors are positive role models and also provide a protective barrier for their newer healthcare professionals. Mentors perform this service by sharing their own transition stories and they can also protect from harmful environmental factors in the workplace (i.e., bullying or incivility) [52].

As a leader, you will serve as either a formal or informal mentor in healthcare. Most enter this relationship as a means to reinforce skills, encourage acclimation to the practice environment, and to ensure functional practice. But this is not the limit to your role when mentoring diverse healthcare workers. All healthcare workers need a voice and a safe place in which to be able to speak freely about their practice experiences. These experiences may not always be positive and if you belong to the majority may not be what you want to hear or understand about your beloved profession, but it is critical that your diverse mentee have you as a confidant to express themselves. However, if your goal as a leader is to support healthcare professionals as they thrive then a part of this goal has to be to serve and mentor in a way that supports the mentee.

An additional aspect to consider if you are a leader who has the formal role of assigning mentee-mentor pairs is to understand how these pairs function properly. The key to a successful relationship is the connection, at times managers are lucky and the pair functions well and in many other instances the dynamics of the pair can be harmful for either or both parties and little positive emerges from the relationship. Leaders must listen and understand personalities and assign mentoring pairs with attention and fully acknowledge the best and worst of the personnel you employ. To assign randomly is to create potential chaos. If you are shorthanded with personnel in your work area then seek ways in which to formally pair a clinical preceptor who can help serve and meet the needs of the transitioning healthcare professionals in regard to practice; but then explore avenues to connect your diverse healthcare professional with someone who is similar to them on another floor to serve as their career mentor. To limit the role of the mentor to that of skills and practice performance is to limit the power that these relationships possess for retention to the organization and the profession overall. As strong leaders, use mentorship as a key tool to socialize and support your diverse healthcare professionals as this will only positively impact their practice and their sense of belonging.

2. **Where You Lead**
   (a) *Diversity, Equity, Inclusion, and Justice Advisors and/or Champions*:

   Just like healthcare systems have specialized staff who have specific certifications, or support staff to help those in challenging settings, diversity, equity, inclusion, and justice needs similar emphasis in the workforce. In answer to this, we recommend developing a role for an individual or individuals in your healthcare systems who can be regarded as diversity, equity, inclusion, and justice advisors or champions. Before you begin thinking about this role, and who should be in this role, please reflect on our discussion on the concepts of tokenism and performative allyship. This is an underdeveloped role in the healthcare workforce, and the person(s) selected for this role needs to be considered critically. You may not feel you are the right person to do this now, and this could be a place in which a diversity mentor could help you make a decision. Lastly, what this role looks like at your institution is up to you, but we suggest the following:

   1. *The Diversity, Equity, Inclusion, and Justice Advisor/Champion will:*
      (a) Help promote a diverse, equitable, inclusive, and just work environment.
      (b) Educate staff on issues related to diversity, equity, inclusion, and justice.
      (c) Identify areas in which the work environment or system needs to improve as it relates to diversity, equity, inclusion, and justice.
      (d) Pledge to continuously engage in self-reflection and learn about evolving issues related to diversity, equity, inclusion, and justice.

   2. *Diversity, Equity, and Inclusion Advisory Committees:*

   Diversity, equity, inclusion, and justice do not materialize in a vacuum. Instead, the conscious and concerted efforts of committed groups are necessary to foster a culture of belonging and build an environment in which diversity, equity, and inclusion is valued and actively fostered. A dedicated steering committee made up of community members, staff as well as formal and informal leaders can serve as an advisory council to guide diversity, equity, and inclusion efforts within an organization. All stakeholders should be involved. This group can serve as a brainstorm sounding board, as accountability partners, as a panel of mentors, and as strategic planning

partners as you build. These committees/councils require openness, account-ability, humility, and tenacity in order to be successfully established and maintained.

15.19 Summary

In this chapter, we have introduced you, the healthcare leader, to the complexities surrounding diversity in healthcare. This has included our perspectives on the words we use as leaders, how our privilege impacts us and those we lead, and the issues we may face. We have asked you to vulnerably check your own privileges and biases, and actively work towards a more diverse, inclusive, and just future for healthcare and those whom we care for. It is time you the leader commit to diversity as a life-long practice both personally and professionally in order to make it meaningful. The maintenance for meaningful diversity will require constant humility, empathy, advocacy, and a commitment to a broad view of social justice for all.

Finally, leaders have a responsibility to advocate for, encourage, and invest in the healthcare professionals they lead. By mindfully creating teams that are diverse, the leader positively impacts the care of patients and their families, no matter the spe-cialty area. However, a key to being mindful and purposeful with building strong, diverse teams, leaders must make a strong commitment to do the work around, assessing, reflecting, and acting on one's own biases, misunderstandings, or short-comings. This work is not easy or comfortable, but it will lead you, the leader, to be sought out as a safe space for diverse nurses to use for both personal and profes-sional encouragement. Using this chapter as a first step to taking the challenge to engage in your development as a nurse leader is one BIG step in the right direction. Please know this chapter is not all encompassing, and is just the beginning of a foundational understanding of the complexities of diversity. We encourage you to continue on your path, thinking of the multiple lives and opportunities you will change positively on the way. You must choose to do this work every day, because ultimately—diversity, and awareness of the complexities that encompass it, makes our organizations better including everyone within, leading *all to thrive.*

Glossary

Ableism Discrimination in favor of able-bodied people.
Affirmative action The practice or policy of favoring individuals belonging to groups known to have been discriminated against previously, as it relates to allo-cation of resources or employment.
Ageism Stereotypes, prejudice, or discrimination against people because of their chronological age.
Antiracist Goes beyond not personally exhibiting racist actions and involves ACTIVELY working against racist actions internally and in the systems within one exists.

BIPOC Short-hand umbrella term for Black, Indigenous, People of Color. This is an inclusive term, which is reasonable to use. It is also okay to use more specific identifiers as the situation allows. Avoid making assumptions about people's identities and respect an individual's self-selected terminology.

Cisheternormativity The tendency to default to the expectation that people will be cisgender.

Classism Prejudice against or in favor of people belonging to a particular social class.

Dehumanization The process of depriving a person or group of positive human qualities; a consequence of oppression.

Demonize The portrayal of a person(s), object, or practice act evil or deserving of disdain.

Diversity A complex concept that encompass a broad range of individual, population, and social characteristics, including but not limited to age; sex; race; ethnicity; sexual orientation; gender identity; family structures; geographic locations; national origin; immigrants and refugees; language; physical, functional, and learning abilities; religious beliefs; and socioeconomic status.

Elitism The advocacy or existence of an elite as a dominating element in a system or society.

Emotional labor Unpaid and invisible work; refers to regulating or managing emotional expressions with others as part of one's professional work role.

Equality Treating everyone the same and giving everyone access to the same opportunities.

Equity The ability to recognize the differences in the resources or knowledge needed to allow individuals to fully participate in society, including access to higher education, with the goal of overcoming obstacles to ensure fairness.

Ethnocentrism Judging other cultural groups in relation to our own culture or holding one's culture as superior to others.

Gaslighting An abusive strategy in which an individual is made to feel as if their concerns are irrational, disproportionate, unreasonable, or misinterpretation in an effort to undermine the confidence of the person being gaslighted, to the point on occasion of question their own sanity.

Gender identity A person's gender, which may or may not correspond with their biological sex.

Health disparity Differences in the quality of healthcare that are not due to access-related factors or clinical needs, preferences, or appropriateness of intervention.

Hegemony Leadership or dominance, especially by one country or social group over others.

Heteronormativity A worldview that promotes heterosexuality as the normal or preferred sexual orientation.

Heteropatriarchy A society or culture dominated by a ruling class of heterosexual males whose characteristic bias is unfavorable to those who are not heterosexual or of male biological sex.

Homophobia Prejudice, discrimination, or antagonism directed against a person or people on the basis of being homosexual.

Human capital A controversial leadership term attached to the deplorable practice of slavery. Centralizes the idea that one's abilities are of more value than the individual themselves.

Inclusion As a culture that encourages collaboration, flexibility, and fairness as well as leverages diversity so that all individuals are able to participate and contribute to their full potential.

Intersectionality The interconnections of different social categorizations such as race, class, gender, as they apply to a given individual or group, that result in an overlapping and interdependent system of dominion and oppression.

Implicit bias Biases we all have by virtue of being reared in a society riddled with normative ideas around race, gender, sexuality, class, ability, religion, and more.

Justice It is a concept that is contested, with many different definitions and applications. When we talk about justice, we can mean many different things. Often we think of fairness and equitable distribution of resources, though there are many dimensions to consider when thinking about justice. Justice looks different depending on the position of its seeker, often, and is dependent on context.

LGBTQ+ An umbrella term used to abbreviate "Lesbian, Gay, Bisexual, Transgender, Queer or Questioning." Often lumped together, within this group there is quite a lot of diversity. This label is assigned to a large and heterogeneous set of identities, behaviors, and gender expressions. More recently, the terminology LGBTQIA has been used to refer to also "Intersex, and Asexual or Allied."

Marginalization The process through which persons are peripheralized based on their identities, associations, experiences, and environment.

Microaggressions Often well-intentioned but patronizing or back-handed comments or actions enacted against members of marginalized groups that are rooted in stereotype, often founded in implicit bias.

Microassaults Verbal or nonverbal attacks meant to hurt the intended victim through name-calling, avoidant behavior, or purposeful discriminatory actions.

Microinsults Communications that convey rudeness and insensitivity and demean a person's racial heritage or identity.

Microinvalidations Communications that exclude, negate, or nullify the psychological thoughts, feelings, or experiential reality of a person of color.

Oppression The dehumanization of individuals of a group.

Paternalism Interference of a state or an individual with another person, against their will, and defended or motivated by a claim that the person interfered with will be better off or protected from harm.

Performative allyship Activism done to increase one's social capital rather than because of one's intention to help a cause. Also referred to as performative wokeness.

Politics Power-structured relationships.

Power A practice, a negotiation that takes place at each interface, relational and exercised within disciplines and between interlocutors

Prejudice A biased or preconceived opinion about someone, or a group of people, not based on reason or actual experience.

Privilege The "unearned benefits and advantages" that have been handed to a group of individuals as a result of a systemic norms and standardizations, the system structures, policies, and practices pave the road for this one group of individuals while creating obstacles for other groups.

Racism Prejudice, discrimination, or antagonism directed against a person or people on the basis of their membership of a particular racial or ethnic group.

Racist A person who has, feels, or shows prejudice, discrimination, or antagonism towards a person or people on the basis of their membership of a particular racial or ethnic group.

Sexism Prejudice, discrimination, or antagonism directed against a person or people on the basis of perceived biological sex.

Stigma A strong feeling of disapproval that most people in a society have about something.

Structural competency Awareness of and fluency in the systems and structures that delimit health and wellness.

Structural racism A system in which public policies, institutional practices, cultural representations, and other norms work in various, often reinforcing ways to perpetuate racial group inequity.

Tokenism The policy of admitting an extremely small number of minorities to work, educational, or social activities to give the impression of being inclusive, when in actuality these groups are not welcome.

Tone-policing A strategy used to set the terms of a conversation by a person in power, often dictating the terms of engagement through an appeal to civility or rationality.

Transphobia The dislike of or prejudice against individuals or groups of individuals who identify as transsexual or transgender.

Ubuntu "Humanity towards others," and "the belief in a universal bond of sharing that connects all humanity."

Vilify The defamation of a person, place, or thing by way of abusive statements, also to lower in importance.

Whataboutisms The reverse engineering a topic or argument, constructing an accusation out of the original statement.

White fragility The discomfort and defensiveness on the part of a white person when confronted by information about racial inequality and injustice.

White privilege The inherent advantages possessed by a white person on the basis of their race in a society characterized by racial inequality and injustice.

White supremacy The belief that white people are superior to those of all other races, especially the Black race, and should therefore dominate society.

Wxman An alternative spelling for "woman." The "a" was replaced with an "x" to resist male-normative language, as well as signify trans-inclusivity and the inclusion of BIPOC.

Xenophobia Prejudice, discrimination, or antagonism directed against a person or people on the basis of being from another country, an immigrant.

Chapter Discussion Questions

Consciousness Raising Discussion Questions

After you have completed the chapter, the following questions are meant to help guide you through the reflection on the consciousness raising activity. We encourage you to complete these questions from a space of non-judgement. Allow yourself time to respond honestly and openly.

1. How did you feel examining your privilege?
2. For part 1 of the consciousness raising activity, what identifiers did you write in your circles?
3. For part 2 of the activity, what identifiers did you not include in your circles?
4. How does the omission of identifiers other than what you selected make you feel?
5. What will you do differently as a result of engaging with this activity?

General Discussion Questions

1. What is diversity?
   (a) Why is diversity a starting place and not an end point?
2. What is the difference between equity and equality?
   (a) Why is understanding the difference between these two concepts important?
3. What is privilege?
   (a) How does your personal privilege impact the environments you work in?
4. What is a diversity issue?
   (a) Why is this terminology problematic?
   (b) What is an example of a "diversity issue"?
   (c) Take a moment to reflect. Have you witnessed one of these issues occurring, or have you experienced one yourself? How can we prevent this from happening in the future?
5. What are two to three areas related to diversity, equity, and inclusion that you as a healthcare provider can learn more about? If you are unsure, take a moment to reflect on the consciousness raising activity. Are there identifiers that you omitted that may be good place to start? What about the implicit bias test? Take a moment to write your thoughts down. If you want to take this a step further, after you write down each area for further learning, take a moment to identify some further resources (e.g., books, articles, and podcasts) that may support you in this journey.

Chapter Discussion Leader Guide

After the reader has completed the chapter, the main focus for the discussion leader should be on guiding the group through a reflection on the consciousness raising activity. The following is a brief script to help the discussion leader promote a supportive environment to complete this reflection.

Discussion Leader Script

The purpose of this activity is to promote a safe space to debrief about your experience examining your privilege with the consciousness raising activity. I am going to ask you a total of five questions. If you want to share your responses or thoughts you are welcome, but it is not required. You are also welcome to sit, listen, and observe. There are no right or wrong answers, but please be thoughtful with the words you choose.

The following questions are for the discussion leader to ask one at a time. Please allow space and time for participants to respond. Expect some periods of silence if participants as it may take some courage for participants to share their personal experiences.

Question 1. How did you feel examining your privilege?

Question 2. For part 1 of the consciousness raising activity, what identifiers did you write in your circles?

Question 3. For part 2 of the activity, what identifiers did you not include in your circles?

Question 4. How does the omission of identifiers other than what you selected make you feel?

Question 5. What will you do differently as a result of engaging with this activity?

If participants are uncomfortable discussing the questions orally, the discussion leader can offer insight from their own experience, only if they are comfortable sharing. Alternatively, the discussion leader can prompt the group through reflective journaling to answer the questions. This means that the discussion leader will ask the questions out loud, or provide a piece of paper with the questions. The participants will then respond to the questions independently in written from. At the end of the journaling experience, the discussion leader can ask if anyone has anything they want to share regarding the experience (e.g., the activity itself, journaling, or in general thoughts). Once again if no participants want to share, the discussion leader can thank all of the participants for their time, and also thank them for creating space in their day to raise their consciousness to promote themselves, as well as all others, to thrive in healthcare.

Video for Discussion - Instructional Video: The online version contains supplementary material available at https://doi.org/10.1007/978-3-031-16983-0_15

References

1. American Nurses Association. Code of ethics for nurses with interpretive statements. 2014.
2. AACN Diversity and Inclusion Advisory Group. Diversity, inclusion, and equity in academic nursing: AACN position statement. 2017.
3. Boateng G, Schuster R, Boateng M. Uncovering a health and wellbeing gap among professional nurses: situated experiences of direct care nurses in two Canadian cities. Soc Sci Med. 2019;242:112568. https://doi.org/10.1016/j.socscimed.2019.112568.
4. Cottingham MD. The missing and needed male nurse: Discursive hybridization in professional nursing texts. Gend Work Organ. 2019;26:197–213. https://doi.org/10.1111/gwao.12333.
5. Doede M. Race as a predictor of job satisfaction and turnover in US nurses. J Nurs Manag. 2017;25:201–14. https://doi.org/10.1111/jonm.12460.
6. Truitt AR, Snyder CR. Racialized experiences of black nursing professionals and certified nursing assistants in long-term care settings. J Transcult Nurs. 2020;31:312–8. https://doi.org/10.1177/1034659619863100.
7. Tobbell DA. Nursing's boundary work: theory development and the making of nursing science, ca. 1950–1980. Nurs Res. 2018;67:63–73. https://doi.org/10.1097/NNR.0000000000000251.
8. Diangelo R. White fragility: why it's so hard for white people to talk about racism. Boston, MA: Beacon Press; 2018.
9. Randall C, Eliason M. Out lesbians in nursing: what would florence say? J Lesbian Stud. 2012;16:65–75. https://doi.org/10.1080/10894160.2011.557644.
10. Barbee EL. Racism in US nursing. Med Anthropol Q. 1993;7:346–62.
11. Hopkins Walsh J, Dillard-Wright J. The case for "structural missingness:" a critical discourse of missed care. Nurs Philos. 2020;21:1–12. https://doi.org/10.1111/nup.12279.
12. Smith KM. Facing history for the future of nursing. J Clin Nurs. 2020;29:1429–31. https://doi.org/10.1111/jocn.15065.
13. Holmes D, Gastaldo D. Nursing as means of governmentality. J Adv Nurs. 2002;38:557–65. https://doi.org/10.1046/j.1365-2648.2002.02222.x.
14. Prescod-Weinstein C. Making black women scientists under white empiricism: the racialization of epistemology in physics. Signs J Women Cult Soc. 2020;45:421–47. https://doi.org/10.1086/704991.
15. De Sousa I, Varcoe C. Centering Black feminist thought in nursing praxis. Nurs Inq. 2021;29(1):e12473. https://doi.org/10.1111/nin.12473.
16. Crenshaw K. Demarginalizing the intersection of race and sex: a black feminist critique of antidiscrimination doctrine, feminist theory and antiracist politics. Univ Chic Leg Forum. 1989;139:139–67.
17. Metzl JM, Hansen H. Structural competency: Theorizing a new medical engagement with stigma and inequality. Soc Sci Med. 2014;103:126–33. https://doi.org/10.1016/j.socscimed.2013.06.032.
18. Metzl JM, Roberts DE. Structural competency meets structural racism: race, politics, and the structure of medical knowledge. AMA J Ethics. 2014;16:674–90. https://doi.org/10.1001/virtualmentor.2014.16.9.spec1-1409.
19. Carmicheal S. Black power. In: Cooper D, editor. Dialectics of liberation. London, UK: Verso; 2015. p. 150–74.
20. Butterfield PGR. Thinking upstream: nurturing a conceptual understanding of the societal context of health behavior. Adv Nurs Sci. 1990;12:1–8.
21. Hill Collins P. Black feminist thought: knowledge, consciousness, and the politics of empowerment. 2nd ed. New York: Routledge; 2009.
22. Prescod-Weinstein C. The rules of the diversity and inclusion racket. In: The Riveter. 2019. https://theriveter.co/voice/the-rules-of-the-diversity-and-inclusion-racket/. Accessed 10 June 2020.
23. Phillips H. Performative Allyship is deadly (here's what to do instead). In: Medium. 2020. https://forge.medium.com/performative-allyship-is-deadly-c900645d9f1f. Accessed 10 June 2020.

24. Papastravrou E, Igoumenidis M, Lemonidou C. Equality as an ethical concept within the context of nursing care rationing. Nurs Philos. 2019;21(1):e12284. https://doi.org/10.1111/nup.12284.
25. Kranich N. Libraries and democracy. Chicago, IL: American Library Association; 2001.
26. Freire P. Pedagogy of the oppressed. New York, NY: The Continuum International Publishing Group Inc; 1970.
27. Eliason MJ, Chinn PL. LGBTQ cultures: what health care professionals need to know about sexual and gender diversity. Philadelphia, PA: Wolters Kluwer; 2018.
28. Dong D, Temple B. Oppression: a concept analysis and implications for nurses and nursing. Nurs Forum (Auckl). 2011;46(3):169–76. https://doi.org/10.1111/j.1744-6198.2011.00228.x.
29. Roberts SJ, Demarco R, Griffin M. The effect of oppressed group behaviours on the culture of the nursing workplace: a review of the evidence and interventions for change. J Nurs Manag. 2009;17(3):288–93. https://doi.org/10.1111/j.1365-2834.2008.00959.x.
30. Millett K. Sexual politics. New York, NY: Columbia University Press; 2016.
31. Foucault M. Prison talk. In: Gordon C, editor. Power/knowledge: selected interviews and other writings. New York, NY: Vintage Books; 1980. p. 1972–7.
32. Murdoch A, McAloney-Kocaman K. Exposure to evidence of white privilege and perceptions of hardships among white UK residents. Race Soc Probl. 2019;11:204–2011. https://doi.org/10.1007/s12552-019-09262-3.
33. Sue DW. Overcoming our racism: the journey to liberation. San Francisco, CA: Wiley; 2003.
34. McIntosh P. White privilege: Unpacking the invisible knapsack. In: Filor AM, editor. Multiculturalism. New York: New York State Teachers United; 1992. p. 30–6.
35. Fontenot J, McMurray P. Decolonizing entry to practice: reconceptualizing methods to facilitate diversity in nursing programs. Teach Learn Nurs. 2020; https://doi.org/10.1016/j.teln.2020.07.002.
36. Laidley D, Bambino D, McIntyre D, et al. Paseo or circles of identity—school reform initiative. 2001. https://www.schoolreforminitiative.org/download/the-paseo-or-circles-of-identity/. Accessed 28 Mar 2022.
37. Carper B. Fundamental patterns of knowing in nursing. Adv Nurs Sci. 1978;1:13–24.
38. Amutah C, Greenidge K, Mante A, et al. Misrepresenting race—the role of medical schools in propagating physician bias. N Engl J Med. 2021;384:872–8. https://doi.org/10.1056/NEJMms2025768.
39. Davis AM, Ernst R. Racial gaslighting. Polit Groups Identities. 2019;7:761–74. https://doi.org/10.1080/21565503.2017.1403934.
40. Pierce C. Offensive mechanisms. In: The black seventies. Boston, MA: Porter Sargent; 1970.
41. Sue DW, Capodilupo CM, Torino GC, et al. Racial microaggressions in everyday life: Implications for clinical practice. Am Psychol. 2007;62:271–86. https://doi.org/10.1037/0003-066X.62.4.271.
42. Nadal KL, Griffin KE, Wong Y, et al. The impact of racial microaggressions on mental health: counseling implications for clients of color. J Couns Dev. 2014;92:57–66. https://doi.org/10.1002/j.1556-6676.2014.00130.x.
43. Overland MK, Zumsteg JM, Lindo EG, et al. Microaggressions in clinical training and practice. PM&R. 2019;11:1004–12. https://doi.org/10.1002/pmrj.12229.
44. Project Implicit. About us. In: Proj. Implicit. 2011. https://implicit.harvard.edu/implicit/aboutus.html. Accessed 23 July 2020.
45. Encyclopedia.com. In: Tokenism. 2020. https://www.encyclopedia.com/social-sciences/encyclopedias-almanacs-transcripts-and-maps/tokenism.
46. Hugs R. No, we won't calm down—tone policing is just another way to protect privilege. In: Everyday fem. 2015. https://everydayfeminism.com/2015/12/tone-policing-and-privilege/. Accessed 8 July 2020.
47. Merriam-Webster. What about "whataboutism"? In: Merriam-Webstercom. 2020. https://www.merriam-webster.com/words-at-play/whataboutism-origin-meaning. Accessed 23 July 2020.
48. Barcelo A. Whataboutisms and inconsistency. Argumentation. 2020. https://doi.org/10.1007/s10503-020-09515-1

49. Ferguson LM. From the perspective of new nurses: what do effective mentors look like in practice? Nurse Educ Pract. 2011;11:119–23. https://doi.org/10.1016/j.nepr.2010.11.003.

50. Gibson T, Heartfield M. Mentoring for nurses in general practice: an Australian study. J Interprof Care. 2005;19:50–62. https://doi.org/10.1080/13561820400021742.

51. Clark CM, Springer PJ. Nurse residents' first-hand accounts on transition to practice. Nurs Outlook. 2012;60:e2–8. https://doi.org/10.1016/j.outlook.2011.08.003.

52. Gazaway SB, Schumacher AM, Anderson L. Mentoring to retain newly hired nurses. Nurs Manag (Harrow). 2016;47:9–13. https://doi.org/10.1097/01.NUMA.0000488861.77193.78.

53. Fawcett DL. Mentoring—what it is and how to make it work. AORN J. 2002;75:950–4. https://doi.org/10.1016/s0001-2092(06)61459-2.

54. Huybrecht S, Loeckx W, Quaeyhaegens Y, et al. Mentoring in nursing education: perceived characteristics of mentors and the consequences of mentorship. Nurse Educ Today. 2011;31:274–8. https://doi.org/10.1016/j.nedt.2010.10.022.

Gender Wellness in the Workplace

16

Roque Anthony F. Velasco and Ashley R. Turner

Abbreviations

AAMC	Association of American Medical Colleges
ACMH	Advisory Committee on Minority Health
AMA	American Medical Association
FMLA	Family and Medical Leave Act
HHS	United States Department of Health and Human Services
LCME	The Liaison Committee on Medical Education
TGD	Transgender and gender-diverse

Learning Objectives
1. Analyze current challenges facing gender equality in healthcare
2. Evaluate the pre-licensure, clinical, and leadership applications of gender inclusivity
3. Establish methods of increasing gender equality and inclusiveness in healthcare

Supplementary Information The online version contains supplementary material available at https://doi.org/10.1007/978-3-031-16983-0_16.

R. A. F. Velasco (✉)
DAP (Desert AIDS Project) Health, Palm Springs, CA, USA
e-mail: avelasco@daphealth.org

A. R. Turner
Denver Health and Hospital Authority, Denver, CO, USA
e-mail: ashley.2.turner@cuanschutz.edu

16.1   Presentation of the Science

Leaders and organizations have promoted diversity across various industries, including healthcare. Strengthening a diverse workforce is crucial to meet the needs of an increasingly diverse America. According to the Advisory Committee on Minority Health (ACMH), a team created to advise the U.S. Department of Health and Human Services (HHS) on interventions and programs that improve the health of minorities in the United States, at least 90% of the American population growth in the next 30 years will be composed of minority groups [1]. To address this, the U.S. Department of Health and Human Services listed strengthening and expanding the healthcare workforce as one of its current strategic objectives [2]. Diversifying the healthcare workforce is critical. And, diversity has been associated with increased healthcare access, accelerated medical advances, increased cultural competence, improved patient satisfaction, decreased cultural barriers, and improved quality of care [1]. While there have been strides in improving diversity within the healthcare workforce, significant gaps remain in addressing gender-related needs among healthcare professionals. In this chapter, we will discuss structural and cultural issues that limit gender diversity within the workplace. We will also be offering concrete solutions to address practices that create and maintain gender-related discrimination. Finally, we will describe the unique needs of transgender and gender-diverse (TGD) healthcare professionals and provide recommendations on how to best support and meet their needs.

16.2   Application of Principles into Wellness Practice

16.2.1   Pre-licensure Application in the Academic Environment

Gender is a social construct that stratifies people into ordered categories that influence their experience within that context [3, 4]. Within the healthcare setting, gender impacts multiple facets of career development, including inter-and intra-professional relationships. Furthermore, gender roles in healthcare affect females and their male and transgender and gender-diverse (TGD) counterparts.

Among female healthcare professionals, gender has been associated with inequities such as occupational biases, inequalities in pay, and underrepresentation in leadership positions [4]. Scholars also argue that these inequities are products of pervasive gender roles in healthcare. Indeed, even in female-dominated fields such as nursing, gender inequality is prevalent. According to the U.S. Census Bureau, while approximately 10% of the nursing workforce are male, they make roughly 10% more than female nurses performing the same job duties [5, 6]. Among female nurses and physicians, traditional gender roles also harm collaboration. In a mixed-methods study exploring perceived gender bias among female physicians, gender played a critical role in inter-professional communication, job satisfaction, wellness, burnout, and self-doubt [7].

Gender roles in healthcare also negatively affect male healthcare professionals. Professional caregiving men such as home health aides and nurses often report experiencing stigma and isolation due to their professional roles [8]. Male nursing students have reported that patients refused care due to their gender and other people questioning their masculinity and sexuality [9]. These gender stereotypes also prevent many male nurses from pursuing a career in nursing [10]. Indeed, while gender stereotypes tend to benefit men in professional caregiving roles, these stereotypes also produce harmful effects.

Efforts have been made at the institutional academic levels to promote inclusion and gender diversity. The Liaison Committee on Medical Education (LCME), a medical education accrediting body, in coordination with medical associations including the Association of American Medical Colleges (AAMC) and the American Medical Association (AMA), has adopted two diversity accreditation standards. The standards mandate that medical schools have systematic efforts to enhance diversity, including gender diversity, amongst their student populations [11]. Since the diversity accreditation standards were implemented in 2012, there has been an increase in the diversity (i.e., sex, ethnicity, and race) of medical students.

While gender diversity has been well supported in other healthcare disciplines, equalization of gender representation remains amiss. For instance, there have been strides to diversify midwifery based on ethnicity and race, but these improvements did not extend in diversifying midwifery based on gender [12]. While more than 70% of midwives felt that men belong in midwifery and that gender does not affect the quality of care, approximately 99% of the midwifery workforce continues to be dominated by women [13, 14]. To address these inequities, we propose the following recommendations pre-licensure:

1. **Structural Changes in the Academic Setting.** Creating structural changes that meaningfully acknowledge and address gender bias and inequality is critical. One of the many ways this can be accomplished is by developing and implementing anti-discrimination policies while fostering an inclusive culture within the organization. An effective strategy to promote gender equality is *gender mainstreaming*. The United Nations described *gender mainstreaming* as a means of integrating viewpoints from all people, regardless of gender, with the goal of having equally represented voices at all levels of the decision-making process [15]. The United Nations also promoted *gender mainstreaming* to ensure that the design, implementation, and evaluation of community programs, policy, and research are informed by equally represented perspectives [15]. Operationalizing this strategy is more than ensuring that various perspectives are represented in critical conversations. *Gender mainstreaming* must also be deployed by understanding relational factors (i.e., cultural gender norms, normalized power imbalances) between men and women, acknowledging the power and privilege men have in society, and addressing these power imbalances by amplifying underrepresented voices. Furthermore, institutional changes that create a safe space for all gender perspectives to be heard in all aspects, such as policy development,

research, and program development, are critical to enculturate this practice in the workplace setting.

2. **Mentorship Programs.** Establishing learning communities is a valuable intervention in improving gender equity. This intervention can be operationalized by developing mentorship programs between students and professors. Involving those who have previously completed these mentorship programs can also serve as future mentors. Developing mentorship programs can be exceptionally beneficial if the mentors are from diverse backgrounds. Several studies indicate that female mentorship dyads improve empowerment, build relationships, increase job satisfaction, and improve representation [16–18].

3. **Negotiation Education.** In a study of salary negotiation across various industries, Stevens and Whelan explained that women are less likely to have the opportunity to negotiate for pay [19]. However, women are likely to negotiate the same rate as their male counterparts when given a chance. This suggests that education about negotiating for salary and benefits during training is critical. Empowering women to initiate salary negotiation can help balance the rates of compensation and benefits.

16.2.2 Clinical Application Post-licensure

Gender-related disparities carry over from the academic environment into the clinical setting. These disparities influence how healthcare professionals experience child-rearing, take parental leave, and experience sexual harassment. Understanding the experience of gender among healthcare professionals is crucial in understanding and creating a healthier gender-diverse workplace.

1. **Child-Rearing and Parental Leave.** Women who have children are often faced with sacrificing either time with their children or their career. In one of the most progressive countries globally, the expectations of the female workforce in the United States often feel antiquated. Giving birth and raising a child are not a disability, yet healthcare treats it as such. Lack of paid parental leave contributes to a divergent work environment where women are forced to choose between career security or advancement and the health and well-being of themselves and their children.

   While granting longer terms of leave for female partners may seem beneficial, this can further engender an expectation of females taking the primary role in childcare [20]. To address this, both parents, regardless of gender, should be granted adequate time to care for their children. Having sufficient paid parental leave is critical in ensuring the health of all healthcare professionals and their families. Patton et al. explained that paid parental leave decreases postnatal mortality rates [21]. Furthermore, the United States is one of the only industrialized countries that does not provide consistent parental leave with job protection [21].

The Family and Medical Leave Act (FMLA) was created in 1993 to support employment protection in single-parent or two-parent households where one or both parents were working [22]. Many U.S. workplaces utilize FMLA as parental leave, which does not have a provision for payment, requires that an employee has worked a minimum of 1250 h in the past year in a company with at least 50 employees, only applies to certain workers, and spans 12 weeks [22]. Paid family leave for parents has been shown to improve child health outcomes and maternal mental health status [23]. Paid, protected parental leave is a step towards gender equality in the workplace.

2. **Breast/ChestFeeding.** Having the ability to breast/chestfeed or pump milk at work is also a crucial step in creating a healthy gender-diverse workplace among birthing people. In a study of healthcare workers in an academic setting (i.e., research/admin staff, nurses, physicians, clinical support staff), breast/chestfeeding support and infrastructure, including space to breast/chestfeeding, distance to lactation space, and access to hospital-grade pumps, led increased breast/chestfeeding amongst healthcare workers [24]. Creating structures that support the biological needs of breast/chestfeeding people to pump is critical to address gender inclusion. Such structures must include developing and implementing policies that allow breast/chestfeeding people to pump privately when needed in a secure and comfortable location.

3. **Sexual Harassment.** A discussion of gender wellness would be incomplete without addressing sexual harassment and its profound impact on gender roles and gender wellness. The prevalence of sexual harassment differs based on demographics, including race, age, and gender. Sexual harassment occurs in various workplace settings, and the prevalence ranges between 20 and 75% among females and around 7% among males [25–27]. Sexual harassment has many forms, including physical, psychological, and verbal. The most prevalent form of sexual harassment is verbal harassment [26].

The prevalence of sexual harassment of female nurses is between 40 and 50% [28, 29]. Nurses experience sexual harassment from patients, family members of patients, and healthcare workers [28]. Deleterious sequela of sexual harassment includes mental health effects, physical harm, social health difficulties, inferior quality of work, and job dissatisfaction. [28, 29]. Furthermore, sexual harassment in the workplace is associated with increased stress, financial burden, and hindrances to career advancement [30]. In contrast, sexual harassment in men was not correlated with financial stress [30]. Promoting gender wellness in the workplace includes addressing sexual harassment and the environments in which it occurs. Sexual harassment prevention training must also be focused on empowering all employees to become active bystanders. This includes promoting allyship, encouraging people to report, and creating a culture of respect. Finally, promoting gender diversity in administrative and leadership roles and developing processes that empower those who have experienced harassment to report are critical.

16.2.3 Leadership Application

1. **Structural Considerations.** Policies need to move beyond reducing exclusion and move towards enhancing inclusion. Leaders within the healthcare field, including healthcare organizations and associations, must set the example and invest in inclusive practices. Such changes begin pre-licensure with inclusive educational opportunities regardless of gender or gender identity. Post-licensure, principles of acceptance and inclusion can be demonstrated through standards in recruitment practices that highlight gender diverse and gender accepting work environments. Inclusive and equal parental leave as well as structural support and protection for those who are breast/chestfeeding begins at the policy level and is integral to promoting gender wellness.
2. **Organizational Considerations.** Gender diversity in leadership positions and equal pay for equal work regardless of gender can help facilitate equality on the organizational level. Educational and workplace engagement and education about gender roles (LGBTQ+ wellness/pronouns) will foster expansive, informed, inclusive, and culturally sensitive environments.

   The creation of an inclusive educational and work environment is a step towards gender wellness and inclusion, limiting or avoiding binary circumstances such as bathrooms, locker rooms, and parenting celebrations with a female focus. Another movement towards gender inclusion in healthcare is administrative support for equal parental leave time, childcare support, and re-entry support for parents regardless of gender. Organizations can support their workers equally to create an inclusive environment.

   Leaders need to address sexual harassment and/or assault from the purview of both the victim and the perpetrator. While there are trained professionals to assist those who have experienced harassment or assault, it is the role of leadership to offer and guide employees towards mental and physical health resources. Leaders must also provide adequate and timely repercussions for the perpetrator. Additionally, routine education is needed for supervisors, faculty, students, and employees about preventing, identifying, and responding to sexual assault.

16.3 Gender Wellness in the Workplace for Transgender and Gender-Diverse People

16.3.1 General Overview

Transgender or gender-diverse (TGD) identity is used to describe people whose gender identity is incongruent with their sex assigned at birth [31]. Recent surveys also indicate that the number of TGD-identifying Americans continues to rise [32–34]. According to the Williams Institute, 1.4 million Americans identified as TGD in 2016 [32]. This was double the number of TGD identifying Americans in 2011 [33]. While some experts report that the increase in TGD identifying adults is attributed to increased social visibility and perceived social acceptance of TGD identities, many argue that the total number of TGD-identifying Americans are likely underestimates of the true population size [32, 33]. Among healthcare professionals, the population estimate of those who are TGD-identifying remains poorly understood. However, several experts argue that the total number of TGD healthcare professionals likely parallels the increasing number of TGD-identifying adults in the United States [32, 33]. Indeed, according to the Association of American Medical Colleges (AAMC), approximately 0.7% of medical students in 2018 identified as TGD [35]. Furthermore, about 1% of physicians in 2011 identified as TGD [36]. While these data are available for our physician colleagues, the number of TGD-identifying nurses and other healthcare professionals remains uncertain. Unfortunately, prior to 2020 the National Nursing Workforce Survey did not include sexual orientation or gender identity (SOGI) data. The survey used a binary option of "male" and "female" when they were really asking for sex assigned at birth/sex (labelled as "gender"). The 2020 report, covering workforce data collected at the end of 2019 and beginning of 2020 with random sampling of nurses throughout the United States, was changed to use three gender identity codes: male (9.4%), female (90.5%), and other (0.1%) [37].

TGD healthcare professionals whose gender identity may not conform to the dominant discourse of the CIS normative binary gender of males and females may have a more complicated time navigating the workplace environment than their cisgender counterparts (i.e., people whose gender identity is congruent to their sex assigned at birth). With the growing number of TGD-identifying healthcare professionals, it is, thus, critical to building a healthier gender-diverse workforce for everyone regardless of gender identity.

16.3.2 In the Academic Environment

TGD students experience significant barriers in the academic environment. According to a 2015 study of almost 6000 lesbian, gay, bisexual, and transgender (LGBT) medical students in the United States and Canada, approximately 60% of TGD-identifying participants reported not disclosing their gender identity at school due to fear [38]. Fear of disclosure is likely related to the high rates of violence TGD people face in the academic environment. According to Rankin et al., TGD students reported higher rates of harassment, experiencing a difficult or hostile campus climate, and feared for their safety due to their gender identity and gender expression [39]. TGD students also reported higher levels of depression, isolation, violence, and microaggressions than their cisgender counterparts [40–42]. Furthermore, TGD students reported poor access to gender-affirming student health and student counselling, experiencing discrimination from university health services staff, and the lack of TGD-related resources and TGD community outreach as significant barriers [40, 42].

In a study of stigma among TGD people, Velasco explained that stigma operates at various levels (i.e., intrapersonal, interpersonal, and structural), and institutional structures can create and maintain stigma [43]. At the intrapersonal level, internalized stigma leads to isolation and marginalization [43]. At the interpersonal level, TGD people experience enacted stigma through verbal harassment, physical violence, and hostility [43]. At the structural level, stigma operates by limiting TGD people from having equitable access to job opportunities and advancement, education, and other critical social domains [43]. Indeed, the discrimination and suboptimal conditions TGD healthcare professionals experience in the workplace are a clear manifestation of structural and systemic issues that create and maintain these barriers. While there has been a positive shift in acknowledging the need for healthcare professionals to be more knowledgeable of TGD-related care, the current academic curriculum is lagging. Indeed, in a survey of medical schools in the United States and Canada, the median number of hours dedicated to LGBT-related topics in the medical curriculum was approximately five hours [44]. Similarly, according to a survey of more than 1000 U.S. nursing faculty members, the average number of hours spent on LGBT-related topics in the nursing curriculum is only 2.12 h [45]. These studies demonstrate the need to improve the current curriculum to create a more culturally and gender-diverse environment in the workplace.

16.3.3 In the Workplace Environment

Several studies report that TGD physicians, nurses, and other healthcare professionals experience unique structural challenges in the workplace, particularly related to stigma and discrimination. In a survey of TGD physicians and medical students in 2019, several respondents reported negative TGD identity-related experiences during medical education and training [46]. Several participants also listed negative experiences such as the lack of mentorship from other TGD healthcare professionals, intrusive interview questions and offensive statements during the application and interview process, and application forms that do not reflect their gender identity [46]. Furthermore, 69% reported hearing colleagues making discriminatory remarks against TGD people, and approximately 33% reported witnessing other colleagues discriminating against or refusing to provide care to TGD patients [46].

   The cis normative context by which most workplace settings are situated in creates and maintains stigma TGD people experience [43]. Stigma is manifested through the well-documented stigma-related experiences TGD healthcare professionals face in the workplace setting. Indeed, healthcare professionals also reported similar negative experiences such as denial of care, harassment, ostracism, and derogatory comments from other healthcare providers when they seek healthcare services themselves [36, 46]. These findings reflect other studies that demonstrated disparities TGD people experience in the workplace, such as the experience of verbal and physical abuse, losing a job, or being denied a promotion due to their gender identity or gender expression [47]. In a landmark survey of more than 27,000 TGD adults in the United States, approximately 77% of TGD people reported hiding their gender identity from co-workers and supervisors, delayed any gender-affirming steps (i.e., social, medical, surgical, or legal transition), or quit their jobs to avoid mistreatment and discrimination in the workplace [47]. Furthermore, 27% reported experiencing other forms of workplace discrimination from their managers or supervisors [47]. These experiences include managers or supervisors disclosing TGD employee's gender identity to other people without their consent and being forced to express a gender or use restrooms that does not align with their gender identity [47].

16.3.4 Implications and Recommendations

There has been an increased discussion of disparities TGD people face in recent years within and across various social contexts. While different sectors have taken steps to improve a gender-diverse workplace environment, healthcare workplaces continue to be unprepared to meet the needs of TGD healthcare professionals. These deficiencies in providing a healthy workplace environment have been associated with increased turnover rate, decreased productivity, poor employee satisfaction, negative job attitudes, increased desire to quit, and underinvestment in human capital [48, 49]. Furthermore, a lack of structures to improve diversity, equity, and inclusion and policies to address discrimination among TGD healthcare professionals in the workplace can lead to poor morale and even litigation [50].

In a recent study of TGD employees in the United States, the experience of discrimination among TGD people in the workplace has been associated with increased hypervigilance, leading to emotional exhaustion during workdays [51]. Approximately 47% of those who reported experiencing discriminatory behaviors from others in the workplace also said that emotional exhaustion contributed to decreased productivity [51]. According to the Center for American Progress, workplace discrimination leads to at least $64 billion loss annually [52]. These financial losses are attributed to retraining new employees to replace those who have quit due to experiencing discrimination in the workplace. Recruitment and retaining healthcare professionals can also be challenging for healthcare settings without anti-discrimination policies [53].

With the significant implications of discrimination TGD healthcare professionals experience in workplace settings, leaders must be actively involved in developing and implementing concrete plans to improve healthier work environments. Addressing the underrepresentation of TGD-identifying healthcare leaders is a critical step organizations must take to address such inequities. Developing mentoring opportunities for TGD healthcare professionals is a strategic way of increasing the number of TGD-identifying leaders. Furthermore, this process facilitates *generativity* or the professional commitment to nurture the next generation of leaders [54]. By being intentional in mentoring underrepresented groups, leaders can empower TGD healthcare professionals and at the same time engage in mentorship that is critical, reflexive, and moves leadership to one that is mutually transformative [54].

Creating healthy work environments for TGD employees involves a two-prong approach: improving policies to protect the rights of TGD employees and creating an inclusive culture in the workplace [55, 56]. In a meta-analysis of contextual support among sexual and gender minorities, the presence of formalized anti-discrimination policies and procedures within the organization were predictive of increased job satisfaction and organizational commitment, decreased psychological strain (e.g., depression and anxiety), and decreased perceived discrimination among TGD employees [56]. These organizational policies should also be strengthened by creating an inclusive culture that supports diversity and leadership that facilitates equity practices [55]. Furthermore, the creation and implementation of these TGD-inclusive policies signal to TGD employees that they are valued members of the organization. Some concrete TGD-inclusive policies are as follows:

1. **Privacy Policies.** Organizations must be explicit in creating privacy policies that create a safe environment for TGD people to disclose their TGD identity. These policies must empower TGD people to decide if, to whom, when, and how to disclose their TGD identity. Other employees and managers should not disclose a TGD employee's gender identity to others without appropriate consent.
2. **Bathroom Access.** Policies that allow TGD people to use bathrooms that align with their gender identity are critical. When desired, TGD people should also be provided access to gender-neutral bathrooms. However, organizations should not require TGD people to use segregated bathrooms. While other employees might be resistant to this, developing programs that educate other employees about gender diversity is essential. This policy should also be applied to locker rooms.
3. **Dress Codes.** Current policies that enforce cis normative gender expression should be revised. Replace restrictive clothing policies based on gender with policies that support gender-neutral dress codes. Similarly, TGD people should have the opportunity to dress in a manner consistent with their gender identity if they choose to.
4. **Names and Pronouns.** All employees should be referred to by their chosen names and pronouns. Encouraging people to have their chosen names and pronouns in their badges and email signatures prevents other people from assuming another person's gender identity. Furthermore, including the employee's chosen name and pronouns in their personnel and administrative files can help affirm TGD employee's gender identity. According to the Transgender Law Center, an intentional refusal to use a TGD employee's chosen name and pronouns can constitute harassment [49].
5. **Transitioning.** Support from managers and human resources is critical when TGD employees transition in the workplace. Similar to when disclosing their gender identity, TGD employees have the authority to decide the process by which they transition. TGD people will be working closely with human resources to ensure a safe and successful transition in the workplace. These steps include establishing mutual expectations and having a thorough discussion of transition plans, updating personnel and administrative records, and communicating the transition process with others [49].
6. **TGD-Specific Diversity Training.** Integrating a TGD-specific diversity training during new employee orientation and at least annually is critical in developing a healthy work environment. Finally, fostering inclusivity through this diversity training also builds allyship, creates a space for self-evaluation of own biases, and develops skills to challenge prejudice actively.

16.4 Opportunities for Future Research

The topics presented in the chapter do not encompass all gender-related issues healthcare professionals experience in academic and clinical settings. However, we hope that this overview provides concrete steps in improving the workplace environment for all healthcare professionals, regardless of their gender. Gender is a complex social construct that operates across several contexts and influences how healthcare professionals experience their work environment. Thus, it is critical to acknowledge gender disparities and create actionable interventions to address these inequities, especially among leaders.

Furthermore, future research is still needed to understand how healthcare professionals experience gender-related issues in the workplace. It is also necessary to explore gender wellness efforts in clinical practice and their impact on patient care and healthcare worker satisfaction and retention. Describing how the regulatory climate and implementation of legislation affect gender diversity in the workforce is crucial. Understanding the lived experience of TGD healthcare workers in clinical settings and their perspective of disclosures can also provide insight into the TGD community's unique needs. Further research in this area would guide future interventions to promote gender wellness in healthcare.

Glossary

Binary gender A gender classification where two distinct and opposite forms of masculine and feminine exist.

Breast/Chestfeeding A process of feeding an infant milk directly from the body.

Cis normative Dominant discourse based on the assumption that everyone is cisgender and privileges this over any form of gender identity.

Cisgender People whose gender identity is congruent with their sex assigned at birth.

Gender equity Presence of fairness, equality, and justice in the distribution of benefits, responsibility, and opportunities for all people, regardless of gender or gender identity.

Gender identity A personal sense of being male, female, a mixture of both, or neither. A person's gender may be the same or different from their sex assigned at birth.

Harassment Any unwelcome conduct or contact.

Transgender and gender-diverse An umbrella term for people whose gender identity is incongruent with their sex assigned at birth.

Transitioning Changing features and characteristics to be more congruent with a person's gender identity. This can be through medical, surgical, social, or legal processes.

Wellness A state of balance and good physical, mental, and spiritual health.

Discussion Questions

1. Think of a time when you were "othered" due to race, sexual orientation, or an interest. How did this affect your ability to do your best?
2. How would the role of parenting change if there was universal paid parental leave for every worker? What if there was equal time for men, women, gender diverse individuals, and adoptive parents?
3. How do you think your perspective of those who are not similar to you would change if you sat with and learned about the lived experience of someone with a different gender identity than you?

Discussion Leader Guide

Suggested Prompts for Discussion
- As we delve into the gender differences in the workplace with a focus on healthcare, what other gender differences or challenges have you experienced in the workplace? Have these experiences affected your work? If so, how?
- In an ideal work environment, how would you envision managing circumstances such as parental leave and gender equality within leadership? Are there other work situations in which gender bias plays a role?
- If you were required to dress in gendered clothing that did not match your gender identity in an academic or work environment, would it affect your school or work performance?
- Does a person's gender identity of sexual orientation impact their ability to be a healthcare worker?

Video for Discussion - Instructional Video: The online version contains supplementary material available at https://doi.org/10.1007/978-3-031-16983-0_16

References

1. Advisory Committee on Minority Health. Reflecting America's population diversifying a competent health care workforce for the 21st century: a statement of principles and recommendations. U.S. Department of Health and Human Services; 2011. Accessed 19 Sept 2021.
2. U.S. Department of Health and Human Services. Strategic goal 1: reform, strengthen, and modernize the nation's healthcare system. U.S. Department of Health and Human Services; 2020. https://www.hhs.gov/about/strategic-plan/strategic-goal-1/index.html. Accessed 19 Sept 2021.
3. Morgan R, George A, Ssali S, Hawkins K, Molyneux S, Theobald S. How to do (or not to do) ... gender analysis in health systems research. Health Policy Plan. 2016;31(8):1069–78. https://doi.org/10.1093/heapol/czw037.
4. Regenold N, Vindrola-Padros C. Gender matters: a gender analysis of healthcare workers' experiences during the first COVID-19 pandemic peak in England. Soc Sci. 2021;10(2):43. https://doi.org/10.3390/socsci10020043.

5. Landivar LC. Men in nursing occupations. United States Census Bureau; 2013. https://www.census.gov/newsroom/blogs/random-samplings/2013/02/men-in-nursing-occupations.html. Accessed 3 Sept 2021

6. Wilson BL, Butler MJ, Butler RJ, Johnson WG. Nursing gender pay differentials in the new millennium. J Nurs Scholarsh. 2018;50(1):102–8. https://doi.org/10.1111/jnu.12356.

7. Cleveland Manchanda E, Chary A, Zanial N, et al. The role of gender in nurse-resident interactions: a mixed-methods study. West J Emerg Med. 2021;22(4):919–30. https://doi.org/10.5811/westjem.2021.3.49770.

8. Hallgren E, Schulte B, Miller R. Professional caregiving men find meaning and pride in their work, but face stigma. Washington, DC: New America; 2021. https://d1y8sb8igg2f8e.cloudfront.net/documents/Professional_Caregiving_Men_find_Meaning_and_Pride_in_their_Work_But_Face_Stigma.pdf. Accessed 20 Sept 2021.

9. Smith JS. Exploring the challenges for nontraditional male students transitioning into a nursing program. J Nurs Educ. 2006;45(7):263–9.

10. Wingfield AH. Caring, curing, and the community: Black masculinity in a feminized profession. In: Williams CL, Dellinger K, editors. Gender and sexuality in the workplace, vol. 20. West Yorkshire: Emerald; 2010. p. 15–37. https://doi.org/10.1108/S0277-2833(2010)0000020004.

11. Stanford FC. The importance of diversity and inclusion in the healthcare workforce. J Natl Med Assoc. 2020;112(3):247–9. https://doi.org/10.1016/j.jnma.2020.03.014.

12. Likis FE, King TL. Gender diversity and inclusion in midwifery. J Midwifery Womens Health. 2020;65(2):193–4. https://doi.org/10.1111/jmwh.13103.

13. Bly KC, Ellis SA, Ritter RJ, Kantrowitz-Gordon I. A survey of midwives' attitudes toward men in midwifery. J Midwifery Womens Health. 2020;65(2):199–207. https://doi.org/10.1111/jmwh.13060.

14. Fullerton J, Sipe TA, Hastings-Tolsma M, et al. The midwifery workforce: ACNM 2012 and AMCB 2013 Core Data. J Midwifery Womens Health. 2015;60(6):751–61. https://doi.org/10.1111/jmwh.12405.

15. Office of the Special Adviser on Gender Issues and Advancement of Women United Nations Supporting gender mainstreaming. United Nations Entity for Gender Equality and the Empowerment of Women; 2001. https://www.un.org/womenwatch/osagi/pdf/report.pdf. Accessed 20 Sept 2021.

16. Farkas AH, Bonifacino E, Turner R, Tilstra SA, Corbelli JA. Mentorship of women in academic medicine: a systematic review. J Gen Intern Med. 2019;34(7):1322–9. https://doi.org/10.1007/s11606-019-04955-2.

17. Gilbert LA, Rossman KM. Gender and the mentoring process for women: implications for professional development. Prof Psychol Res Pract. 1992;23(3):233–8. https://doi.org/10.1037/0735-7028.23.3.233.

18. Henry-Noel N, Bishop M, Gwede CK, Petkova E, Szumacher E. Mentorship in medicine and other health professions. J Cancer Educ. 2019;34(4):629–37. https://doi.org/10.1007/s13187-018-1360-6.

19. Stevens K, Whelan S. Negotiating the gender wage gap. Indust Relat J Econ Soc. 2019;58(2):141–88. https://doi.org/10.1111/irel.12228.

20. Kaufman G, Petts RJ. Gendered parental leave policies among Fortune 500 companies. Community Work Fam 2020; 1-21. https://doi.org/10.1080/13668803.2020.1804324

21. Patton D, Costich JF, Lidströmer N. Paid parental leave policies and infant mortality rates in OECD countries: policy implications for the United States. World Med Health Pol. 2017;9(1):6–23.

22. U.S. Department of Labor. The Family and Medical Leave Act of 1993, as amended. U.S. Department of Labor. https://www.dol.gov/agencies/whd/fmla/law. Accessed 31 Aug 2021.

23. Bullinger LR. The effect of paid family leave on infant and parental health in the United States. J Health Econ. 2019;66:101–16. https://doi.org/10.1016/j.jhealeco.2019.05.006.

24. Henry-Moss D, Abbuhl S, Bellini L, Spatz D. Lactation space experiences and preferences among health care workers in an academic medical center. Breastfeed Med. 2018;13(9):607–13. https://doi.org/10.1089/bfm.2018.0101.
25. Aycock LM, Hazari Z, Brewe E, Clancy KBH, Hodapp T, Goertzen RM. Sexual harassment reported by undergraduate female physicists. Phys Rev Phys Educ Res. 2019;15(1):010121. https://doi.org/10.1103/PhysRevPhysEducRes.15.010121.
26. Jenner S, Djermester P, Prügl J, Kurmeyer C, Oertelt-Prigione S. Prevalence of sexual harassment in academic medicine. JAMA Intern Med. 2019;179(1):108–11.
27. La Lopa JM, Gong Z. Sexual harassment of hospitality interns. J Hosp Tour Educ. 2020;32(2):88–101. https://doi.org/10.1080/10963758.2020.1726767.
28. Kahsay WG, Negarandeh R, Dehghan Nayeri N, Hasanpour M. Sexual harassment against female nurses: a systematic review. BMC Nurs. 2020;19(1):58. https://doi.org/10.1186/s12912-020-00450-w.
29. Lu L, Dong M, Lok GKI, et al. Worldwide prevalence of sexual harassment towards nurses: a comprehensive meta-analysis of observational studies. J Adv Nurs. 2020;76(4):980–90. https://doi.org/10.1111/jan.14296.
30. McLaughlin H, Uggen C, Blackstone A. The economic and career effects of sexual harassment on working women. Gend Soc. 2017;31(3):333–58. https://doi.org/10.1177/0891243217704631.
31. Transgender Law Center. Model transgender employment policy: negotiating for inclusive workplaces. Transgender Law Center; 2013. http://transgenderlawcenter.org/wp-content/uploads/2013/12/model-workplace-employment-policy-Updated1.pdf. Accessed 17 Aug 2021.
32. Flores AR, Herman JL, Gates GJ, Brown TNT. How many adults identify as transgender in the United States? Los Angeles: The Williams Institute; 2016.
33. Gates GJ. How many people are lesbian, gay, bisexual, and transgender? Los Angeles: The Williams Institute; 2011.
34. Jones JM. LGBT identification rises to 5.6% in latest U.S. estimate. Gallup; 2021. https://news.gallup.com/poll/329708/lgbt-identification-rises-latest-estimate.aspx. Accessed 6 July 2021.
35. Association of American Medical Colleges. Association of American Medical Colleges: Matriculating student questionnaire 2018 all schools summary report. Washington, DC: Association of American Medical Colleges; 2018.
36. Eliason MJ, Dibble SL, Robertson PA. Lesbian, gay, bisexual, and transgender (LGBT) physicians' experiences in the workplace. J Homosex. 2011;58(10):1355–71. https://doi.org/10.1080/00918369.2011.614902.
37. Smiley RA, Ruttinger C, Oliveira CM, Hudson LR, Allgeyer R, Reneau KA, Silvestre JH, Alexander M. The 2020 national nursing workforce survey. J Nurs Regul. 2021;12(1):S1–S96.
38. Mansh M, White W, Gee-Tong L, et al. Sexual and gender minority identity disclosure during undergraduate medical education: "in the closet" in medical school. Acad Med. 2015;90(5):634–44. https://doi.org/10.1097/ACM.0000000000000657.
39. Rankin S, Weber G, Blumenfeld W, Frazer S. 2010 state of higher education for lesbian, gay, bisexual, and transgender people. Campus Pride; 2010. https://www.campuspride.org/wp-content/uploads/campuspride2010lgbtreportssummary.pdf. Accessed 2 Sept 2021.
40. Hood L, Sherrell D, Pfeffer CA, Mann ES. LGBTQ college students' experiences with university health services: an exploratory study. J Homosex. 2019;66(6):797–814. https://doi.org/10.1080/00918369.2018.1484234.
41. Lapinski J, Sexton P. Still in the closet: the invisible minority in medical education. BMC Med Educ. 2014;14:171. https://doi.org/10.1186/1472-6920-14-171.
42. Santos TC, Mann ES, Pfeffer CA. Are university health services meeting the needs of transgender college students? A qualitative assessment of a public university. J Am Coll Health. 2021;69(1):59–66. https://doi.org/10.1080/07448481.2019.1652181.
43. Velasco RAF. Stigma among transgender and gender-diverse people accessing healthcare: a concept analysis. J Adv Nurs. 2022;78(3):698–708. https://doi.org/10.1111/jan.15040.

44. Obedin-Maliver J, Goldsmith ES, Stewart L, et al. Lesbian, gay, bisexual, and transgender-related content in undergraduate medical education. JAMA. 2011;306(9):971–7. https://doi.org/10.1001/jama.2011.1255.
45. Lim F, Johnson M, Eliason M. A national survey of faculty knowledge, experience, and readiness for teaching lesbian, gay, bisexual, and transgender health in baccalaureate programs. Nurs Ed Perspect. 2015;36(3):144–52. https://doi.org/10.5480/14-1355.
46. Dimant OE, Cook TE, Greene RE, Radix AE. Experiences of transgender and gender non-binary medical students and physicians. Transgend Health. 2019;4(1):209–16. https://doi.org/10.1089/trgh.2019.0021.
47. James SE, Herman JL, Rankin S, Keisling M, Mottet L, Anafi M. The report of the 2015 U.S. transgender survey. National Center for Transgender Equality; 2016. https://transequality.org/sites/default/files/docs/usts/USTS-Full-Report-Dec17.pdf. Accessed 18 June 2021.
48. Lee Badgett MV, Waaldijk L, van der Meulen RY. The relationship between LGBT inclusion and economic development: macro-level evidence. World Dev. 2019;120:1–14. https://doi.org/10.1016/j.worlddev.2019.03.011.
49. Thoroughgood CN, Sawyer KB, Webster JR. Finding calm in the storm: a daily investigation of how trait mindfulness buffers against paranoid cognition and emotional exhaustion following perceived discrimination at work. Organ Behav Hum Decis Process. 2020;159:49–63. https://doi.org/10.1016/j.obhdp.2019.02.004.
50. Transgender Law Center. Tools for transgender people to address discrimination. Transgender Law Center; 2021. http://transgenderlawcenter.org/wp-content/uploads/2021/04/Tools-for-Transgender-People-to-Address-Discrimination.pdf. Accessed 18 Sept 2021.
51. Thoroughgood CN, Sawyer KB, Webster JR. What lies beneath: how paranoid cognition explains the relations between transgender employees' perceptions of discrimination at work and their job attitudes and wellbeing. J Vocat Behav. 2017;103:99–112. https://doi.org/10.1016/j.jvb.2017.07.009.
52. Burns C. The costly business discrimination: the economic cost of discrimination and the financial benefits of gay and transgender equality in the workplace. Center for American Progress; 2012. https://cdn.americanprogress.org/wp-content/uploads/issues/2012/03/pdf/lgbt_biz_discrimination.pdf. Accessed 18 Sept 2021.
53. Human Rights Campaign. A workplace divided: understanding the climate for LGBTQ workers nationwide. Human Rights Campaign; 2018. https://assets2.hrc.org/files/assets/resources/AWorkplaceDivided-2018.pdf?_ga=2.238641216.1183728143.1632012663-1977614411.1632012663. Accessed 18 Sept 2021.
54. Velasco RAF. Critical mentorship: empowering mentor-mentee relationships toward transformative learning. HIV Specialist Mag. 2021;13(2):48–9. https://aahivm.org/wp-content/uploads/2021/06/FINAL-MAGAZINE-1.pdf
55. Ruggs EN, Martinez LR, Hebl MR, Law CL. Workplace "trans"-actions: how organizations, coworkers, and individual openness influence perceived gender identity discrimination. Psychol Sex Orientat Gend Divers. 2015;2(4):404–12. https://doi.org/10.1037/sgd0000112.
56. Webster JR, Adams GA, Maranto CL, Sawyer K, Thoroughgood C. Workplace contextual support for LGBT employees: a review, meta-analysis, and agenda for future research. Hum Resour Manage. 2017;57(1):193–210. https://doi.org/10.1002/hrm.21873.

Patient Violence: Providing More than Duck and Cover Training to Protect Employees

17

Danisha Jenkins and Vanessa Lauzon

Abbreviations

HCW Healthcare worker
WPV Workplace violence

Learning Objectives
1. The reader will identify the ways in which trauma-informed communication is necessary for safety.
2. The reader will identify the importance of addressing the pathology in preventing aggressive behavior
3. The leader will identify structural and societal contributors to violence in the workplace.

17.1 Presentation of the Science

Healthcare workers, particularly those working in acute care settings, are the most vulnerable professionals to workplace violence [1]. While violence in the workplace may be experienced in many forms, such as lateral violence and bullying; for the purposes of this chapter, we define workplace violence (WPV) as any act or threat of physical violence, harassment, intimidation, or other threatening disruptive behavior that occurs at the work site, and may include threats and verbal abuse to

D. Jenkins (✉)
University of California, Irvine, CA, USA
e-mail: danishj@uci.edu

V. Lauzon
Department of Psychiatry, University of California, San Diego, San Diego, CA, USA

© The Author(s), under exclusive license to Springer Nature
Switzerland AG 2023
J. E. Davidson, M. Richardson (eds.), *Workplace Wellness: From Resiliency to Suicide Prevention and Grief Management*, https://doi.org/10.1007/978-3-031-16983-0_17

physical assaults and homicide [2]. Meta-analysis of rates of workplace violence demonstrates 61.9% of HCW reported exposure to any form of WPV, 42.5% reported exposure to nonphysical violence, and 24.4% reported experiencing physical violence in the past year. Verbal abuse is the most common form of nonphysical violence, followed by threats and sexual harassment [3]. Across occupations, studies have demonstrated that nurses have the highest exposure to any form of WPV, followed by physicians and other healthcare professionals [3]. It is important to note that this data is frequently based on reported incidences of WPV, and both underreporting and lack of processes for reporting WPV are both prevalent barriers to fully understanding the extent of this phenomenon [4]. Significant physical violence is experienced most frequently in emergency and psychiatric departments, and the sequalae to healthcare workers is profound, including anxiety, anger, depression; all of which present direct impacts to workforce retention and engagement [5].

The National Institute for Occupational Safety and Health (NIOSH) groups risk factors that lead to violence in healthcare are clinical (pain, fear, anger, altered mental status, history of violence, and the influence of drugs and alcohol), environmental (department layout and design), and organizational (understaffing, long work shifts, inadequate security procedures and protocols, discouragement to report and difficulty in reporting violent incidents, acceptance by management and staff that violence is "part of the job," and lack of staff training and preparedness) [6]. Despite the known complexities of socioecological and environmental conditions leading to WPV, training, if provided at all, often heavily prioritizes self-defense training, placing the onus on an individual to be able to physically protect themselves in the face of physical violence. While such training has shown value in the imminent response to physical harm [7], in this chapter, we attempt to shift the focus to the *upstream* contributors to workplace violence, to move beyond duck-and-cover toward resources, and processes that humanize both healthcare workers and patients in the prevention of violence in the workplace occurring at all.

17.2 Application of Principles into Wellness Practice

17.2.1 Pre-licensure Application in the Academic Environment

In the pre-licensure environment, it is critical that burgeoning healthcare workers are enculturated through education to understand that violence in the workplace should never be accepted as "part of the job." It is the responsibility of the individual, the community, and the institution to protect healthcare workers and patients. Assure that students are educated to the multitude of evidence-based interventions proven to reduce risk of workplace violence in the care setting and are prepared to assess and advocate for including early identification of prodromal symptoms, environmental safety considerations, de-escalation techniques, and trauma-informed communication. Pre-licensure curricula must aide in fostering foundational understanding of not only disease processes but also the structural violence that potentiates such risk factors for agitated and potentially violent behavior including unaddressed pain, substance dependence, mental illness, and racism. Introduce students early to the appropriate use and the dangers of restraint utilization, and an early emphasis on respect for autonomy and trauma-informed communication are essential.

17.2.2 Clinical Application Post-licensure

In exploring the causes of agitated and potentially violent behavior, be curious about the underlying etiology. All behavior is a form of communication, and healthcare workers must ask "what is being communicated?" Focus on identifying the behaviors, and refrain from clouding one's assessment with judgements of motives, character, or morality. Critical for safety is the simultaneous setting of appropriate and clear limits regarding behavior and enforcing safety mechanisms.

There are a multitude of clinical issues that may underlie aggressive behavior, including traumatic brain injuries, strokes, neurodegenerative disorders, seizures, and central nervous system infections, hypoxic injury, and cognitive impairment and disability. Medical and nursing assessment may inform considerations regarding patient's level of legal responsibility for behavior, including awareness of right and wrong, appreciation of consequences, and the ability to regulate behavior accordingly. Assessing a patient's cognitive capacity, or ability to understand their own current behaviors and potential consequences to those behaviors, is a necessary and often overlooked step in developing an interdisciplinary safety and care plan. Psychiatric issues, substance intoxication and withdrawal, history of psychological trauma, and maladaptive responses to stress may also potentiate violent behavior, and few of these etiologies can successfully be managed in the same way. However, setting clear limits, redirecting in developmentally and clinically appropriate ways, consistency across time and team members, and leadership support for front-line clinicians is universally critical in managing agitation and preventing violence and injury.

To illustrate the importance of patient and pathology specific interventions, the following two examples are of patients who hit and scratch when being touched:

Case 1: A patient with hepatic encephalopathy hits and scratches the nurse when touched. The patient is being treated with lactulose. They are intermittently alert, extremely agitated upon arousal, and not oriented to person, place, or time.

Case 2: A patient with an acute traumatic frontal lobe injury hits and scratches the nurse when touched. The patient is alert, oriented to self, and intermittently oriented to place, and is extremely agitated and impulsive upon arousal.

In both cases, the healthcare worker can employ similar tactics to reduce agitation, potential injury, and harm such as clustering care to reduce interruptions in rest, maintaining distance if needing to wake the patient up, setting boundaries, and eliciting permission before touching. In the first case, however, given the patient's orientation status, it is unlikely that the patient has the cognitive capacity to consider consequences of actions, and will be unable to engage in providing consent. Addressing the pathology is imminently critical, and lowering the ammonia levels and aggressively managing hypernatremia are necessary to manage aggression. In this case it will be important that the healthcare worker not be alone providing care during periods of high agitation, and to create a coordinated plan to provide for safety (e.g., considering the use of mittens) prior to further care. A thoughtful plan shared with all those who have direct contact with the patient can prevent injury when engaging in activities such as waking the patient to provide necessary care or perform assessments.

For the second case, it will be especially important to keep the patient surroundings clear of objects that can be thrown, as the HCW knows that the highest risk period of agitation and impulsive behavior is immediately upon awakening. Additionally, this patient is somewhat oriented, so it will likely be valuable for the HCW to reorient the patient, explain what the HCW is there to accomplish, and elicit permission before approaching the bed. This might sound like "Hi Steve, I am your nurse Ray, and you are in the hospital right now. Can you tell me where you are right now?" After validating that the patient is oriented to the place, the nurse can continue, "It is time for me to take your blood pressure, may I come close to your bed and touch your arm? When I come close to you, I need to make sure we are both safe, can you please tell me that you are not going to hit or scratch me?" If the patient exhibits agitation, or threatens to hurt the HCW, do not approach the bedside at that time.

These examples illustrate just some of the ways in which managing behavior requires addressing the pathology. There is unlikely to be one clinical pathway or predetermined set of resources and interventions that will meet the needs of the patient, or the safety of the care team.

17.2.3 Respect for Personhood

Respect for autonomy and trauma-informed approaches are underutilized, and yet powerful tools. Simple processes such as eliciting permission before touching, explaining roles, explaining what will happen before doing it, giving choices, being consistent, and respecting personhood are essential. Healthcare workers must have a strong understanding of the high prevalence of trauma, especially for patients that live in intentionally marginalized communities. There are many experiences in the healthcare setting that can be re-traumatizing, and these experiences will impact how a person responds to healthcare interventions. Frequently throughout the course of healthcare interventions and services, patients will experience a lack of control, vulnerability, feeling frightened, or ashamed. These experiences are key triggers to re-traumatization and may elicit a self-defense response that can be dangerous for healthcare workers and the patient alike. Providing for safety, establishing trust, offering choice, preserving autonomy and dignity, and empowering patients to decide what is best for them are critical trauma-informed approaches, and must be preserved despite perceived inconveniences or individual clinicians' perceptions of what is best. Healthcare workers must work diligently to create an experience in which the patient makes their own choices, feels safe, and understood. In participating in trauma-informed approaches, we must acknowledge that healthcare institutions are historically very unsafe and traumatizing environments for many patients, particularly Black, Indigenous, persons of color, and people living with physical and mental disabilities. Historical and current data demonstrates that the feelings of mistrust and corresponding need to defend oneself is often a matter of survival, particularly in a hospital. Acknowledging and understanding such realities create space for empathy and open the door for working toward an authentic human connection. Such connections may lay a framework for trust and safety for patient and healthcare worker alike.

Healthcare workers caring for patient populations that are at high risk of agitated behavior, and therefore violence, face challenges. Such environments often include trauma departments, acute drug and alcohol detoxification units, and psychiatric intensive care units. In such departments, it is especially critical that healthcare workers identify and advocate for the resources needed to safely provide ethical and complete care. Additionally, HCWs frequently working in these settings must set boundaries for care for themselves including taking time off, advocating for rotating patient assignments when appropriate, and utilizing employee assistance programs (EAP) consistently. Many "evidence-based" policies and guidelines are not created to support the HCW in engaging in truly patient-centered care that offers autonomy, and the rigidity of hospital schedules and protocols may lead to increased frustration.

HCW's must collaborate to meet the patient's needs in ways that prioritize patient and HCW safety, even when this may not be the most productive or protocolized method of providing care. To help illustrate this recommendation, a case study will be discussed:

A patient who suffered a severe traumatic brain injury after their camp site was hit by an intoxicated driver. The patient had ben unhoused for over a decade, and was accustomed to sleeping on the ground. Due to a combination of the brain injury and underlying psychiatric illness, the patient often moved very slowly, and would not take medication until all of their food was eaten, and their "camp" was organized, which would often take over an hour. The nurses would often attempt to pull the patient up off the floor. They were concerned the floor was dirty and would cause pressure injury, that the behavior disruptive the unit, and that they did not have time to wait an hour for every morning med pass. When being forcefully removed from the ground, the patient would become extremely combative, leading to security being called, four-point restraints being placed, and chemical sedation administered. The chemical sedation would render the patient unable to participate in therapies, increased delirium, and prolonged periods restrained.

When debriefing with the team after both a nurse and the patient were injured, the team discussed the top priority, which was to provide for safety. When asking the nurses what being safe looked like, they said not being hit when trying to provide care, and they requested security presence on the floor. When asking the patient what safety looked like, they stated, "Why can't I be on the floor? Leave my stuff alone and let me eat my food in peace!" Collectively, the team devised a plan to meet the needs of the patient and the nurses, although it required some additional resources and operated outside of the usual confines of the standard protocols. Safety for the patient first meant having their environment arranged in a certain way. The nurses obtained a floor mattress for the patient, and removed the bed. The psychiatrist evaluated the patient's medications, and made adjustments secondary to the agitation and impulsive behavior that was exhibited. Physical and occupational therapy set their schedules to see the patient during the hour every morning when the patient insisted on organizing the "camp." The patient was incentivized with ice cream outside in the wheelchair after medications were taken. While the new plan was being trialed, security maintained a presence outside of the patient's room, but by the end of the first day, the nurses stated that they did not need security any longer. Although there continued to be challenging moments, after the implementation of the patient-centered plan, there was not another instance in which security had to be called, and there was no further injury.

17.3 Leadership Application

The Joint Commission (TJC) mandates healthcare organizations to both assess for and address violence [8]. Despite regulatory standards, there is a continued lack of attention to facility and department-specific risk assessment and policies [7]. Although TJC specifically requires training in de-escalation, nonphysical intervention skills, physical intervention techniques, and response to emergency incidents [8], leaders must diligently strive to develop and provide systems, processes, and resources that prevent workplace violence. Leaders must recognize the significant challenges that clinical staff face in caring for communities in which trauma, untreated mental illness, substance dependence, and violence has become increasingly common. In many locations, healthcare workers are in danger when caring for their patients. It is not reasonable to expect that support for clinicians, including the provision of resources, would look the same as what was required even just five years ago. Leaders must provide for adequate education, specialists, and human and material resources with the understanding that different situations require different experts and interventions. In conducting annual assessments of workplace violence events, leaders must identify areas of high risk of violence, and collaborate with the caregivers in identifying what safety provisions are necessary. It is unlikely that online learning modules are sufficient, and interdisciplinary subject matter experts must be involved in designing structures and processes that account for the patient population, knowledge, and experience of the HCWs, and environmental limitations.

When WPV occurs, leaders must also engage in trauma-informed approaches to address the issue. It is never a HCW's fault that they were assaulted, and any such incident must be viewed as a systems failure. In response to a WPV event, providing for both physical and psychological safety for the victim must be the first priority, as well as implementing immediate measures to prevent further harm. Offer the employee access to psychological and medical support services, as well as time off from work. Conduct an interdisciplinary briefing with every major incident of WPV, and prioritize providing authentic support for the HCW's who are tasked to navigate providing care to a person that presents a credible risk to their physical safety. Actively empower all members of the team to express concerns, identify problems, identify early warning signs, and collaborate expeditiously to address these issues.

Many incidences of WPV could have been prevented had the appropriate resources been provided and utilized. Too often, leaders engage in addressing workplace violence only after a series of major incidences have occurred. Equitable and proactive attention must be given to all of the NIOSH domains of risk factors for workplace violence, and leaders must move beyond "duck and cover" training for these high-risk staff. Addressing the clinical risk factors requires investing in appropriate screening tools, clinical experts such as psychiatry and chemical dependence specialists, and establishing community resources to implement upstream interventions to prevent acute hospital admissions. Addressing organizational contributors requires repairing staffing models that pervasively leave departments understaffed and unable to meet the needs of the patients, and radically changing the idea and messaging that violence is an expected part of the job. Environmental modifications may be required, including reducing noise and overcrowding, as well as designing safe spaces for HCWs. Lastly, staff training must be robust and appropriate for the specific needs of the work that a HCW is performing. There is WPV prevention training that everyone in healthcare needs; however, a healthcare professional working in a trauma unit will need specialized training in the understanding and treating the behaviors of a patient with a frontal lobe versus occipital lobe injury, whereas a neurology healthcare professional may need additional treatment in post-epileptic safety. The resounding message is that the required tools to prevent WPV are as individualized and complex as the patients themselves. The time, space, and resources must be allotted to create a care delivery environment and processes that meets the needs of the patients and the HCWs doing the work.

17.4   Opportunities for Future Research

Many healthcare institutions have implemented training for HCWs in *response* to workplace violence, but the impact of these training programs on *preventing* workplace violence is unclear. There is little research on the impact of upstream, or preventative interventions on workplace violence in healthcare. The HCW in direct contact with the patient, particularly those in acute care where a patient is likely in crisis, is at the end of a long line of opportunity for intervention and prevention. There is an opportunity to study how community substance abuse and mental health services, housing support, economic equity, and mutual aid impact the rates and severity of violence in the workplace. Until the healthcare system and society addresses structural inequities and the dearth of public and community health resources, the institution is responsible for the provision of enhanced resources to mitigate, prevent, manage, respond to, and recover from violence in the workplace.

References

1. Mento C, Silvestri MC, Bruno A, Muscatello MRA, Cedro C, Pandolfo G, Zoccali RA. Workplace violence against healthcare professionals: a systematic review. Aggress Violent Behav. 2020;51:101381. https://doi.org/10.1016/j.avb.2020.101381.
2. OSHA. Guidelines to preventing worplace violence for healthcare and social service workers. (OSHA 3148-06R 2016). Washington, DC: Occupational Safety and Health Administration; 2015. https://www.osha.gov/sites/default/files/publications/osha3148.pdf.
3. Liu J, Gan Y, Jiang H, Li L, Dwyer R, Kai L, Yan S, Sampson O, Hongbin X, Wang C, Zhu Y, Chang Y, Yang Y, Yang T, Chen Y, Song F, Zuxun L. Prevalence of workplace violence against healthcare workers: a systematic review and meta-analysis. Occup Environ Med. 2019;76(12):927–37. https://doi.org/10.1136/oemed-2019-105849.
4. Copeland D, Henry M. Workplace violence and perceptions of safety among emergency department staff members: experiences, expectations, tolerance, reporting, and recommendations. J Trauma Nurs. 2017;24(2):65–77. https://journals.lww.com/journaloftraumanursing/Fulltext/2017/03000/Workplace_Violence_and_Perceptions_of_Safety_Among.3.aspx.
5. Rosenthal LJ, Byerly A, Taylor AD, Martinovich Z. Impact and prevalence of physical and verbal violence toward healthcare workers. Psychosomatics. 2018;59(6):584–90. https://doi.org/10.1016/j.psym.2018.04.007.
6. NIOSH. Workplace violence prevention for nurses. Washington, DC: The National Institute for Occupational Safety and Health; 2013.
7. Arbury S, Hodgson M, Zankowski D, Lipscomb J. Workplace violence training programs for health care workers: an analysis of program elements. Workplace Health Saf. 2017;65(6):266–72. https://doi.org/10.1177/2165079916671534.
8. The Joint Commission. 2021. https://www.jointcommission.org/-/media/tjc/documents/resources/workplace-violence/ts_10_2021_preventing-workplace-violence.pdf.

Shifting Culture Through Structured Organizational Second Victim Support

18

Susan D. Scott

Abbreviations

HCP   Healthcare professional
MUHC   University of Missouri Health Care
SV   Second victim
SVP   Second victim phenomenon

Learning Objectives
1. Explain the second victim phenomenon and describe high-risk clinical events that elicit a second victim response.
2. Describe the importance of knowing the second victim's healing trajectory when designing institutional support plans.
3. Describe the deployment of a comprehensive three-tiered model of interventional support to address the emotional well-being needs of healthcare professionals.

Note: The common descriptors used to describe the second victim experience (second victim, second victim phenomenon, second victim syndrome, distressed clinician) are *not* recognized as Medical Subject Headings.

Supplementary Information The online version contains supplementary material available at https://doi.org/10.1007/978-3-031-16983-0_18.

S. D. Scott (✉)
University of Missouri Health Care, Columbia, MO, USA

Sinclair School of Nursing, University of Missouri, Columbia, MO, USA
e-mail: scotts@health.missouri.edu

J. E. Davidson, M. Richardson (eds.), *Workplace Wellness: From Resiliency to Suicide Prevention and Grief Management*, https://doi.org/10.1007/978-3-031-16983-0_18

18.1 Presentation of the Science

The second victim phenomenon (SVP) is a unique professional/personal trauma experienced by an HCP in the aftermath of a clinically complex event/case. The term "second victim" (SV) was initially introduced by Albert Wu, who described his observations of a fellow resident intimately involved in a serious medical error and the resultant negative impact on the individual, both professionally and personally [1]. Years later, a formal definition of the SV was offered as HCPs "who are involved in an unanticipated patient event, in a medical error, or a patient-related injury and became victimized in the sense that the provider is traumatized by the event" [2].

Despite professional role, gender, age, or tenure as a healthcare professional, research participants in a seminal University of Missouri Health Care study were able to instantaneously recall the initial and enduring influence of their respective challenging clinical event on its impact on their professional and personal lives [2]. In a vast majority of the cases, participants could describe specific details in exquisite detail even many years (sometimes decades later). Individuals suffering from the SVP frequently describe mild-to-severe physical, emotional, cognitive, or behavioral responses during their healing.

Common psychological symptoms include troubling memories, anxiety, anger toward oneself, panic, embarrassment, guilt, self-doubt, flashbacks, overwhelming feelings of inadequacy, and suicidal ideation [3–6]. Frequent physiologic symptoms include extreme fatigue, sleeping difficulties, digestive difficulties, inability to concentrate/focus, increased agitation, and withdrawal [2, 6, 7]. The psychological burden can be immense. The experienced psychosocial/physical tsunami can be professionally debilitating and potentially career-ending. Some experiences are so profound that it leads the clinician to leave their beloved profession, consider self-harm, or even contemplate suicide [5, 6, 8].

In today's healthcare environment, the extent of clinical events potentially evoking an SV response extends well beyond the initial focus on medical error-related events and unanticipated clinical outcomes. Additional high-risk events identified for inducing an SV response can include unanticipated patient decline/death, failure to rescue cases, first death experiences, exposure to workplace violence, death of a co-worker, and pandemic exposures [9–12]. Based on the current understanding of the SVP, it is appropriate to broaden the original definition. Second victims are now recognized as individuals working within an environment offering/providing care and are professionally/personally traumatized by exposure to a challenging clinical case/event.

Individuals experiencing an SV response use unique coping mechanisms, yet each transcends a predictable six-stage recovery trajectory of healing [2]. This healing trajectory includes (1) chaos and accident response, (2) intrusive reflections, (3) restoring personal integrity, (4) enduring the inquisition, (5) obtaining emotional first aid, and (6) moving on. Stage six, "moving on," describes the individual's healing and recovery from that event. It is important to understand that this stage does not indicate an individual's potential success or failure in future professional roles. Instead, it is genuinely an evaluation of the healthcare entities' provision of adequate support.

The sixth stage of recovery offers three distinct potential outcomes within the recovery pathway—drop out, survive, or thrive. The idyllic recovery from an SV exposure is thriving. Thriving occurs when the HCP learns from the event, continues their work, and assists with practice modifications to benefit future patients/clinicians, thus experiencing a form of post-traumatic growth. Surviving, sometimes referred to as presenteeism, occurs when HCPs continue their roles within the same clinical specialty/environment. The individual typically suffers from a decline in performing their professional functions, notably contrasting with pre-event baseline performance. Dropping out refers to the HCP that transitions careers due to one specific challenging clinical event. This unexpected career shift for an individual clinician will commonly result in the individual realizing a decreased fulfillment in the new role. If clinician support needs are not adequately addressed, it is quite possible that exceptional clinicians will become a dropout and hastily leave their beloved profession. One of the prominent reasons for an individual to consider dropping out is the perception of inadequate support from departmental and institutional leaders [13].

A key objective for an institution's plan for SV support is to concentrate on clinicians that experience healing as thrivers or survivors therefore minimizing or even eliminating the dropouts Achieving a clear understanding of the healing trajectory and the unique clinician needs/desires within each stage offers valuable insights into designing a comprehensive and holistic supportive approach within the context of a healing environment. Develop effective interventions to address the individual HCP's immediate needs and desires.

18.1.1 Restorative Second Victim Support: Influencing Recovery

With emerging research on second victimization, it has become an ethical responsibility to alter healthcare's previous culture of inattentiveness for suffering HCPs to one of nurturing and support [3]. In the aftermath of emotionally challenging clinical events, specific support needs identified included talking to someone about the experience, validating decisions made and care provided, receiving professional reaffirmation of professional capabilities, and assurances to regain a sense of self-worth [14]. These needs can be addressed within the organization's supportive infrastructure design by integrating two basic interventional strategies—one-on-one peer support offered by a skilled colleague and group briefings when a problematic case affects an entire team.

Collectively, research regarding effective SV recovery proposes that healthcare organizations design an infrastructure of social support for HCPs suffering professionally and personally [3, 5, 6]. Social support is a critical factor that positively influences a SVs professional/personal recovery [15]. The individual's professional network plays a pivotal role in helping ensure the HCP's positive recovery. Two key factors have been identified as essential for a healthcare organization's work environment. First, overall awareness of the SVP and its traumatic impact on the individual with the potential long-term effects is needed. A detailed understanding of the SVP is the first intervention that any organization can deploy. Second, the existence of a comprehensive institutional response plan to meet the unique needs of SVs has the capability of strongly influencing the individual's overall healing. Broadly convey this response plan to every member of the respective healthcare team [16].

At the organizational level, focus efforts to minimize the emotional toll on the individual by formalizing holistic, comprehensive support strategies across every worksite to guarantee that all individuals are observed for potential SV reactions [11]. Create support interventions concentrating on various SV reactions, from fundamental supportive interactions to expert assistance for the more severe responses. Include the institution's commitment to providing a rapid internal response that offers a supportive presence on a 24/7 basis within the support plan. Support provided by peers, confidentiality, timeliness of services, accessibility ease, a nonjudgmental approach and promotion of a blame-free, non-punitive culture, quality review regarding care rendered, and predictable staff follow-up are desirable features of a model SV support infrastructure [17–19]. These confidential support conversations create a "safe zone" for the HCP to share insights into their experience. Minimize the human toll experienced by the HCP in the aftermath of any potentially stressful patient-related events through these carefully planned supportive strategies.

18.1.2 A Framework for Support: The forYOU Team

In 2007, University of Missouri Health Care (MUHC) implemented an evidence-based response strategy to address the diverse needs of its healthcare workforce experiencing SVI. Known as the forYOU Team, this rapid response team offers SVs emotional and social support by promptly delivering a wide range of comprehensive services for the HCP [12, 19, 20]. The team mission includes increasing SVP awareness, providing continual surveillance for possible SVs wherever they may work within the healthcare system, and providing prompt emotional support once a potential SV has been identified [12]. The forYOU Team utilizes the Scott Three-Tiered Interventional Model of Support that addresses diverse SV needs by delivering various support strategies based on the individual HCP's unique needs [19].

To help aid in SV recovery, each tier within the interventional model offers complementary resources. Tier One support engages department-based leaders and colleagues ready to render initial support for the HCP requiring assistance. HCP support occurs most commonly within this tier. Department-based leaders can offer distinctive aid to the HCP, ranging from arranging flex time off to assisting with healthcare record documentation or adverse event reporting to providing an objective review of care decisions made and care rendered.

Tier Two offers two distinct forms of interventional support—one-on-one peer support and team debriefings when a challenging clinical event/case impacts an entire team. Peer supporters embedded throughout MUHC monitor colleagues during their assigned shifts for symptoms suggestive of an SV response following a potentially challenging clinical event. Capitalizing on the HCPs professional social network, peer support delivered by a skilled colleague is a critical, evidence-based intervention that can reduce SV stress and promote healing [12, 21–23]. Skilled peer supporters are a vital component of the forYOU Team and offer instantaneous one-on-one support if indicated. Peers, especially those who have previously endured the SVP, can provide support and compelling healing words to the suffering colleagues. A skilled peer responder's well-timed emotional support can positively influence the individual clinician's ultimate recovery. For most HCPs, the department-based leaders (Tier One) and peer supporters (Tier Two) are vital elements of a supportive healing environment for the recovering SV.

Complimenting the one-on-one peer conversations in Tier Two are team debriefings. These debriefings, facilitated by two individuals trained explicitly on working with groups in crisis, are offered when an emotionally challenging case/event adversely impacts an entire team. Approximately one hour in length, team debriefings provide an opportunity for the involved HCPs to acknowledge their shared lived experience. The experience frequently aids in an enhanced understanding and appreciation of case complexities, supports team healing, and often stimulates a sense of overall camaraderie and team resilience.

Tier Three resources guarantee the availability of mental health professional services for those individuals who have support needs that exceed the capabilities of a department-based leader or skilled peer supporter. Between 10 and 15% of suffering SVs will require this advanced level of interventional support. The experts capable of rendering support within Tier Three are frequently employed within healthcare organizations in varying capacities. These include clinical psychologists, social workers, chaplains, holistic nurses, wellness officers, and employee assistance programs. Harnessing the talents of these skilled mental health well-being experts into a comprehensive network of supportive presence are hallmarks of a robust interventional program that can address even the most complex SV needs.

18.2 Application of Principles into Wellness Practice

18.2.1 Pre-licensure Application in the Academic Environment

Understanding that the SVP can affect anyone working in the healthcare environment, especially the student learner, multiple interventions can be proactively designed and implemented at the academic and host healthcare institutions. Trainees are not exempt from experiencing the potential negative professional and personal influence of the SVP. Our increasing knowledge of the SVP includes specific implications for the adequate preparation of student learners. The HCP student learner can be subjected to various clinical scenarios that can trigger an SV response. These clinical exposures could evoke an SV response and even cause the student learner to question their resolve to join the healthcare profession. Anticipating that stressful clinical events will occur during training, design preemptive conversations regarding emotions commonly experienced during stressful situations within the healthcare environment as standard part of your faculty role functions [24]. These candid discussions allow the student to understand the normalcy of these emotions among both student learners and practicing clinicians and enhance their working knowledge of the SVP.

Assure faculty members and additional resources for support are readily available when an upsetting situation occurs. Some HCP students may be subdued about revealing true feelings and fear that any displayed vulnerability could be viewed as a sign of weakness impacting their student learner reputations. Awareness of the SVP is vital for the student learner to develop strategies to lessen the damaging effect. Proactive approaches, such as offering student debriefings after challenging clinical events or those caring for patient populations who could evoke an SV response, encourage a conversation about the SVP within the context of a safe learning environment. Incorporate the realization of the true impact of the SVP on the practicing clinician as a core competency for guiding student experiences. Integrating didactic content on the SVP, such as faculty seminars relating to their SV experiences, simulations, self-care wellness toolkits, assigned readings, and self-paced modules, can effectively complement the lived experiences of the student learner and assist in preparing the student learner [7, 24–27].

The host healthcare environment where the student learns the art and science of their chosen profession has distinct responsibilities in offering a safe and effective learning environment. The host organization considers the student learner within the design of response teams to ensure a holistic approach of supportive care for any individual working within that environment, including the student learner. Monitor closely individuals learning within your organization who are involved in a clinical event that could evoke an SV response, including potential student learner involvement and follow-up care.

Preparing the HCP student to enter the healthcare workforce successfully is the most fundamental objective of any academic program and the associated healthcare host institutions. Incorporating the necessary knowledge, skills, and attitudes regarding the SV experience and insights into restorative, supportive care in the aftermath of the experience are key survival tactics for the future HCP. In addition to promoting their own sustainability, the new HCP will understand and recognize high-risk clinical situations. By becoming knowledgeable about the SVP while in training, the HCP will have the skills and knowledge necessary to offer supportive care for future colleagues experiencing the adverse professional consequences of challenging clinical events.

18.2.2 Clinical Application Post-licensure

The newly licensed HCP is quite vulnerable during early career years and needs to understand how to process stressful patient-related events effectively. Being aware of the SVP and potential implications on professional/personal lives gained during their professional training encourages healthy recovery. However, if SVP conceptual analysis is deficient from professional training, a knowledgeable and experienced mentor may help to facilitate both the individuals' transition into the healthcare profession and role model effective processing of challenging case events. This peer mentor can offer supportive and confidential guidance during some of the most challenging career events ahead.

18.2.3 Leadership Application (Structural and Organizational Considerations)

Organizational leaders play a pivotal role in ensuring restorative professional support services are delivered within their respective institutions. Broadly publicize an executive leader endorsed SV social support structure so that every HCP is aware of the SVP, responsive to assistance, and familiar with resources to access in times of need for themselves or others. Although researchers continue to explore the SVP and evaluate optimum tactics for team deployment and the most meaningful services provided, there is ample understanding to recognize the variety of benefits for implementing a formal institutional support plan. The evidence-based Scott Three-Tiered Model of Clinician Support can serve as the basic framework for institutional design of a support system to ensure a comprehensive, holistic support team capable of addressing all identified SV needs. Incorporating readily available internal resources addresses various SV reactions, ranging from simple "check-ins" and leadership reassurances to protracted professional help when more severe responses are identified.

Build clear guidelines on the institution's SV emotional support response plan. Widely publicize the project plan with basic considerations that HCPs have explicit knowledge of the SVP, understand the organizational-specific plan, and know steps to activate support services when needed. Develop broad educational campaigns (for both organizational/departmental leaders and HCPs) regarding SV and available supports. Execute various mechanisms for the prompt identification of a colleague experiencing a potential SV reaction. Closely monitor potentially challenging clinical cases with department-based leadership to identify potential SVs proactively. Open dialogue with leaders sharing their own SV experiences will promote internal cultural acceptance for assistance.

The design and effective deployment of formal support processes will serve both providers and patients well in the future. The most prevalent SV response involves stress and related anxieties. Stressed and distracted HCPs can potentially create unsafe care environments. The holistic design of a formal support infrastructure for a healthcare organization benefits the individual SV by proactively addressing the professional/personal influence of the SVP, ultimately reducing unplanned absences, decreasing turnover intent, and promoting productive future healthcare careers [28–30]. Institutional SV support has been demonstrated to improve healthcare quality, influences stronger relationships between HCPs and their leadership, significantly impact joy and meaning in the work environment, and augments the general patient safety culture of the organization [3, 5, 31].

As a healthcare community, we are only now beginning to fully appreciate the provision of reliable and predictable emotional support. It is now understood that clinician support can serve as a lifeline for the suffering HCP. In addition to career-saving support for the workforce following a stressful patient event, the infrastructure of a formal support team can also offer alternatives to other organizational needs. Some existing peer support programs are now serving as an essential bedrock for overall well-being initiatives by assisting the institution's workforce as it faces the many challenges associated with the pandemic and associated stressors [10, 11].

18.3 Opportunities for Future Research

Since 2010, research on the topic of second victimization has become abundant. Yet, there remains an opportunity to continue our collective understanding of the SVP. It is important to continue learning about the various aspects of second victimization and the restorative support required for healthy recovery to define SV peer-support program efficacy.

Focus future research on five distinct areas that remain unanswered including: earlier SV detection, the relationship between SV and other distressed clinician concepts, SV supportive intervention analysis, primary factors associated with acceptance of peer support, and overall peer support program outcomes. Table 18.1 includes specific research questions for future exploration of these essential elements.

Table 18.1 Future second victim research topics

Research Topic	Research Questions
Distressed Clinician Concepts	– Is there a relationship between SVP and other distressed clinician conditions (such as compassion fatigue, moral injury, burnout, post-traumatic stress disorder)? – Can SV interventional support also serve as interventions for other distressed clinician conditions? – What are desired support interventions for the other distressed clinician conditions? – What are the critical elements of a comprehensive support structure to address all distressed clinician conditions?
Early Second Victim Identification	– Can predictive modeling within an electronic medical record identify patients at high risk for evoking an SV response from their care team? – Can a real-time warning system be designed to notify department-based leaders of potential stressful patient events? – Can an acuity tool be devised to determine SV effect and identify associated supportive care requisites? – Can patient safety culture assessments identify high-risk units/departments populations vulnerable to becoming an SV?

Table 18.1 (continued)

Research Topic	Research Questions
Second Victim Support Interventions	– What are the necessary qualities of a peer support training program? – What additional complementary support services should be considered when designing a system-wide SV support structure of the future? – How can we reliably identify when an SV requires additional support? – Can individual risk factors be identified to assist with earlier referral to mental health practitioners? – What standards should be developed that address the timing of SV support interventions?
Acceptance of Peer Support	– Are there generational considerations when designing strategies to encourage an SV's acceptance of peer support? – Are there generational influences or considerations for peer supporters when offering support to a clinician?
Peer Support Outcomes	– Does the presence of a formal SV support structure influence an organization's unplanned absences, turnover, and churnover rates? – What are the most meaningful organizational metrics to evaluate the effectiveness of formal SV support infrastructures? – What are gold standard metrics of peer support performance when evaluating individual SV recovery? – What criteria should be considered when determining if a clinician is safe to continue patient care?

18.4 Conclusion

Today's HCP faces an unprecedented clinically complex, demanding, and uniquely intense work environment. Well-meaning HCPs who work in these conditions face the harsh reality of clinical complexity that may evoke an SV response. Regrettably, a substantial percentage of the workforce has been enduring professional and personal struggles in relative silence. Current research offers keen insights into the potential harm suffered by the HCP experiencing acute occupational stress, the SVP.

Evidence-based support infrastructures have been successfully deployed to address the aftershock of emotionally challenging clinical events. Healthcare facilities can use these programs as a blueprint to create their comprehensive plan that supports any HCP experiencing the SV. Supportive intervention begins the moment HCP duress is realized. Create supportive presence as a predictable component of the healthcare organization's response plan to emotionally distressing clinical events.

The presence of an institutional response plan is a necessary step in protecting our most valuable resource, our healthcare professionals. These individuals have the primary focus on rendering care to others. The promotion of a healing environment for our healers is a key priority for healthcare leaders in both academic and service environments.

Glossary

Second victim (SV) Individuals working within an environment offering/providing care and are professionally/personally traumatized by exposure to a challenging clinical case/event.

Second victim phenomenon (SVP) A unique professional/personal trauma experienced by a healthcare professional in the aftermath of acute or chronic clinically complex clinical events.

Discussion Questions

1. Before this reading assignment, were you aware of the second victim phenomenon?
2. Has anyone experienced the second victim phenomenon OR identified a colleague who was suffering? What were your observations about the experience? What type of clinical event evoked the response?
3. Peer support—what would be important personal attributes for the peer supporter to render care?
4. What would you perceive as potential barriers to receiving peer support?

Discussion Leader Guide

1. Sadly, the second victim phenomenon is one that no one wants to experience, yet almost every practicing healthcare professional has experienced the second victim phenomenon—personally or witnessed a suffering colleague. Most clinicians will have this response 3–4 times (or more) during their clinical years of practice. When it does occur, many healthcare professionals are unsure of what they are experiencing. Many will internalize their emotional responses and suffer in relative silence. Most professional colleagues do not know how to respond or assist the suffering co-worker, which further confounds the suffering and eventual healing. Awareness and an understanding of the second victim phenomenon are the first interventions to address this concern. *What does the student learner understand about the second victim phenomenon and how will that apply to their future careers?*
2. Facilitate a conversation about first-hand experiences with the second victim phenomenon. It is helpful if the leader is willing to share their personal story to start the conversations. To facilitate these conversations, encourage a basic overview of the patient scenario in a de-identified manner. Next, describe your emotional responses/feelings and what support you needed and may have received. What helped? What did not? If no support was received, describe tips on how you processed the event. Once shared, ask others in the group to share their stories.

3. Peer support is the most desired form of supportive intervention by second victims. The peer supporter is crucial in helping the second victim recover. Some individuals describe an efficient peer supporter as someone who has high emotional intelligence. Individuals who have the respect and trust of their peers are perfect candidates to become a peer supporter.

A successful one-on-one peer conversation relies heavily on the interpersonal relationships that the peer can form. Peers should have an empathic and non-judgmental approach to discussions. Active listening skills and the ability to keep confidence are essential. *What does the student learner think is the most crucial attribute of peer supporter?*

4. Several significant barriers within the healthcare environment have been identified for healthcare professionals not to receive the support they desperately need and desire. The most notable is the fact that there is a stigma associated with reaching out for help. As healthcare professionals, we are amazing helpers, but when we need help, that is quite different. Many do not seek help on their own behalf because they fewar that it could be a sign of professional weakness. In addition, high acuity areas have little time to integrate what has transpired under the team's watch. Frequently, these teams disband, and each move independently in different directions of the healthcare organization. Fear of loss of professional integrity is profound, with specific worries about loss of licensure, compromise of collegial relationships, and future legal woes. Lack of confidentiality and access to support services are also considered barriers to receiving support. *What does the student learner think is a barrier for a student to receive help?*

What are some ideas for an organization to overcome these barriers?

Video for Discussion - Instructional Video: The online version contains supplementary material available at https://doi.org/10.1007/978-3-031-16983-0_18

References

1. Wu AW. Medical error: the second victim. The doctor who makes the mistake needs help too. BMJ. 2000;320:726–7.
2. Scott SD, Hirschinger LE, Cox KR, et al. The natural history of recovery for the healthcare provider second victim after adverse patient events. J Qual Saf Health Care. 2009;18:325–30.
3. White R, Delacroix R. Second victim phenomenon: is 'just culture' a reality? An integrative review: App Nursing Res; 2020. https://doi.org/10.1016/j.apnr.2020.151319.
4. Schroder K, Janssens A, Hvidt E. Adverse events as transitional markers: using liminality to understand experiences of second victims. Soc Sci Med. 2020;268:113598. https://doi.org/10.1016/j.socscimed.2020.113598.
5. Coughlan B, Powell D, Higgins M. The second victim: a review. Eur J Obstet Gynecol Reprod Biol. 2017;213:11–6. https://doi.org/10.1016/j.ejogrb.2017.04.0020301-2115.
6. Busch I, Scott SD, Connors C, et al. The role of institution-based peer support for healthcare workers emotionally affected by workplace violence. Jt Comm J Qual Patient Saf. 2021;47(3):146–56. https://doi.org/10.1016/j.jcjq2020.11.005.
7. Ozeke O, Ozeke V, Coskun O, et al. Second victims in health care: current perspectives. Adv Med Educ Pract. 2019;10:593–603. https://doi.org/10.2147/AMEP.S185912.

8. Seys D, Scott S, Wu AW, et al. Supporting involved health care professionals (second victims) following an adverse health event: a literature review. Int J Nurs Stud. 2013;50(5):678–87. https://doi.org/10.1016/j.ijnurstu.2012.07.006.
9. Busch IM, Moretti F, Purgato M, Barbui C, Wu AW, Rimondini M. Psychological and psychosomatic symptoms of second victims of adverse events: a systematic review and meta-analysis. J Patient Saf. 2020;16(2):e61–74. https://doi.org/10.1097/PTS.0000000000000589.
10. Godfrey K, Scott SD. At the heart of the pandemic: nursing peer support. Nurse Lead. 2021;19:188–93. https://doi.org/10.1016/j.mnl.2020.09.006.
11. Scott SD. The pandemic's toll—a case for clinician support. Mo Med. 2021;118(1):45–50.
12. Hirschinger LE, Scott SD, Hahn-Cover K. Clinician support: five years of lessons learned. Patient Saf Qual Healthcare. 2015;12(2):26–31.
13. Rodriquez J, Scott SD. When clinicians drop out and start over after adverse events. Jt Comm J Qual Patient Saf. 2018;44(3):137–45. https://doi.org/10.1016/j.jcjq.2017.08.008.
14. Newman MC. The emotional impact of mistakes on family physicians. Arch Fam Med. 1996;5:71–5.
15. Dekker S. Second victim - error, guilt, trauma and resilience. Boca Raton: CRC; 2013.
16. Connors CA, Dukhanin V, March AL, et al. Peer support for nurses as second victims: resilience, burnout, and job satisfaction. J Patient Saf Risk Manag. 2019;25(1):22–8. https://doi.org/10.1177/2516043519882517.
17. Dukhanin V, Edrees H, Connors CA, et al. Case: a second victim support program in pediatrics – successes and challenges to implementation. J Pediatr Nurs. 2018;41:54–9.
18. Edrees HH, Morlock L, Wu AW. Do hospitals support second victims? Collective insights from patient safety leaders in Maryland. Jt Comm J Qual Saf. 2017;43(9):471–83.
19. Scott SD, Hirschinger LE, Cox KR, et al. Caring for our own: deployment of a second victim rapid response system. Jt Comm J Qual Saf. 2010;36(5):233–40.
20. Scott SD, Hirschinger LE, McCoig MM. The second victim. In: DeVita M, Hillman K, Bellomo M, editors. Textbook of rapid response systems. New York: Springer; 2011. p. 321–30.
21. Stone M. Second victim support programs for healthcare organizations. Nurs Manage. 2020;202051(6):38–45.
22. Lane MA, Newman BM, Taylor MZ, et al. Supporting clinicians after adverse events: development of a clinician peer support program. J Patient Saf. 2018;14(3):e56–60.
23. Merandi J, Liao N, Lewe D, et al. Deployment of a second victim peer support program: a replication study. Pediatr Qual Saf. 2017;2(4):e031.
24. Hall LW, Scott SD. The second victim of adverse health care events. Nurs Clin North Am. 2012;47(3):383–93.
25. Kennesaw State University. Just culture, medication error prevention, and second victim support: a better prescription for preparing nursing students for practice. Georgia: WellStar College of Health and Human Services; 2021.
26. Chung AS, Smart J, Zdradzinkski M, et al. Educator toolkits on second victim syndrome, mindfulness, and meditation, and positive psychology: the 2017 resident wellness consensus summit. West J Emerg Med. 2018;19(2):327–31.
27. Jones J, Treiber LA. More than 1 million potential second victims: how could nursing education prevent? Nurse Educ. 2018;43(3):154–7. https://doi.org/10.1097/NNE.0000000000000437.
28. Miller C, Scott SD, Beck M. Second victims and mindfulness: a systematic review. J Patient Saf Risk Manage. 2019;24(3):108–17. https://doi.org/10.1177/2516043519838176.
29. Quillivan RR, Burlison JD, Browne EK, et al. Patient safety culture and the second victim phenomenon: connecting culture to staff distress in nurses. Jt Comm J Qual Saf. 2016;42(8):377–86.
30. Burlison JD, Quillivan RR, Scott SD, et al. The effects of the second victim phenomenon on work-related outcomes: connecting caregiver distress to turnover intentions and absenteeism. J Patient Saf. 2016;17(3):195–9. https://doi.org/10.1097/PTS.0000000000000301.
31. Sexton J, Adair K, Profit J, et al. Perceptions of institutional support for "second victims" are associated with safety culture and workforce well-being. Jt Comm J Qual Patient Saf. 2021;47(5):306–12. https://doi.org/10.1016/j.jcjq.2020.12.001.

Bullying and Lateral Violence: Building a Process to Address Root Causes

19

Karen M. O'Connell

Abbreviation

TJC   The Joint Commission

Learning Objectives
1. Identify the reasons lateral violence occurs in healthcare
2. Describe methods to prevent or mitigate lateral violence
3. Discuss reasons why zero tolerance policies are not effective

19.1   Presentation of the Science

Bullying in healthcare has occurred for over a century. In 1909, *The New York Times* reported on the bullying of student nurses by head nurses in the hospitals [1]. While the solution proposed by the physician cited in the article is outdated, the despotism described was unacceptable then as it is now. Unfortunately, bullying continues in healthcare. In 2008, The Joint Commission (TJC) issued a Sentinel Event Alert describing disruptive behaviors that affect teamwork and result in poor patient outcomes. The alert announced a new requirement for organizations to have a code of conduct to outline acceptable and unacceptable behaviors and leaders need to have a procedure to address inappropriate behaviors [2]. Even with this TJC requirement in effect, bullying continued in healthcare facilities. TJC issued a Quick Safety publication on bullying in 2016. The publication reviewed what bullying is, its prevalence, and effects on the workplace. Actions suggested in the 2008 TJC alert are

K. M. O'Connell (✉)
Northern Kentucky University, Highland Heights, KY, USA
e-mail: oconnellk@nku.edu

© The Author(s), under exclusive license to Springer Nature   275
Switzerland AG 2023
J. E. Davidson, M. Richardson (eds.), *Workplace Wellness: From Resiliency to Suicide Prevention and Grief Management*, https://doi.org/10.1007/978-3-031-16983-0_19

reinforced along with additional recommendations [3]. A pre-publication standard, effective in January 2022, described on the TJC website addresses workplace violence, [4] a sign bullying still occurs in healthcare.

Bullying, incivility, and lateral violence are often used interchangeably in the literature. All describe the same type of behavior but differ in the intensity of the behavior. Additional terms used are horizontal violence, disruptive behavior, and mobbing. Any repeated negative behavior found offensive and/or intimidating by the target from a peer is considered lateral violence. Negative behaviors are overt to covert and include: eye rolling, gossiping, breaking confidences, intentional withholding of information, and rude or demeaning remarks [5]. This behavior is intended to demean and humiliate the target [6]. Healthcare providers that are new to practice or new to a practice area are most often targeted by bullies [7].

Lateral violence effects are seen in the target, bystanders, patients, and organizations. Targets often suffer from physiological and psychological symptoms. These symptoms include dry mouth, nausea, diarrhea, migraine headaches, sleep disturbances, weight loss, lethargy, anxiety, panic attacks, fear of making mistakes or asking questions, loss of confidence, and post-traumatic stress symptoms. Studies report bystanders to the violence also suffer from similar symptoms [8, 9].

Patient care is affected by lateral violence. TJC, in their 2008 alert, identified teamwork as vital to patient safety [2]. Targets have lower self-confidence which impacts their critical thinking and clinical judgement skills leading to medication errors, missed care, and patient harm or death [5, 10, 11]. Lastly, providers that are targeted often leave their positions. Replacing a healthcare provider is expensive for institutions and the cost is often passed on to the consumer. Other costs include poor outcomes of patients. In one report from 2001, an estimated $23.8 billion was spent on the cost of disruptive behaviors annually [5].

Why does this negative behavior persist in healthcare, among providers believed to be caring? Multiple causes of this negative behavior have been cited. Healthcare is a stressful environment and poor staff cohesiveness can contribute to the behavior [6]. In a recent literature review, Shorey and En Wong [8] identified causes of bullying as the intergenerational differences between providers and as a way to maintain power. Although most facilities have introduced policies on disruptive behavior as directed by TJC [2, 3], these have not been effective in preventing or mitigating bullying. Multiple authors have called for leadership to enforce these policies and address the behavior immediately [6, 12, 13].

Bullying in healthcare must stop. Providers who are targeted may make preventable mistakes and often leave their positions or career. Our patients deserve the best efforts of the healthcare team.

19.2 Application of Principles into Wellness Practice

19.2.1 Pre-licensure Application in the Academic Environment

To stop bullying behaviors in the workplace, educate students early in their studies on the concept, causes, and ways to respond or intervene. Several studies have suggested methods to educate healthcare provider students. Presenting the negative behaviors that may be experienced in a lecture or computer-based format has been examined. Another method is a virtual reality simulation. Finally, the use of cognitive rehearsal training has reported positive outcomes. Educating students early on the behaviors will allow them to recognize and report to their clinical instructors. Introducing effective responses to the behavior can be accomplished by cognitive rehearsal training and/or simulation

Cognitive rehearsal training is based in cognitive behavioral training (CBT). It is a strategy to allow individuals to rehearse their reactions to problematic interactions with others. CBT has been used to assist with understanding and changing thinking patterns or behavior [14]. Griffin (2004) [15] described a cognitive rehearsal training intervention that included didactic and practical components. Education on what lateral violence is and theories why it occurs was presented. Following this, individuals were presented with cards listing the ten most frequent lateral violence behaviors (Table 19.1) and potential responses. Individuals were then allowed time to rehearse their responses to the identified behaviors in small groups. The participants in this study who reported experiencing lateral violence responded using the suggested phrases and found this stopped further lateral violence directed against them.

Table 19.1 Ten most frequent lateral violence behaviors	
	Non-verbal innuendo (raising eyebrows, rolling eyes, making faces)
	Verbal affront (snide remarks, short responses)
	Undermining activities (not available to assist)
	Withholding information (patient or practice)
	Sabotage (deliberately setting up others for failure)
	Infighting (arguing with peers in public)
	Scapegoating
	Backstabbing
	Failure to respect privacy
	Broken confidences

An example of the education in the training includes identification of lateral violence behaviors and their prevalence, effects, and root causes. Review policies from accreditation agencies and the facility to assure they include mitigation/prevention strategies. For the rehearsal portion, participants are divided into groups of four to five with a facilitator lead. The facilitator presents a lateral violence behavior and asks a group member to respond. The group then discusses the positive and negative aspects of the response. An example scenario might be: A nurse is discussing information with you about another nurse who is not present. A potential response could be: I do not feel comfortable speaking about (the absent nurse) without her being here.

Provide clinical instructors with the same training as the students. At the beginning of the clinical rotation, educate students on the facility's policy regarding disruptive behavior. Bring to the attention of the unit manager any negative behaviors encountered in the clinical setting as outlined in the facility policy. Role model the appropriate actions and response to negative behavior on the unit when serving as a clinical instructor. As the student gains confidence in their clinical abilities, encourage students to address the behaviors themselves.

19.2.2 Clinical Application Post-licensure

Educate healthcare professionals in clinical practice on the appearance of bullying, methods to address/prevent bullying; and how to recognize if they are the bully. Many of the methods used in the academic environment can be used in clinical application. It is important to include education on what specific behaviors are considered negative. Often the providers using these negative behaviors do not recognize the negativity of their actions. Many feel that since this is how they were treated; it is an appropriate behavior. Providing the education and an opportunity to practice responses is very effective.

Targeted individuals often do not know how to respond to the behavior. Most targets are new to practice or new to the practice area and may not feel confident. Some targets may "freeze" when confronted with the behavior, similar to opossums when confronted with danger. Educate the workforce to the role of bystander. Bystanders who witness lateral violence behaviors need to be informed regarding how to respond to the situation. The bystander can either support the target in their response or respond for the target.

One way to raise awareness of lateral violence is to create an environment where the behavior is not tolerated. If bystanders do nothing, the provider may feel empowered to continue the behavior. Educate all personnel in the healthcare system on lateral violence behaviors and how to respond as a bystander. One method that has been successful is "Green Dot" training. Green Dot training was originally developed to help prevent sexual or domestic violence, and stalking on college campuses; however, the training can be applied to lateral violence situations [16].

There are three ways to intervene according to Green Dot training.

First: Direct—stepping into the situation to handle it. For example, addressing the provider and pointing out the unacceptable behavior.
Second: Distract—creating a distraction that interrupts the unacceptable behavior. Asking the provider or target to assist with a task is an example of distraction.
Third: Delegate—enlisting someone else, a manager or supervisor, to intervene. Calling for additional assistance from security or police is an example of delegating [17].

19.2.3 Leadership Application (Structural and Organizational Considerations)

TJC requires policies against bullying; however, the existence of a policy is not enough. Leadership needs to enforce the policies equally. TJC has published two safety statements related to lateral violence. Both have called for zero tolerance policies in healthcare facilities. The fact that TJC has had to publish a second call for these policies suggest that either they are not in place or they are not effective.

Leaders who do not take action related to bullying behaviors implicitly approve it. Staff who have reported or seen offenses reported with no action will not report again. Other targets and bystanders will not report because no action was taken and/or they fear retaliation for reporting.

Leaders must commit to not tolerating these behaviors and following through on any reports received. Individuals need to feel safe in their work environment and safe to report lateral violence behaviors. First the current culture of their environment must be assessed. From this assessment, the type and amount of training needed are determined. Types of training that may be directed are communication training, diversity training, emotional intelligence training, problem resolution training, and training on identification and response to lateral violence including facility policy review. Include specific examples of lateral violence behavior in the training [18].

If the inappropriate behavior is not corrected following discussion and time for correction, discipline is warranted. Disciplinary procedures must be included in the disruptive behavior policies and must be enforced. Leaders often do not discipline the offender because they are uncomfortable with the process. Leadership training in responding to lateral violence is indicated. Writing a zero-tolerance policy for disruptive behavior is useless without an implementation plan. Include education, specific steps to report behavior, and a disciplinary policy within the implementation plan.

Reporting procedures need to be outlined in the facility policy. Report episodes of lateral violence through chain of command. Notify the appropriate law enforcement officials if the behavior includes threats of or physical assault. Including an anonymous option to report may increase reports as bystanders may fear retaliation from the offender. Every report must be investigated by the leadership. Notify the alleged offender of the reported behavior and provide an opportunity to present their side of the incident. As an example, after receiving a report that a provider made a disparaging comment about a newly graduated nurse's ability to complete their assessments in a timely manner, the leader schedules a private conversation with the provider. The leader may convey concern regarding the behavior with a statement such as, "I understand you feel the newly graduated nurses are not prepared for practice on our unit. Could you tell me more about why you feel this way?" Remain non-accusatory and non-defensive during the conversation. Should the alleged offender ask who reported the behavior, do not disclose this information.

Individuals may engage in lateral violence behaviors for several reasons. Attempt to identify the root cause of the behavior. Often, individuals who are experiencing stress lash out in frustration at those around them. Individuals who feel threatened by others may make disparaging comments about or attempt to sabotage others to make themselves appear superior. Burnout and/or depression in healthcare providers can decrease patience with others and surface as irritability, generating complaints from coworkers. Employees with symptoms of burnout or depression may benefit from mental health assessment and referral through the employee assistance program or other offerings available through the organization. Bullying may also occur when the offender has a lack of confidence in skills. Therefore, assessing the root cause of the behavior is important when creating an action plan.

Raising awareness through a transparent discussion on why the behavior is considered lateral violence may be sufficient action for an isolated event. Include within the discussion empathic communication inquiring about events that might have led to the outburst or behavior. However, if the behavior continues, in refractory cases progressive counseling and discipline may be needed. The exact progression of discipline related to the behavior is normally clearly outlined in the facility policy [18].

When working in a leadership position, investigate internal resources ahead of time and keep them readily available when the situation occurs. Resources to assist with stress or burnout as well as mental health resources are often provided through the human resources (HR) department. Leaders are often required to work with HR representatives when dealing with suspected harassment in the workplace. Investigate institutional policies outlining your role and responsibilities.

19.3   Opportunities for Future Research

There is minimal intervention research into the reasons for lateral violence. Authors have advanced theories on the root cause; however, no known studies have asked the question of the offenders. The stigma of being singled out as the offender may contribute to this lack of study.

Interventional research studying best prevention practices is needed. Current evidence has the limitations of small sample sizes resulting in a lack of generalizability. Larger, system-wide studies are needed to support the implementation of new strategies to irradicate bullying in the workplace.

Glossary

Bullying Any repeated negative behavior from a peer that is found offensive and/or intimidating and intended to demean or humiliate the target [5, 6].

Burnout A state of emotional, mental, and physical exhaustion resulting from continued excessive stress.

Cognitive rehearsal training A method to allow individuals to recognize bullying behavior, manage personal emotional reactions, and rehearse responses in a safe environment to increase confidence and skill; based in cognitive behavioral therapy [19].

Incivility Rude or unsociable behavior.

Lateral violence Any repeated negative behavior found offensive and/or intimidating by the target by a peer.

Stress A feeling of emotional tension.

Discussion Questions (With Leader Guide)

1. Discuss the reasons why bullying behaviors occur in healthcare?

   (Encourage discussion of what causes stress in healthcare providers? Do bullies know they are bullying others?)

2. Have you experienced bullying behaviors as a target? As a bystander? What was your response? How would you respond now?

   (Encourage those who wish to share to give examples. If no one volunteers, begin with a story of your own. Let participants know it is ok if they did not intervene; they know better and will in the future. Be alert for anyone who is triggered by the discussion.)

3. Have you ever displayed bullying behaviors to someone else? Why do you think you behaved that way?

   (Let participants know it is ok if they have committed these—a lot of us have. Remember going forward to monitor yourself for these behaviors.)

4. What are the key ingredients in preventing or mitigating bullying behaviors?

   (Ensure leadership commitment to eradicating bullying behaviors is vital.)

References

1. The hospital tyrants and their victims, the nurses: what doctors say of the oppression of young women in these institutions. New York Times. 22 August 1909.
2. The Joint Commission. Sentinel event alert: behaviors that undermine a culture of safety. 2008. https://www.jointcommission.org/-/media/tjc/documents/resources/patient-safety-topics/sentinel-event/sea-40-intimidating-disruptive-behaviors-final2.pdf
3. The Joint Commission. Bullying has no place in healthcare. 2016. https://www.jointcommission.org/-/media/tjc/newsletters/quick-safety-issue-24-june-2016-6-2-21-update.pdf
4. The Joint Commission. New and revised workplace violence prevention requirements. 2021. https://www.jointcommission.org/standards/prepublication-standards/new-and-revised-workplace-violence-prevention-requirements/

5. Kile D, Eaton M, deValpine M, Gilbert R. The effects of education and cognitive rehearsal in managing nurse-to-nurse incivility: a pilot study. J Nurs Manag. 2019;27:543–52.
6. Anthony MR, Brett AL. Nurse leaders as problem solvers: addressing lateral and horizontal violence. Nurs Manage. 2020;51(8):12–9. https://doi.org/10.1097/01.NUMA.0000688928.78513.86.
7. Castronovo MA, Pullizzi A, Evans S. Nurse bullying: a review and a proposed solution. Nurs Outlook. 2016;64(3):208–14. https://doi.org/10.1016/j.outlook.2015.008.
8. Shorey S, En Wong PZ. A qualitative systematic review on nurses' experiences of workplace bullying and implications for nursing practice. J Adv Nurs. 2021;2021(00):1–15. https://doi.org/10.1111/jan.14912.
9. Rutherford DE, Gillespie GL, Smith CR. Interventions against bullying of prelicensure students and nursing professionals: an integrative review. Nurs Forum. 2018;54:84–90. https://doi.org/10.1111/nuf.12301.
10. Clark CM. Combining cognitive rehearsal, simulation, and evidence-based scripting to address incivility. Nurse Educ. 2018;44(2):64–8.
11. Gosselin TK, Ireland AM. Addressing incivility and bullying in the practice environment. Semin Oncol Nurs. 2020;36:151023. https://doi.org/10.1016/j.soncn.2020.15023.
12. Hopkinson SG, Dickinson CM, Dumayas JY, Jarzombek SL, Blackman VS. A multicenter study of horizontal violence in the United States military nursing. Nurse Educ Pract. 2020;47:102838. https://doi.org/10.1016/j.nepr.2020.102838.
13. Vessey JA, Williams L. Addressing bullying and lateral violence in the workplace. J Nurs Care Qual. 2020;36(1):20–4.
14. American Psychological Association (APA). What is cognitive behavioral therapy? 2017. https://www.apa.org/ptsd-guideline/patients-and-families/cognitive-behavioral
15. Griffin M. Teaching cognitive rehearsal as a shield for lateral violence: an intervention for newly licensed nurses. J Contin Educ Nurs. 2004;35(6):257–63.
16. Alteristic Social accelerators. https://alteristic.org/story/
17. Eastern Kentucky University. What is a green dot? https://greendot.eku.edu/what-green-dot
18. Lassiter BJ, Bostain NS, Lentz C. Best practices for early bystander training on workplace intimate partner violence and workplace bullying. J Interpers Violence. 2021;36(11-12):5813–37.
19. Fehr FC, Seibel LM. Cognitive rehearsal training for upskilling undergraduate nursing students against bullying: a qualitative pilot study. QANE-AFI. 2016;2(1):article 5. https://doi.org/10.17483/2368-6669.1058.

Preventing and Addressing Moral Distress

20

Beth Epstein, Phyllis Whitehead, Dea Mahanes,
Vanessa Amos, and Ashley Hurst

Abbreviations

HCO   Healthcare organization
HCP   Healthcare provider
RVU   Relative value units

Learning Objectives
1. Explain the concept of moral community and how it applies to the experience of moral distress and well-being.
2. Apply the categories of moral distress to your own academic, clinical, or leadership experience.
3. Construct a set of actions you intend to take to address moral distress in your workplace.

Supplementary Information The online version contains supplementary material available at https://doi.org/10.1007/978-3-031-16983-0_20.

B. Epstein (✉) · V. Amos · A. Hurst
University of Virginia School of Nursing, Charlottesville, VA, USA
e-mail: meg4u@virginia.edu; vka7q@virginia.edu; arh7kz@virginia.edu

P. Whitehead
Carilion Clinic, Roanoke, VA, USA
e-mail: pbwhitehead@carilionclinic.org

D. Mahanes
University of Virginia Health, Charlottesville, VA, USA
e-mail: sdm4e@hscmail.mcc.virginia.edu

20.1   Presentation of the Science

Healthcare providers (HCPs) can certainly promote their own well-being through mindfulness practices, balancing work and family, and healthy eating and living. We contend, however, that no matter how emotionally strong or resilient a HCP is, placing her in a system that routinely demoralizes, exhausts, and confounds her will eventually overwhelms her ability to be resilient and cause psychological harm. Thus, in this chapter, we shift the focus from individual providers to organizational systems, addressing their role in preventing burnout and moral distress in HCPs.

Healthcare organizations (HCO) are communities. Those who work within them serve a common purpose of providing high quality, safe care for people. The many stakeholders in this community, although they do very different work, serve this common purpose. Pharmaceutical suppliers, high-level administrators, cafeteria staff, nurses, housekeeping staff, physicians, social workers, pharmacists, therapists such as respiratory, physical and occupational, transport staff, and laboratory technicians are all present to provide high quality, safe patient care. Importantly, HCOs are *moral* communities because achieving the common purpose requires morally relevant factors such as respecting autonomy, considering best interests, telling the truth, ensuring safety, and preventing unnecessary suffering [1]. Further, these moral issues are bound up in a complex context of high-stakes patient care decisions, teams composed of professions with different codes of ethics, high levels of regulation and monitoring, and extreme financial pressures. Because the work within an HCO is so morally complex, everyone in this moral community is obligated to commit to the central mission *and* sustain a culture that dignifies those who work and visit with the respect, recognition, and empowerment they deserve.

Many of the problems HCOs and HCPs face today—poor clinician well-being, disempowerment, burnout, risk for suicide, turnover, moral distress, dysfunctional teamwork, poor organizational leadership—can be understood using the grounding principle that HCOs are moral communities. Burnout, for example, is associated with the burdens of working in healthcare systems such as excessive documentation requirements, pressure to increase relative value units (RVU), and lack of control over one's work [2, 3]. Organizations that struggle to address these burdens or allow problems like bullying and incivility to go unaddressed put themselves at risk of staff burnout and turnover [4–7] and poor patient outcomes [8, 9]. Shanafelt and Noseworthy [10] urge HCO leaders to recognize that reducing clinician burnout is not an individual responsibility, but an organizational one.

The goal of this chapter is to focus on one factor identified as a predictor of burnout, moral distress. In this chapter, we outline for educators, students, clinicians, and administrators, ways to prepare for and recognize it, understand its impact on HCPs, and consider interventions to mitigate it.

20.1.1 Moral Distress Defined

Over the years, several definitions of moral distress have emerged [11]. In our work with morally distressed clinicians and HCO leaders, the "standard account" [12] of moral distress: *moral distress occurs when HCPs believe they know a correct ethical action to take based on their professional ethical obligations but cannot take it due to constraints that impede action* [12–14] has always fit best. The range of moral and ethical experiences HCPs encounter during their careers is broad. To identify and address them effectively, HCPs and HCO leaders need to understand what they are up against. For example, HCPs face situations in which they truly do not know which option would be best for a patient. This is an ethical dilemma, and the remedy might be to evaluate the range of options and determine which would be the better "right" actions. HCPs face situations where, if they only had a bit more information, they would be able to see realistic options more clearly. This is moral uncertainty—gathering additional information is needed. HCPs face situations in which they watch as their colleagues are treated disrespectfully by team members or patients. This is unprofessional behavior. They face situations in which patients have no resources or make "bad" decisions, families are torn apart by disagreement, or well-intended treatments go awry. If any of these situations is called moral distress, measuring moral distress, conducting rigorous research, and identifying interventions to address it become difficult because the boundaries of what moral distress is and is not so unclear. Thus, we advocate for using the narrower definition, moral distress applies when (a) the HCP believes he/she knows a professional ethical action to take, (b) the action cannot be taken due to constraints (often but not always) beyond the HCP's control, and (c) the HCP feels complicit in doing something wrong.

20.1.2 Moral Distress Among HCPs

Moral distress was first characterized in nurses in the 1980s [14]. Since then, multiple studies have identified moral distress in other healthcare professions including medicine [15–19], nurse practitioners [20–22], respiratory therapy [23], pharmacy [24], social work [25], nurse managers [26–28], and occupational therapy [29]. In short, experiencing moral distress is a widespread phenomenon among HCPs across disciplines. Further, moral distress is not confined to any healthcare setting. Although first identified in critical care [30, 31], many studies have confirmed the presence of moral distress in primary care [20], emergency departments [22], acute care, and long-term acute care [32–35]. Recognizing and (importantly) addressing moral distress, then, is an organization-wide, multi-professional objective.

20.1.3 Categories and Causes of Moral Distress

Moral distress has long been known to be associated with the organizational climate. For HCPs practicing in climates perceived to be supportive and to practice ethically, moral distress levels tend to be lower than those who perceive their practice environment to be more troubled [16, 17, 32, 36–39]. Discrete causes of moral distress have been identified and categorized as patient-level, unit/team-level, and organization-level causes [18, 40]. From several studies, patient-level causes such as nonbeneficial treatment, treatment not in a patient's best interest, prolonged dying, and unit-level causes such as poor care quality due to a lack of provider continuity or poor team collaboration are the highest ranked causes of moral distress [17, 41–44]. A leading cause of moral distress among HCPs is excessive documentation requirements that interview with patient care; a systems-level issue that applies to HCOs nationally [15, 18]. Another oft identified cause of moral distress, exacerbated by the COVID-19 pandemic, is caring for more patients than is safe; another systems level issue impacting HCOs nationally [15, 17]. Thus, the causes of moral distress may arise at the patient, unit and systems levels and require different responses. Validated tools such as the Moral Distress Scale-Revised (MDS-R) and the updated Measure of Moral Distress for Healthcare Professionals (MMD-HP) measure moral distress levels and highlight the categories (patient, unit, system). Using these tools can be helpful in implementing interventions to address the most morally distressing problems [18].

20.1.4 Links Between Moral Distress and Intention to Leave or Burnout

A link between moral distress and intention to leave is commonly reported [16–18, 38, 45–47] with between 10 and 25% of HCPs surveyed considering leaving their current position due to moral distress. A worrisome finding is that intention to leave due to burnout has been found among those new to their professions such as medical residents [15, 48]. Not surprisingly, burnout is also associated with moral distress. Long before the COVID-19 pandemic, HCPs experiencing high levels of moral distress also reported higher levels of burnout [49–52], but there is great concern about the impact of the pandemic on physician and nurse burnout [53, 54].

20.1.5 Interventions for Moral Distress

Given the prevalence of moral distress, many have recognized the need to intervene [55, 56]. However, recent reviews of interventions [57, 58] revealed most of these interventions were unit-based and focused on nurses rather than broader populations. Fortunately, interventions are generally well-received [39, 59, 60] and some show measurable differences in moral distress levels [59, 61]. The most common interventions are educational workshops and reflective practice programs [62–65] designed to address moral distress in a particular setting (e.g., intensive care) or cause of moral distress (e.g., end-of-life decision making). Because different groups within HCOs such as staff, unit leaders, and medical residency directors can recognize when and why moral distress tends to occur in their populations, targeted interventions make good sense in many situations. A different approach that applies across settings and professions, specifically moral distress consultation, has been implemented at multiple HCOs [66]. This hospital-wide intervention recognizes that morally distressing situations can occur in any healthcare setting and that more than one profession can be impacted by any particular situation. Although how moral distress consultation is carried out can vary, the basic process of identifying the sources of moral distress and working with teams to resolve the situation is foundational [39, 40]. For such a service to be successful, HCO leaders, ethics consultation service leaders, unit leaders, and others must be willing to collaborate. Further, the environment of the HCO must be one where system-related problems, for example, dealing with unprofessional behavior and dysfunctional teams, are invited to be brought forward and dealt with, not hidden away or ignored. The end goal of interventions for moral distress is to provide high quality, safe, equitable care for patients and to improve the ability of HCPs to practice ethically and at the top of their ability. HCO leaders are critical to setting the tone and environment to make that happen.

20.2 Application of Principles to HCP Well-Being

Understanding what moral distress is and how it impacts clinician well-being is the first step. To use this knowledge to improve clinician well-being is the next. Although eradicating moral distress completely is likely an impossible goal, educating and empowering HCPs in combatting moral distress are not. As described below, education and action in the academic, clinical, and leadership settings are critical to combatting moral distress's pernicious effects.

20.2.1 Application in the Academic Setting

As noted above, moral distress negatively affects the well-being of HCPs and can lead to burnout and intent to leave. Alarmingly, moral distress and burnout are on the rise in new clinicians [3], jeopardizing their well-being and the well-being of a nation dependent on them. Indeed, recent research shows that residents experience high levels of moral distress and express intent to leave their positions due to moral distress [15, 48]. Nurses are most at risk of leaving the profession in their first five years of practice and this is especially true due to the COVID-19 pandemic [67]. Many interventions are needed to address this phenomenon plaguing our newest clinicians, and education about moral distress within academic settings preparing the next generation of healthcare professionals.

Along with the technical training provided to future healthcare professionals, education about what moral distress is, what causes it, and what needs to be done to address it at the patient, unit and systems levels are needed in clinical curricula. Many academic settings have added resiliency and mindfulness-based practices into their core curricula or as electives, seeking to highlight for students the importance of well-being practices to aid them in their future careers [68]. However, it is important that these practices are taught within the context of specific situations within modern healthcare practice that might challenge their well-being. Long hours, excessive documentation requirements, complex systems, and much more require healthy practices best developed early. Some environmental stressors are inherent and inevitable in HCOs. All the same, it is unfair to expect HCPs to function well in work environments that assume that because these problems are inherent, they can be ignored or that retaliation may be used as a weapon against those who raise concerns. Students must learn that situations will arise that challenge their moral agency and integrity and may leave them feeling they did not do the right thing by their patients, themselves, or their teams. As highlighted by Epstein's and Hamric's work, the residue left by morally distressing experiences builds up over time, potentially leading to a crescendo of negative effects [69]. Encourage students to report concerning situations to you as their faculty for discussion and remediation. As the student's advocate, develop a strategy for mediating these situations with the host clinical institution.

Creating resilient future HCPs must include comprehensive instruction about:

- Moral distress—its causes, its residue, and negative downstream effects.
- The importance of the work environment on the ability to practice ethically. In the pre-licensure phase, tips and hints for recognizing healthy and unhealthy environments during job searches and interviews are useful [70].
- Advocacy skills at the patient, unit, and system level. This includes chains of command and resources for support and problem-solving.
- Systems-generated problems. The key causes of moral distress and burnout are dysfunctions of the system, not the self. Thus, a systems response is needed [10].

20.2.2 Application in the Practice Setting

Many of the health professions include, as an entry point into independent practice, a residency program. During this time, developing a deep understanding of roles within the organization, resources for support and problem-solving, and moral distress are as vital as honing technical and critical thinking skills. In their study of pediatric residents and hospitalists, Beck et al. [15] found that while only 5% of residents ($n = 288$) were currently considering leaving their position due to moral distress, more than 20% had considered it at some point. Additionally, in a secondary analysis of three datasets, 10% of residents were currently considering leaving their position [48]. Encountering moral distress occurs early so from the very beginning of one's career, acknowledgement of this phenomenon as real helps to set two expectations; (1) morally distressing problems will arise and (2) it is not a sign of weakness to feel morally distressed. HCOs that have a mechanism to address moral distress set an additional expectation—that HCOs value their HCPs and seek various ways to improve patient care.

In the clinical setting, HCPs can experience moral distress at any of the three levels: patient (e.g., inappropriate/nonbeneficial treatments), team (e.g., lack of care continuity), system (e.g., chronic understaffing and overemphasis on quality metrics and other regulations) [28, 33, 40, 44, 69, 71, 72]. Recognizing moral distress when it occurs is important, but not enough. It is important because HCPs know their concerns are legitimate and that the experience of moral distress is an indicator of their astuteness to the situation, not their weakness. It is not enough because simply talking about how distressing a situation is does not resolve it. Seeking ways to resolve what is causing distress not only helps resolve the current problem but also shows HCPs that morally distressing situations can and should be acted upon.

Examples of actions that may prevent or resolve moral distress:

- Implementing interprofessional rounds, team meetings, and routing HCP-family meetings can help resolve or prevent moral distress related to poor intra-team or team-family communication.
- Developing a unit or system-based plan for addressing aggressive patient behaviors. When exhibited by patients and families, such behavior is disturbing, but the more significant contributor to moral distress is when the organizational leadership response fails to support clinicians. In fact, experiencing a "lack of administrative action or support for a problem that is compromising patient care" was ranked fifth (of 27 distinct causes of moral distress) by physicians in one recent study [18]. When such behavior is exhibited by staff and goes unaddressed, failure to address the behavior erodes trust in the leadership and, ultimately, the moral community in which clinicians practice.
- Creating an open and honest work environment that invites HCPs to shed light on problems so they can be addressed [73].
- Preventing retaliation.
- Developing a unit-based system for recognizing and acting on morally distressing situations when they occur.

20.2.3 Application in the Leadership Setting

As exposed by the COVID-19 pandemic, many of the key areas negatively impacting HCP well-being and contributing to moral distress are organizational or systems level issues. Thus, organizations have a moral obligation to promote HCPs' well-being and address moral distress by providing resources to individuals and teams, and by building systems and processes that create a moral and ethical practice environment. HCOs have begun promoting or adopting wellness and resiliency programs for their HCPs. However, these interventions are ineffective unless coupled with concrete efforts to address the system level causes of moral distress. In fact, focusing on wellness and resiliency alone, while leaving organizational issues unaddressed, can have the unintended impact of victim-blaming and thus may contribute to burnout.

HCPs consistently identify structural challenges that decrease patient care and safety as top causes of moral distress [17, 18]. Compromised patient care due to lack of staff, uncoordinated care, and poor administrative responsiveness and resources [18] are HCO leadership level concerns and require a leadership response. Addressing these issues is certainly in the best interest of the organization as a whole. In today's healthcare environment, success depends on listening to and engaging those on the front-line in identifying problems and developing solutions. Insights from those experiencing the problems increase the likelihood that solutions will be effective and also promote HCP engagement in their implementation. Further, HCPs are more resilient and able to adapt when they are engaged in creating change. Addressing contributors to moral distress is both a moral imperative and good business. Moral distress is highly linked to turnover which ultimately compromises the quality of care delivered and increases organization costs for hiring and training. Whereas the "Triple Aim" focuses on patients through improved outcomes, patient experience, and cost of care, the "Quadruple Aim" expands to include the clinician experience [74]. Achieving the first three aims is unlikely to occur without attention to the fourth aim. Preventing and mitigating moral distress is an essential element of improving the clinician experience.

Strategies for healthcare leaders:

- "Walk the talk". Leaders' actions, even more than their words, set the tone for the HCO as a moral community.
- Be visible and open to understanding the experience of clinicians.
- Promptly address gaps in respect and professionalism by *any* team member, with attention to power differentials.
- Provide resources to address patient/family conflict that supports clinicians (examples: behavioral contracts, psychiatric liaisons).
- Ensure adequate staffing with staffing plans based on acuity and necessary staff mix.
- Develop policies, procedures, and processes that support ethical practice (examples: policies related to resuscitation, non-beneficial treatment, and decision-making).
- Provide conflict resolution resources to address communication breakdown between and within teams.
- Seek healthcare provider feedback regarding implementation of regulatory requirements and advocate for clarification or changes that align with high-quality clinical care.
- Promote early ethics consultation by any healthcare provider to address patient/family, unit, and system contributors to moral distress (can be accomplished even when a specific moral distress consultation service is not available). Ethics committees and consultation services may also serve as a support to address organizational ethics concerns.
- Provide resources for addressing moral distress when it occurs (examples: development of a moral distress consultation service, educating Employee Assistance staff on the differences between emotional and moral distress).

20.3   Opportunities for Future Research

While much is known now about the experience of moral distress among HCPs, there is still much work to be done. Collaborative work between HCPs and HCO leaders to create effective avenues for bringing problems forward and to discuss honestly the kinds of problems that keep people up at night would go far toward creating the moral community so many HCPs and leaders desire. Future studies should focus on innovative organizational interventions that reward HCPs who speak up and target moral distress at the patient, team/unit, and systems levels. Evaluation of these interventions is also an area of current and future work. Focusing on interventions aimed at alleviating the *causes* of moral distress rather than attempting to alleviate the feelings of moral distress will not only prevent moral distress but also improve patient care. At the end of the day, being able to provide high quality, safe, and equitable patient care is the goal of HCOs as moral communities. Striving toward this goal will achieve an important secondary outcome, HCP well-being.

Glossary

Burnout A syndrome of emotional exhaustion, depersonalization, and diminished personal achievement [75].

Moral community Groups of people bound together for a common moral purpose that transcends personal interests and promotes the well-being of others [76].

Moral distress A phenomenon occurring when healthcare providers are constrained from taking what they believe to be ethically appropriate actions or are forced to take actions they believe are ethically inappropriate. As a result, they feel complicit in acting unethically and are unable to fulfill important professional obligations.

Discussion Questions

1. Does the concept of moral distress resonate with you? Would you be willing to describe a situation of moral distress you have encountered?
2. As a student, what might have helped prepare you for the workplace?
3. In your current practice setting, what do you see as the most common or troubling causes of moral distress? How does your organization act on them?
4. What does moral community mean to you? What kind of environment exemplifies a moral community?
5. What do you wish your organizational leaders knew that would make your professional life more fulfilling?

Discussion Leader Guide

Many healthcare providers who participate in discussion on this topic will have encountered moral distress at some point in their career. Because the causes of moral distress tend to lie with the system, discussions can easily become "venting" or "gripe" sessions. While it is helpful to let off steam, ensuring a productive dialogue may require some redirection and focus. Suggestions for redirection include:

- Requesting a pause in conversation to identify whether a common cause for moral distress is apparent (e.g., insufficient staffing, problems with the supply chain, problems with escalation pathways). If so, direct conversation to how those present might suggest fixes for the problem (e.g., documenting near-misses in patient safety when staffing is low or documenting the impact that problems in the supply chain have on patient care). Decide as a group how you might want to act on this list of resolutions. If no common cause is present, list the causes the group has identified and help the group determine which might be the most important or easiest to address.
- Avoid doctor or nurse bashing.
- Everyone at the table has an equal voice. Enter the conversation with curiosity and an assumption of good will intended.

Questions 3–5 could yield potentially useful information and feedback for administrative leaders. Discuss with the group whether they would be willing to take the product of their conversation forward, gather additional information, or construct a response for the leadership with an offer to assist in working on resolutions to morally distressing problems.

Question 2 may yield potentially useful information for educators. Assess the interest of the group in taking ideas, suggestions, and information to educators. Two additional ideas are to identify what HCPs wish they had been taught about ethics and moral distress during training, or to write a paper outlining the group's discussion (and publish it!).

Video for Discussion - Instructional Video: The online version contains supplementary material available at https://doi.org/10.1007/978-3-031-16983-0_20

References

1. Liaschenko J, Peter E. Fostering nurses' moral agency and moral identity: the importance of moral community. Hastings Cent Rep. 2016;46:S18–21.
2. Dyrbye LN, Shanafelt TD, Sinsky CA, et al. Burnout among health care professionals: a call to explore and address this underrecognized threat to safe, high-quality care. NAM perspectives, discussion paper. Washington, DC: National Academy of Medicine; 2017. https://doi.org/10.31478/201707b.
3. National Academies of Sciences, Engineering, and Medicine, National Academy of Medicine; Committee on Systems Approaches to Improve Patient Care by Supporting Clinician Well-

Being. Taking action against clinician burnout: a systems approach to professional well-being. Washington, DC: National Academies Press; 2019. https://www.ncbi.nlm.nih.gov/books/ NBK552618/ Accessed 17 Oct 2021.

4. Quick Safety 24: Bullying has no place in health care. The Joint Commission. Updated June 2021. https://www.jointcommission.org/resources/news-and-multimedia/newsletters/newsletters/quick-safety/quick-safety-issue-24-bullying-has-no-place-in-health-care/bullying-has-no-place-in-health-care/ Accessed 11 Oct 2021.
5. Simons S. Workplace bullying experienced by massachusetts registered nurses and the relationship to intention to leave the organization. ANS Adv Nurs Sci. 2008;31:E48.
6. Swamy L, Mohr D, Blok A, et al. Impact of workplace climate on burnout among critical care nurses in the Veterans Health Administration. Am J Crit Care. 2020;29:380–9.
7. Phillips JP. Workplace violence against health care workers in the United States. N Engl J Med. 2016;374:1661–9.
8. Aiken LH, Clarke SP, Sloane DM, et al. Effects of hospital care environment on patient mortality and nurse outcomes. J Nurs Adm. 2009;39:S45–51.
9. Institute of Medicine (US) Committee on the Work Environment for Nurses and Patient Safety. Keeping patients safe: transforming the work environment of nurses. Washington, DC: National Academies Press; 2004. https://www.ncbi.nlm.nih.gov/books/NBK216190/ Accessed 11 Oct 2021.
10. Shanafelt TD, Noseworthy JH. Executive leadership and physician well-being: nine organizational strategies to promote engagement and reduce burnout. Mayo Clin Proc. 2017;92:129–46.
11. Campbell SM, Ulrich CM, Grady C. A broader understanding of moral distress. Am J Bioeth. 2016;16:2–9.
12. McCarthy J, Monteverde S. The standard account of moral distress and why we should keep it. HEC Forum. 2018;30:319–28.
13. Pauly BM, Varcoe C, Storch J. Framing the issues: moral distress in health care. HEC Forum. 2012;24:1–11.
14. Jameton A. Nursing practice: the ethical issues. Englewood Cliffs: Prentice-Hall; 1984.
15. Beck J, Randall CL, Bassett HK, et al. Moral distress in pediatric residents and pediatric hospitalists: sources and association with burnout. Acad Pediatr. 2020;20:1198–205.
16. Hamric AB, Blackhall LJ. Nurse-physician perspectives on the care of dying patients in intensive care units: collaboration, moral distress, and ethical climate. Crit Care Med. 2007;35:422–9.
17. Whitehead PB, Herbertson RK, Hamric AB, et al. Moral distress among healthcare professionals: report of an institution-wide survey. J Nurs Scholarsh. 2015;47:117–25.
18. Epstein EG, Whitehead PB, Prompahakul C, et al. Enhancing understanding of moral distress: the measure of moral distress for health care professionals. AJOB Empir Bioeth. 2019;10:113–24.
19. Dodek PM, Norena M, Ayas N, et al. Moral distress is associated with general workplace distress in intensive care unit personnel. J Crit Care. 2019;50:122–5.
20. Bourne DW, Epstein E. The experience of moral distress in an academic family medicine clinic. HEC Forum. https://doi.org/10.1007/s10730-021-09453-9. [Epub ahead of print 29 May 2021].
21. Laabs CA. Moral problems and distress among nurse practitioners in primary care. J Am Acad Nurse Pract. 2005;17:76–84.
22. Trautmann J, Epstein E, Rovnyak V, et al. Relationships among moral distress, level of practice independence, and intent to leave of nurse practitioners in emergency departments: results from a national survey. Adv Emerg Nurs J. 2015;37:134–45.
23. Schwenzer KJ, Wang L. Assessing moral distress in respiratory care practitioners. Crit Care Med. 2006;34:2967–73.
24. Sporrong SK, Hoglund AT, Hansson MG, et al. 'We are white coats whirling round'—moral distress in Swedish pharmacies. Pharm World Sci. 2005;27:223–9.
25. Fantus S, Greenberg RA, Muskat B, et al. Exploring moral distress for hospital social workers. Br J Soc Work. 2017;47:2273–90.

26. Mitton C, Peacock S, Storch J, et al. Moral distress among healthcare managers: conditions, consequences and potential responses. Healthc Policy. 2010;6:99–112.
27. Ganz FD, Wagner N, Toren O. Nurse middle manager ethical dilemmas and moral distress. Nurs Ethics. 2015;22:43–51.
28. Whitehead PB, Carter KF, Garber JS, et al. The nurse manager's experience of moral distress. J Nurs Adm. 2021;51:334–9.
29. Penny NH, Bires SJ, Bonn EA, et al. Moral distress scale for occupational therapists: Part 1. Instrument development and content validity. Am J Occup Ther. 2016;70:7004300020.
30. Wilkinson JM. Moral distress in nursing practice: experience and effect. Nurs Forum. 1987;23:16–29.
31. Corley MC. Moral distress of critical care nurses. Am J Crit Care. 1995;4:280–5.
32. Corley MC, Minick P, Elswick RK, et al. Nurse moral distress and ethical work environment. Nurs Ethics. 2005;12:381–90.
33. Henrich NJ, Dodek PM, Alden L, et al. Causes of moral distress in the intensive care unit: a qualitative study. J Crit Care. 2016;35:57–62.
34. Rice EM, Rady MY, Hamrick A, et al. Determinants of moral distress in medical and surgical nurses at an adult acute tertiary care hospital. J Nurs Manag. 2008;16:360–73.
35. Pauly B, Varcoe C, Storch J, et al. Registered nurses' perceptions of moral distress and ethical climate. Nurs Ethics. 2009;16:561–73.
36. Altaker KW, Howie-Esquivel J, Cataldo JK. Relationships among palliative care, ethical climate, empowerment, and moral distress in intensive care unit nurses. Am J Crit Care. 2018;27:295–302.
37. Asgari S, Shafipour V, Taraghi Z, et al. Relationship between moral distress and ethical climate with job satisfaction in nurses. Nurs Ethics. 2019;26:346–56.
38. Hamric AB, Borchers CT, Epstein EG. Development and testing of an instrument to measure moral distress in healthcare professionals. AJOB Prim Res. 2012;3:1–9.
39. Epstein E, Shah R, Marshall MF. Effect of a moral distress consultation service on moral distress, empowerment, and a healthy work environment. HEC Forum. 2021; https://doi.org/10.1007/s10730-021-09449-5. [Epub ahead of print 3 Apr 2021].
40. Hamric A, Epstein E, et al. A health system-wide moral distress consultation service: development and evaluation. HEC Forum. 2017;29:127–43.
41. Allen R, Judkins-Cohn T, deVelasco R, et al. Moral distress among healthcare professionals at a health system. JONAS Healthc Law Ethics Regul. 2013;15:111–8.
42. Epstein EG. End-of-life experiences of nurses and physicians in the newborn intensive care unit. J Perinatol. 2008;28:771–8.
43. Dodek PM, Wong H, Norena M, et al. Moral distress in intensive care unit professionals is associated with profession, age, and years of experience. J Crit Care. 2016;31:178–82.
44. Bruce CR, Miller SM, Zimmerman JL. A qualitative study exploring moral distress in the ICU team: the importance of unit functionality and intrateam dynamics. Crit Care Med. 2015;43:823–31.
45. Fujii T, Katayama S, Miyazaki K, et al. Translation and validation of the Japanese version of the measure of moral distress for healthcare professionals. Health Qual Life Outcomes. 2021;19:120.
46. Laurs L, Blaževičienė A, Capezuti E, et al. Moral distress and intention to leave the profession: Lithuanian nurses in municipal hospitals. J Nurs Scholarsh. 2020;52:201–9.
47. Sajjadi S, Norena M, Wong H, et al. Moral distress and burnout in internal medicine residents. Can Med Educ J. 2017;8:e36–43.
48. Hurst A, Esptein EG, Chiota-McCollum N. Moral distress among graduate medical education trainees. Abstract presented at the American Society for Bioethics and Humanities, Oct 2020.
49. Neumann JL, Mau L-W, Virani S, et al. Burnout, moral distress, work-life balance, and career satisfaction among hematopoietic cell transplantation professionals. Biol Blood Marrow Transplant. 2018;24:849–60.

50. Fumis RRL, Junqueira Amarante GA, de Fátima NA, et al. Moral distress and its contribution to the development of burnout syndrome among critical care providers. Ann Intensive Care. 2017;7:71.
51. Johnson-Coyle L, Opgenorth D, Bellows M, et al. Moral distress and burnout among cardiovascular surgery intensive care unit healthcare professionals: a prospective cross-sectional survey. Can J Crit Care Nurs. 2016;27:27–36.
52. Austin CL, Saylor R, Finley PJ. Moral distress in physicians and nurses: impact on professional quality of life and turnover. Psychol Trauma. 2017;9:399–406.
53. Physician retention and engagement survey results. Jackson Physician Search. https://www.jacksonphysiciansearch.com/physician-retention-and-engagement-survey-results/ Accessed 11 Oct 2021.
54. NSI Nursing Solutions. 2022 NSI National health care retention & RN staffing report. https://www.nsinursingsolutions.com/Documents/Library/NSI_National_Health_Care_Retention_Report.pdf. Accessed 4 March 2021.
55. Meese KA, Colón-López A, Singh JA, et al. Healthcare is a team sport: stress, resilience, and correlates of well-being among health system employees in a crisis. J Healthc Manag. 2021;66:304–22.
56. Perni S. Moral distress: a call to action. AMA J Ethics. 2017;19:533–6.
57. Dacar SL, Covell CL, Papathanassoglou E. Addressing moral distress in critical care nurses: a systemized literature review of intervention studies. CONNECT World Crit Care Nurs. 2019;13:71–89.
58. Amos V, Epstein E. Moral distress interventions: an integrative literature review. Nurs Ethics. 2022;29(3):582–607. https://doi.org/10.1177/09697330211035489.
59. Chiafery MC, Hopkins P, Norton SA, et al. Nursing ethics huddles to decrease moral distress among nurses in the intensive care unit. J Clin Ethics. 2018;29:217–26.
60. Davis M, Batcheller J. Managing moral distress in the workplace: creating a resiliency bundle. Nurse Lead. 2020;18(6):604–8. https://doi.org/10.1016/j.mnl.2020.06.007.
61. Robinson EM, Lee SM, Zollfrank A, et al. Enhancing moral agency: clinical ethics residency for nurses. Hastings Cent Rep. 2014;44:12–20.
62. Allen R, Butler E. Addressing moral distress in critical care nurses: a pilot study. Int J Crit Care Emerg Med. 2016;2(1):1–6. https://doi.org/10.23937/2474-3674/1510015.
63. Bevan NA, Emerson AM. Freirean conscientization with critical care nurses to reduce moral distress and increase perceived empowerment: a pilot study. ANS Adv Nurs Sci. 2020;43:E131–46.
64. Meziane D, Ramirez-Garcia MP, Fortin M-L. A reflective practice intervention to act on the moral distress of nurses providing end-of-life care on acute care units. Int J Palliat Nurs. 2018;24:444–51.
65. Brandon D, Ryan D, Sloane R, et al. Impact of a pediatric quality of life program on providers' moral distress. MCN Am J Matern Child Nurs. 2014;39:189–97.
66. Moral Distress Consultation Collaborative. Center for Health Humanities & Ethics. https://med.virginia.edu/biomedical-ethics/moral-distress-collaborative/ Accessed 17 Oct 2021.
67. Raso R, Fitzpatrick JJ, Masick K. Nurses' intent to leave their position and the profession during the COVID-19 pandemic. J Nurs Adm. 2021;51:488–94.
68. Dyrbye LN, Thomas MR, Eacker A, et al. Race, ethnicity, and medical student well-being in the United States. Arch Intern Med. 2007;167:2103–9.
69. Epstein EG, Hamric AB. Moral distress, moral residue, and the crescendo effect. J Clin Ethics. 2009;20:330–42.
70. Fontaine DK, Cunningham T, May N. Self-care for new and student nurses. 1st ed. Indianapolis: SIGMA Theta Tau International; 2021.
71. Davidson JE, Chechel L, Chavez J, Olff C, Rincon T. Thematic analysis of nurses' experiences with the Joint Commission's medication management titration standards. Am J Crit Care. 2021;30(5):375–84.

72. Davidon JE, Doran N, Petty A, Arellano DL, Henneman EA, Hanneman SD, et al. Survey of nurses' experiences applying the Joint Commission's medication management titration standards. Am J Crit Care. 2021;30(5):365–74.
73. Brach C. Creating psychological safety in teams: handout. Washington, DC: Agency for Healthcare Research and Quality; 2018. https://www.ahrq.gov/evidencenow/tools/psychological-safety.html. Accessed 17 Oct 2021.
74. Bodenheimer T, Sinsky C. From triple to quadruple aim: care of the patient requires care of the provider. Ann Fam Med. 2014;12:573–6.
75. Maslach C, Jackson SE, Leiter MP. Maslach burnout inventory manual. In: Zalaquett CP, Wood RJ, editors. Evaluating stress: a book of resources. 3rd ed. Lanham: Scarecrow Press; 1997. p. 191–218.
76. Volbrecht RM. Nursing ethics: communities in dialogue. 1st ed. Upper Saddle River: Pearson; 2001.

Preventing and Identifying Risky Substance Use in the Health Professions

21

Amanda Choflet

Learning Objectives
1. Analyze frameworks of risky substance and addiction in the context of the health professions.
2. Apply principles of harm reduction to risky substance use in the health professions.
3. Develop individual and institutional strategies to reduce risky substance use and promote healthy coping strategies among health professionals.

21.1 Presentation of the Science

21.1.1 Substance Use in the Health Professions

Since the publication of the landmark Surgeon General's Report ("Facing Addiction in America") in 2016, calls have been increasing to adopt a social-medical framework for managing risky substance use behaviors [1]. Rather than understanding addiction as a personality defect or moral issue, the scientific community urges clinicians and the public to adopt an understanding of substance use along a continuum of risky behaviors, where moderate and heavy use can lead to the neurobiological changes that characterize addiction [1]. Substance use in the United States is a major public health risk, with 60% of the population reporting past-month substance use and at least 8% meeting criteria for a substance use disorder [2]. It is estimated that only about 10% of the population with active substance use disorders, or addictions, actually received any kind of substance use treatment in the United States, leaving the overwhelming majority of those affected without resources or

A. Choflet (✉)
School of Nursing, Northeastern University, Boston, MA, USA
e-mail: a.choflet@northeastern.edu

support to manage their disease [1]. Not all substances are used equally; of those diagnosed with a substance use disorder, the majority of people struggle primarily with alcohol [2].

Substance use disorder is best understood as the uncontrolled use of one or more substances despite harmful consequences and, when present, places the individual at risk of immediate harm, a problem even more acutely felt when that individual is charged with caring for others in a clinical setting. Less discussed but equally as important is risky substance use, which includes any use of substances above recommended guidelines and always precedes the development of addictive behaviors. Substance use is best understood along a continuum, with no use and no harm from substances at one end and substance use disorder with harmful consequences up to and including death at the other end. Most people find themselves somewhere in the middle of the continuum, engaging in internal benefit/risk negotiations on a routine basis when choosing whether or not to use substances (Fig. 21.1). Many people may engage in increasingly harmful behaviors as substance use becomes more prevalent

Positive Physical, Social, and Mental Health	Substance Misuse	Substance Use Disorder
A state of physical, mental, and social well-being, free from substance misuse, in which an individual is able to realize his or her abilities, cope with the normal stresses of life, work productively and fruitfully, and make a contribution to his or her community.	The use of any substance in a manner, situation, amount, or frequency that can cause harm to the user and/or to those around them.	Clinically and functionally significant impairment caused by substance use, including health problems, disability, and failure to meet major responsibilities at work, school, or home; substance use disorders are measured on a continuum from mild, moderate, to severe based on a person's number of symptoms.

Substance Use Status Continuum

⟵――――――――――――――――――――――――――――――――――⟶

Substance Use Care Continuum

Enhancing Health	Primary Prevention	Early Intervention	Treatment	Recovery Support
Promoting optimum physical and mental health and well-being, free from substance misuse, through health mmunications and access to health care services, income and economic security, and workplace certainty.	Addressing individual and environmental risk factors for substance use through evidence-based programs, policies, and strategies.	Screening and detecting substance use problems at an early stage and providing brief intervention, as needed.	Intervening through medication, counseling, and other supportive services to eliminate symptoms and achieve and maintain sobriety, physical, spiritual, and mental health and maximum functional ability. Levels of care include: • Outpatient services; • Intensive Outpatient/ Partial Hospitalization Services; • Residential/ Inpatient Services; and • Medically Managed Intensive Inpatient Services.	Removing barriers and providing supports to aid the long-term recovery process. Includes a range of social, educational, legal, and other services that facilitate recovery, wellness, and improved quality of life.

Fig. 21.1 Substance use continuum. (Substance Abuse and Mental Health Services Administration (US); Office of the Surgeon General (US). Facing Addiction in America: The Surgeon General's Report on Alcohol, Drugs, and Health [Internet]. Washington (DC): US Department of Health and Human Services; 2016 Nov. Figure 4.1, Substance Use Status and Substance Use Care Continuum. Available from: https://www.ncbi.nlm.nih.gov/books/NBK424859/figure/ch4.f1/ HHS Vulnerability Disclosure)

or relied upon as a coping mechanism, resulting in the neurobiological changes that characterize the disease of addiction [1]. It is critical to remember that addiction follows a disease model of treatment and recovery, and there are also risky substance use behaviors that precede substance use dependence and addiction that may represent opportunities for intervention to prevent fulminant disease.

In the healthcare setting, much of the historical discussions around substance use in clinicians have focused on a legal or moral model with issues such as drug diversion and work impairment centered. It is believed that clinicians have similar substance use disorder rates as the general population [3], although further characterization of the problem is complicated by legal and employment risks to nurses, which likely reduces self-report [4, 5]. Alcohol and drug use among health professionals has the potential to harm individual nurses, the nursing workforce, and the provision of care to patients. Even at levels reported by the general public, it is believed that somewhere between one in five and one in seven working nurses actively uses substances in a risky way [6].

Another factor in the specific nature of risky substance use among clinicians is a cultural phenomenon that normalizes the casual overuse of substances while simultaneously vilifying clinicians who succumb to addiction [7]. Nurses, in particular, are acculturated into a professional environment that does not prepare them for the risks of substance use and focuses instead on reporting deviant or criminal behaviors rather than viewing substance use and addiction as health issues. Such a process undermines help-seeking behavior and makes it more difficult for clinicians in crisis to receive the help they need.

21.1.2 Substance Use in the Pre-licensure Setting

Several studies have been completed regarding substance use behaviors of college students, most utilizing anonymous surveys and targeting either undergraduate or graduate cohorts [8, 9]. Outcomes of these studies indicate that, for many people, substance use patterns are established early in adulthood [10]. The impact of the state-by-state legalization of marijuana and state-specific responses to the opioid crisis has complicated the understanding of substance use patterns within this vulnerable group. Regardless, there is some evidence that health sciences students may be especially vulnerable to dangerous substance use patterns during their pre-licensure academic experience [11]. Recently, researchers have noted a lack of data regarding the influence of the legalization of marijuana on substance use decision-making by college students [12], while also finding that the use of marijuana is correlated with use of illicit substances [13].

Aiming interventions at college students may be an effective strategy for understanding and preventing risky substance use in licensed nurses [3, 8]. Risky substance use decisions among college students may influence long-term substance use behaviors, and intervening at that point may be key to stopping the addiction cycle [10]. Nursing students have been shown in limited studies to display a unique set of risky substance use behaviors that require further exploration [8], such as less drug use than the general population but increased alcohol use. Additionally, increased anxiety and depressive symptomatology have been shown to correlate with increased harmful alcohol and drug use among college students in general [9, 14] and health professions students in particular [15].

21.2 Application of Principles into Wellness Practice

The good news about risky substance use and addiction is that they are preventable and treatable. Whether a clinician or student is misusing substances to treat underlying mental health issues, to create or maintain social relationships that involve risky substance use, or is facing the burden of active addiction, every phase of the risky substance use continuum is amenable to specific, individualized interventions. Promoting help-seeking behaviors, normalizing the process of openly discussing substance use and mental health concerns, and providing material resources for individuals in need are all evidence-based approaches to substance use disorders. A comprehensive strategy consisting of community-level resources designed to increase universal education around risky substance use paired with individualized risk assessment opportunities and advocacy efforts to promote help-seeking behaviors is likely to result in the most positive outcomes.

21.2.1 Pre-licensure Application in the Academic Environment

Some students will arrive at college in the throes of active addiction, while others may develop risky substance use behaviors that lead to addiction during the context of college. For students entering college during late adolescence or early adulthood, the opportunity to prevent future substance use disorders is robust. Preventing or even delaying substance use by young people will reduce their risk of developing a substance use disorder later in life [1]. While all college students are at risk of substance misuse, it is important to understand that healthcare students may be at increased risk of substance use issues and design interventions specifically designed to reach them.

   While developing resources for clinically focused students, remember that while they may be at increased risk of substance issues, they also carry many of the same issues and concerns as their non-clinical counterparts. It is important to strike a balance between clinically specific resources that also tie in academic-based programs that are already available through the larger university. Faculty engaged in wellness initiatives may also consider creating long-term bridge programs for new graduates and alumni to ensure support as students transition from the pre-licensure to the professional work environment. Bridge programs can provide ongoing social outlets and emotional support for students as they enter professional practice. For students with pre-existing substance use disorders, it is vital that a transition plan is put into place as they move into professional practice. It is also critical that faculty behaviors, attitudes, and knowledge are addressed as part of the overall intervention plan. Just like every other aspect of teaching, faculty members must hold themselves accountable to the same standards they are instilling in the students.

21.2.1.1 Community-Level Interventions

One of the most substantial transitions a school can make is to reduce the stigma associated with help-seeking for risky substance use. Programs specifically designed to decrease stigma associated with substance use disorders have been shown to be effective at improving therapeutic attitudes among pre-licensure students [16]. Pair a strategy of community-level education, screening, and training with access to individualized self-assessment tools and treatment opportunities for students. Student leaders have an opportunity to set the tone for socialization opportunities that do not rely on alcohol or drugs and embracing healthy coping strategies [17]. Most importantly, these interventions can lead to reduced stigma and increased awareness of a range of risky substance use behaviors, which can increase help-seeking among pre-licensure students.

21.2.1.2 Universal Education

Many colleges and universities are actively engaged in substance use education for all new students, though the impact of this education is not always well understood in terms of decreasing actual substance use. One promising approach is the use of consistent and routine education addressing the substance use continuum by building information into the curricula of future health professionals. Ideally this eduction would include at least one teaching opportunity per semester. Universal education can take the form of substance-focused simulated patients, modules regarding clinician risk for substance use issues, guest speakers, and readings to increase overall understanding of risky substance use and addiction among health professionals. Students must understand that they are at risk of substance use disorders, just like anyone else.

21.2.1.3 Faculty Education

Universal education must be provided by faculty who embrace both the continuum model of risky substance use and the disease model of addiction; therefore, faculty training is also required in order to effectively deliver universal education regarding risky substance use. Faculty education can involve formal training programs such as in-services and third-party consultation, or a series of discussions and readings shared by faculty in an effort to promote self-education. The Surgeon General's report on addiction is an excellent place to start a discussion among faculty regarding substance use risk and addiction (Fig. 21.1).

21.2.1.4 Individual-Level Interventions

Periodic and routine risk screening can be incorporated into the pre-licensure academic environment as an adjunct to community-level interventions. Many universities have already adopted measures that allow for confidential self-assessments for substance use and for alcohol in particular. One such example is the "eCheckUpToGo" program at San Diego State University, in which students follow substance-specific modules to receive personalized screening and risk-based interventions with referrals for those who need it [18]. The best risk screening programs will link participants directly to referral resources such as counseling, crisis intervention, and even inpatient treatment options. Most academic settings offer counseling and psychological support services as part of the package of student services. Offering these services onsite and with flexible scheduling will reduce barriers as much as possible and increase the uptake and effectiveness of the programs. For students with chemical dependency issues, medication-assisted treatment may be indicated. Access to care may be enhanced by having these services available on campus or through campus-based resources or by becoming a collegiate recovery program [19].

21.2.2 Clinical Application Post-licensure

Once an individual crosses into the licensed phase of their clinical career, help-seeking for risky substance use can become more complicated. This is partly due to variability in regulatory response to clinician substance use issues, the overwhelming stigma involved with accessing substance use resources, and a failure to recognize a worsening substance use issue on the part of the individual. Similar to the strategy for pre-licensure clinicians, a multi-faceted approach that combines community-level interventions with individualized resources will result in the most effective outcomes.

21.2.2.1 Community-Level Interventions

At the hospital or organizational setting, shifting the culture of risky substance use will likely require an ongoing and proactive effort. Many clinicians are simply unaware of substance use recommendations and do not routinely apply the same level of scrutiny to their own lives that they apply to patient assessments. Organizations would benefit from adopting an ongoing substance use education process that incorporates a scientific understanding of pre-addictive and addictive behaviors. This education can take the form of annual training modules, bringing in speakers for in-service training, posting educational materials on organizational units or as screensavers on computers, and hosting a journal club that incorporates substance-associated discussions. Most importantly, clinicians need to build an understanding of themselves as vulnerable to risky substance use and subsequent addiction so that they can participate in ongoing self-assessment of their own behaviors.

Many clinical organizations use alcohol as a social outlet, offering "happy hours," openly discussing or joking about using substances as coping mechanisms, and ignoring "red flag" language about the consequences of substance misuse, such as discussions in the break room about being hungover or telling positive stories about drunkenness or "partying." While being careful not to squash open discussion or becoming judgmental of social activities, consider offering substance-free or at least substance-neutral social outlets and bonding opportunities. Moving social activities out of a substance-dependent setting sends a strong message about positive coping skills and helps to build a culture of empathy and resilience. One way to ensure inclusivity is by asking yourself whether a given social opportunity would be safe for colleagues in recovery from a substance use addiction; if the answer is no, reconsider the components of the situation that are unsafe.

21.2.2.2 Individual-Level Interventions

While many individuals will respond positively to increased education about risky substance use and self-limit their intake based on new information, some will require additional support in order to understand their risk and change their behaviors. For this reason, it is imperative that community-level interventions are paired with individualized screening and assessment opportunities as well. Consider offering routine, proactive, confidential risk screening regarding substance use to all clinicians within the healthcare organization. The Healer Education Assessment and Referral Program (HEAR) at the University of California San Diego is an excellent example of individualized risk screening for clinicians with immediate access to individualized, professional resources based on the needs of the participants. The benefit to this program is that the healthcare professional can access services through encryption and not be identified by anyone in the workplace. This overcomes the risk of loss of license or employment while seeking treatment [20]. The employee assistance program can also be used as referral sources for employees who require additional support.

21.2.2.3 Community Engagement Beyond the Hospital

Because of stigma and the fear of disciplinary action, many clinicians will never feel comfortable disclosing their risky substance use behaviors or addiction to a work-based program, even one that promises confidentiality. For this reason, develop a list of community-based resources for clinicians based outside of an employment relationship. An independent peer support program, such as the Nurses Peer Support Network in Minnesota (https://www.npsnetwork-mn.org/), has shown effectiveness in providing a platform for peer support to help clinicians with addiction maintain sobriety and find specific support for healthcare professionals. Some mental health providers have even offered their services free of charge for healthcare workers through a program called the Emotional PPE Project (https://emotionalppe.org/).

21.2.3 Leadership Application

Organizational leaders have a profound effect on the culture and practices of a workplace. Proactive leadership training focused on best practices for managing substance use issues can make a difference in establishing a positive work environment for those in active recovery as well as those who are working with unrecognized risky substance use [21]. Once a leadership team has established a thoughtful and consistent approach to addressing substance use among staff members, consider additional interventions as described below.

21.2.3.1 Community-Level Interventions

At the hospital or organizational level, clinical leaders can make a significant impact by destigmatizing help-seeking behaviors among health professionals. As leaders, feel empowered to openly discuss the risks of substance use among health professionals and emphasize the resources that are available both within the employment environment and outside of it. Many clinicians are ashamed of talking about their risky substance use except to attempt to normalize it as a necessary coping mechanism for the grueling work of patient care. It is important to remember that most of the clinicians working with a substance use disorder are "flying under the radar" and not receiving help for their addiction. Leaders can set a tone of empathy, humility, and resourcefulness among the clinical team in engaging substance use help when it is needed.

When an organization has committed to universal substance use education and the clinical teams maintain a level of understanding of the disease model of substance use, it is much easier to welcome back colleagues who have received treatment for addiction. Another method to reduce the stigma associated with help-seeking behaviors for substance use addiction is to consistently and lovingly provide a pathway to return to work and thrive in the clinical setting. Leaders set the tone in this area, by supporting clinicians with restricted practice requirements, educating and supporting staff who will be working with the returning employee, and setting up ongoing access to support services for the employee. Treat addiction just like any other chronic disease, where employees can often return to the clinical environment with certain safeguards put into place to ensure their success and safety. Treat disciplinary actions related to substance use issues with much care. Actively encourage those who are willing to pursue substance use treatment to benefit from ongoing support and access to available resources. Researchers have found that, at least for some, disciplinary action related to substance use may place an individual at increased risk of harm, including suicide [22].

21.2.3.2 Policy and Advocacy

The issue of risky substance use and addiction in the healthcare environment is complex. Many organizations have adopted an approach to substance use that centers issues like medication diversion and the risks associated with working while intoxicated, responding from a disciplinary or law enforcement rather than sociomedical perspective when issues arise. While these are indeed serious problems, they are much less common than risky substance use and addiction that occur completely outside of the work environment. In fact, diversion and working while intoxicated represent end-stage or fulminant addiction and a continued focus on that end of the continuum ignores the far more common and insidious issue of risky substance use. Leaders are encouraged to advocate for the use of a disease-based approach to substance use disorders rather than a law enforcement approach in the professional environment, understanding that addiction is more like diabetes (medical) than murder (criminal). To the extent that clinical leaders are able to influence hospital or organizational policy, advocate for HR policies that prioritize medical referrals, alternative to discipline programs, and pathways to return to work within the frameworks provided by the state licensing boards. From a broader policy perspective, advocacy at the state and national level regarding these policies is desperately needed. Clinical leaders are encouraged to volunteer to serve on substance use-oriented committees for your state licensing boards, hospitals, and professional organizations.

21.3   Opportunities for Future Research

Research regarding substance use in the health professions is desperately needed, from prevalence studies to help characterize risky substance use among clinicians to treatment efficacy studies to document best practices in long-term substance use treatment for this at-risk population. Some of the biggest barriers to completing this research are the stigma associated with reporting substance use issues as well as barriers to help-seeking behaviors that run rampant in the clinical environment. Given the opportunity, some of the research questions that should be addressed include:

- When do substance use problems begin for health professionals and is the trajectory different than the general population?
- Is there something unique about the specific education health professionals receive about substances, including the presumed safety of narcotic and other mind-altering substances, that leads to dangerous attitudes towards substance use?
- How prevalent is risky substance use (across the spectrum) in the health professions?
- What interventions are effective in preventing the progression of risky substance use to addiction in the health professions?
- What role can health providing institutions play in reducing risky substance use? What resources are currently being used and how can they be used more effectively?
- What are the best ways to treat addiction among health professionals?
- What are the ideal relationships between regulatory bodies, healthcare institutions, addictions treatment providers, and individuals in need?

Glossary

Risky substance use Any use of substances above recommended guidelines.
Substance use disorder The uncontrolled use of one or more substances despite harmful consequences which places the individual at risk of immediate harm.

Discussion Questions

- What kind of information did you receive about substance use risk for yourself and other health providers in school or in your professional environment?
- Have you witnessed concerning substance use behaviors by peers or even in yourself?
- What messages have you received about drinking from your peers in the health professions?
- What kinds of resources are you aware of to help clinicians who have substance use problems?
- Do you have an impression of how your work environment would respond to a person with a substance use problem? What do you think would happen? Would your organization's response empower you to reach out for help if you needed it or would it encourage you to remain silent?

Discussion Leader Guide

- *What kind of information did you receive about substance use risk for yourself and other health providers in school or in your professional environment?*
  Many participants will report little to no education regarding substance use risk, especially as it relates to the health professions in particular. Encourage the group to talk through why this might be and how education might be applied or adapted in the future. It is never too early or too late to provide information about risky substance use behaviors and addiction.
- *Have you witnessed concerning substance use behaviors by peers or even in yourself?*
  Participants will be more likely to report concerning behaviors by peers than by themselves. Respond in a non-judgmental manner and hold others accountable to that approach as well. Ask the participants how they've responded to their peers in the past: did they remain silent, did they have a conversation with their friend, did they stop spending time with their friend, did they join in? How would they respond in the future? What would a conversation based in empathy and concern look like?
- *What messages have you received about drinking from your peers in the health professions?*
  Given the prevalence of casual reference to alcohol overuse in particular, participants may note a social tendency among health professionals to use substances as coping mechanisms, norming risky behaviors. Follow the conversation wherever it leads and, if there is variability among the participants in terms of messaging, call out any examples of best practices around substance use messaging. Use this part of the discussion as an opportunity to highlight positive environments or role-play/talk through alternative responses to unhealthy social norms.

- *What kinds of resources are you aware of to help clinicians who have substance use problems?*

  Hopefully, participants will name at least 1–2 resources they are aware of, though you may hear crickets in response to this question. Come prepared with a list of both organizationally based and community-based resources to share with the group. If participants are able to name specific resources, use this as a brainstorming session and record the ideas for future distribution to the group.

- *Do you have an impression of how your work environment would respond to a person with a substance use problem? What do you think would happen? Would your organization's response empower you to reach out for help if you needed it or would it encourage you to remain silent?*

  Hopefully, by the time you get to this question, participants will feel enough trust among the group to openly share their feelings about perceived organizational responses to substance use issues. Some may have witnessed a colleague go through a disciplinary process and share their experiences in that role. Others may have strong feelings that follow a moralistic framework. If the conversation veers towards moralism, re-orient the participants by focusing on the disease model of addiction and continuum model of risky substance use. Remind participants of their shared vulnerability to risky behaviors and utilize a humble and empathetic approach to guide the discussion.

References

1. U.S. Department of Health and Human Services (HHS). Office of the Surgeon General, Facing Addiction in America: The Surgeon General's report on alcohol, drugs, and health. Washington, DC: HHS; November 2016.
2. Substance Abuse and Mental Health Services Administration (SAMHSA). Key substance use and mental health indicators in the United States: Results from the 2018 National Survey on Drug Use and Health (HHS Publication No. PEP19-5068, NSDUH Series H-54). Rockville: Center for Behavioral Health Statistics and Quality, Substance Abuse and Mental Health Services Administration; 2019. https://www.samhsa.gov/data/
3. Worley J. Nurses with substance use disorders: where we are and what needs to be done. J Psychosoc Nurs Ment Health Serv. 2017;55(12):11–4. https://doi.org/10.3928/02793695-20171113-02.
4. Foli KJ, Reddick B, Zhang L, Krcelich K. Substance use in registered nurses: "I Heard About a Nurse Who …". J Am Psychiatr Nurses Assoc. 2020;26(1):65–76. https://doi.org/10.1177/1078390319886369. Epub 2019 Nov 21
5. Monroe TB, Kenaga H, Dietrich MS, Carter MA, Cowan RL. The prevalence of employed nurses identified or enrolled in substance use monitoring programs. Nurs Res. 2013;62(1):10–5. https://doi.org/10.1097/NNR.0b013e31826ba3ca.
6. Starr KT. The sneaky prevalence of substance abuse in nursing. Nursing. 2015;45(3):16–7. https://doi.org/10.1097/01.NURSE.0000460727.34118.6a.
7. Ross CA, Jakubec SL, Berry NS, Smye V. "A two glass of wine shift": dominant discourses and the social organization of nurses' substance use. Glob Qual Nurs Res. 2018;5:2333393618810655. https://doi.org/10.1177/2333393618810655.

8. Boulton M, O'Connell K. Past year substance use by student nurses. J Addict Nurs. 2017;28(4):179–87.
9. Skidmore C, Kaufman E, Crowell S. Substance use among college students. Child Adolesc Psychiatr Clin N Am. 2016;25(2016):735–53.
10. Jang J, Schulerb M, Evans-Polcec R, Patrick M. College attendance type and subsequent alcohol and marijuana use in the U.S. Drug Alcohol Depend. 2019;204:107580.
11. Ayala EE, Roseman D, Winseman JS, Mason HRC. Prevalence, perceptions, and consequences of substance use in medical students. Med Educ Online. 2017;22(1):1392824. https://doi.org/10.1080/10872981.2017.1392824.
12. Alley Z, Kerra D, Bae H. Trends in college students' alcohol, nicotine, prescription opioid and other drug use after recreational marijuana legalization: 2008–2018. Addict Behav. 2020;102(2020):106212.
13. Kollath-Cattanoa C, Hattebergb S, Kooper A. Illicit drug use among college students: The role of social norms and risk perceptions. Addict Behav. 2020;105(2020):106289.
14. Paulus D, Zvolensky M. The prevalence and impact of elevated anxiety sensitivity among hazardous drinking college students. Drug Alcohol Depend. 2020;209(2020):107922.
15. Sainz M, Nagy G, Mohedano G, Véleza N, García S, Cisneros D, Rey G. The association between substance use and depressive symptomatology in nursing university students in Mexico. Nurse Educ Pract. 2019;36(2019):114–20.
16. Dion K, Griggs S. Teaching those who care how to care for a person with substance use disorder. Nurse Educ. 2020;45(6):321–5. https://doi.org/10.1097/NNE.0000000000000808.
17. Balthazar EB, Gaino LV, Almeida LY, Oliveira JL, Souza J. Risk factors for substance use: perception of student leaders [Article in English, Portuguese]. Rev Bras Enferm. 2018;71(Suppl 5):2116–22. https://doi.org/10.1590/0034-7167-2017-0587.
18. Counseling & Psychological Services, San Diego State University. eCheckUpToGo. 2021. http://www.echeckuptogo.com/ Accessed 27 Sept 2021.
19. Association of Recovery in Higher Education. Standards and Recommendations. 2021. https://collegiaterecovery.org/standards-recommendations/ Accessed 27 Sept 2021.
20. Martinez S, Tal I, Norcross W, Newton IG, Downs N, Seay K, McGuire T, Kirby B, Chidley B, Tiamson-Kassab M, Lee D, Hadley A, Doran N, Jong P, Lee K, Moutier C, Norman M, Zisook S. Alcohol use in an academic medical school environment: A UC San Diego Healer Education Assessment and Referral (HEAR) Report. Ann Clin Psychiatry. 2016;28(2):85–94.
21. O'Neill C, Schroeder S. Supervisor training makes a difference with a tough issue. Nurse Lead. 2014;12(2):67–9. https://doi.org/10.1016/j.mnl.2013.12.006.
22. Davidson J, Ye G, Parra M, Choflet A, Lee K, Barnes A, Zisook S. Job-related problems prior to nurse suicide 2003-2017: A longitudinal mixed methods analysis. J Nurs Regul. 2021;12(1):28–39. https://doi.org/10.1016/S2155-8256(21)00017-X.

Substance Use Disorder: From Moral Failure to Disease Management

22

Cadie Ayers, Marie Manthey, and Amanda Choflet

Learning Objectives
1. Participants will explain the impact the myth has on the capacity of individuals to effectively engage in treatment.
2. Healthcare workers will apply appropriate skills to create a culture of openness regarding substance use disorder.
3. Participants will be able to define and describe the MYTH of substance use disorder as a moral failure rather than a treatable disease.

22.1 Introduction

The question of whether addiction is caused by choice or a brain disease is one of lingering debates. On the one hand, thinking about addictive behaviors from the framework of choice offers a potential post-addiction freedom to the individual suffering from addiction. On the other hand, the framing of addiction as choice frequently leads those unafflicted to a question of morality rife with judgment. One may ask, "How could one who seemingly has it all, throw it all away for drugs and or alcohol or?" Most of society believes that professionals with substance

Supplementary Information The online version contains supplementary material available at https://doi.org/10.1007/978-3-031-16983-0_22.

C. Ayers (✉)
Department of Veterans Affairs, FRESNO, CA, USA

M. Manthey
Creative Health Care Management, Minneapolis, MN, USA

A. Choflet
School of Nursing, San Diego State University, San Diego, CA, USA

309

J. E. Davidson, M. Richardson (eds.), *Workplace Wellness: From Resiliency to Suicide Prevention and Grief Management*, https://doi.org/10.1007/978-3-031-16983-0_22

addictions are weak and morally inferior [1]. Many remain staunchly supportive of the theory that addiction is a moral failure by the individual [2]. While there has been widespread education to guide patient care explaining the genetic, physiologic, social, and environmental root causes of addiction, when it comes to understanding the problem within our own professions too many continue to support views that stigmatize those with substance use disorders (SUD).

An alternative perspective has been offered by addiction specialists framing addictive behaviors as a result of changes within the human brain that occur over time. These changes become permanent with repeated exposures to the substances in question. Patterns of addictive behaviors that follow family genealogies add weight to this theory. The question is then obvious; how can an individual who is predisposed to addictive behaviors be blamed for succumbing to their genetic recipe?

While it is important to note that the majority of health professionals who exhibit risky substance use behaviors do not have addiction, those who are suffering from addiction require support. Addiction has been defined as a medical disorder that causes deep alterations within the brain after repeated exposure [2]. These alterations affect the reward processing system, thus disrupting self-regulation and mood [2]. The well-being of the individual is ultimately disturbed creating catastrophic effects on the individual's life [2]. One key feature of addiction is denial, where the individual suffering from addiction may be (and usually is) unable to accept the reality of their addictive behaviors or the consequences of those behaviors. Because of this component of addiction, it can be very challenging to encourage an addicted person to reach out for help on their own. Workplace wellness strategies that include supporting a colleague into treatment are necessary [3]. However, these efforts are thwarted by structural issues within health systems and the profession as described below.

22.2   Treatment of Substance Use Disorder Among Health Professionals

Though this book is written for all healthcare professionals, the issue of inequitable treatment of professionals with substance use disorder is pronounced among nurses. The context of the social contract between nurses and the public complicates the situation. According to the nursing scope and standards of practice [4] and Code of Ethics [4], nurses can be held accountable for actions and behaviors outside the workplace. An example of this is when a nurse's license is revoked or suspended for being found impaired driving under the influence of substances on a day off from work. When a nurse is found to have a substance use issue, it has been historically viewed that they have broken the social contract and can no longer serve with integrity in the profession [4].

The treatment of healthcare professionals (HCPs) with substance use disorder varies from profession to profession and state to state. Because physicians are often independent contractors to the organization and/or due to the revenue-producing nature of their employment, they are generally able to work and retain their position while receiving treatment. The actions against a physician's license for issues such as driving under the influence are often more lenient than a nurse. For instance, after reviewing Performance Measure 4: Formal Discipline on the department of consumer affairs website, https://www.dca.ca.gov/publications/2021_annrpt.pdf, authors have found discrepancies between how nurses vs. physicians are regulated including cost of licensure, fines, and citations. Nursing seems to receive a disproportionate burden while regaining sobriety. Given this history, nurses may feel the need to go underground and hide their disease to prevent loss of employment or loss of license [4]. The involvement of legal, licensure, social, and financial consequences because of addiction leads to devastating outcomes including depression and suicide [4].

However, moving past the disparity among nurses, all licensed healthcare professionals (pharmacists, physicians, and nurses) suffer in many states from the impact of mandatory reporting of mental health problems (including substance use disorder) with licensing and accreditation. The requirement of questions regarding treatment for mental health concerns on licensure and accreditation was once created with the good intention of protecting the public but is now known to thwart health-seeking behaviors. Those with mental health problems who are untreated may self-treat with drugs and alcohol [1]. The American Medical Association has taken action to encourage dismantling these outdated processes to reduce harm, stigma, and improve access to care (https://www.ama-assn.org/print/pdf/node/77416).

Best practices in SUD treatment among health professionals have produced improved results to both the individual and the public. The state of Colorado has taken an all-professions approach to case management for health professionals referred for treatment of substance use disorder. In this state, peer support is required to help nurses, physicians, and other allied health providers navigate their recovery from substance use disorder, even including access to integrated mental health support and evidence-based best recovery practices.

Such a program operates in stark contrast to the situation described by Diane Kunyk (2015) who found that Canada's punishment-centered approach focused on punishment rather than recovery [2]. Similarly, in the United States, many organizations take a very conservative approach to managing the addicted health professional, often firing medical professionals when identified with substance use disorder or diversion of medications.

22.3 Alternative to Discipline Programs

"Alternative to discipline" is a term used to describe a non-punitive approach to treatment for substance use disorder. Many state boards of nursing in the United States state that they are "alternative to discipline" in their approach to substance use disorder amongst nurses. However, the definition of "alternative to discipline" is often limited to not reporting the nurse for criminal activity. The nurse's employment or license may be suspended while in mandatory treatment in a program selected by the board of nursing and paid for at the nurse's expense [2]. At the time of this writing, there are no standards between or within professions on the way that alternative to discipline programs is structured or monitored. There are no standard metrics for measuring success of these programs. Return to work following treatment and monitoring is not included as a national standard workforce metric. There are public-facing datasets of those convicted of felonies related to substance use, but no public-facing data of successes of treatment and exemplary treatment programs. The situation is ripe for future research and quality improvement strategies at the local, state, and national levels.

22.4 The Stigma of Substance Use Disorder Among Health Professionals

Recognizing addiction as a treatable, chronic disease instead of labeling it as a moral failure is imperative, not just for the average patient, but to those who work in healthcare [2, 5]. Education is readily available to support this concept, but our standards have yet to change amongst those who carry a license. It is time to look within the healthcare community to how we treat each other and use the same health-directed principles used for patients within and among ourselves.

22.5 Learning Through Example: A Testimony and Exemplar

In the remaining portion of this chapter, we present an interview with Marie Manthey (h)PhD RN, designated Living Legend in the American Academy of Nursing, because of her contributions to the profession, and expertise in the support of those with substance use disorder.

Myth: *Addiction is a moral failure.*
Truth: *Addiction is a brain disease*

Manthey: The simple answer to what is moral failure is that moral failure is an act or thought that is carried out when one knows that one should not carry it out. Not carry it out, or the converse, an act or thought that is not carried out when it should be. Personally, I believe that our confusion comes from the fact that when a person is in the throes of addiction, one loses one's access to one's own moral values. I know that I did. I've heard people talk about it in meetings for years. People who cracked up cars because they were driving while drunk, people will do all kinds of things that were against their own morality that they thought they would never do. As a sponsor of women in recovery, sometimes there is an issue about restitution, for example, if someone stole money or stole something of value. We need to be prepared to risk or refund that item or give back in whatever way we possibly can. Like I said, it's not that we don't have morals, it's that we lose the capacity, the brain power, the willpower to live according to our values, because there's nothing more important than getting the next fix, the next drink. In terms of moral failure and nursing, there has been an issue with this idea, and I think it stems between nurses and the public that places us in a position of trust. And when we violate that trust, the public considers that a moral failure.

The definition of chronic disease is that it is a disease, like diabetes, that lasts for a long time or for the rest of your life.

22.5.1 Denial is Common and Complex

Manthey: *To be perfectly honest, it really started with my own experience in becoming an addicted alcoholic. It wasn't part of my game plan. My goal was always to be a very good nurse with a lot of focus on nurse–patient relationships. Unfortunately, in the middle of my career I found myself fired from one of the most prestigious hospitals in the world, where I had been holding a high-level position within the executive staff. My alcoholism had become a terrible problem, and it was insisted by my employers that I enter treatment. I did, but in the end, that is what caused them to terminate my position. Fortunately, I was able to get into a strong recovery program; I spent the next 30–40 years in recovery.*

It was from this position I entered treatment at their insistence. I was told that if I completed full inpatient treatment, I could save my job.

Myth: *Nurses who use substances are impaired, and it will be obvious that they are in trouble.*
Truth: *Substance use often affects the "best and brightest"*

Interviewer: *I understand that you created the concept of Primary Nursing and were in a very high-level position at the time of your intervention at Yale. Is that right?*
Manthey: *Yes, 10 years earlier I oversaw a project that resulted in the development of primary nursing which brought about a change in the organizational dynamics of the nursing care unit. Eventually the idea spread organically throughout the United States as well as other countries. Those 10 years, from the inception of primary nursing until the time I was fired from my position, were years of enormous growth and opportunity. I was speaking all over the world on Primary Nursing. But I was also holding down two different high-level positions. One as Head of Clinical services at United Hospital in St. Paul, Minnesota, and the other for Yale in New Haven, Connecticut. At Yale, I had the responsibility for all clinical departments, including pharmacy, respiratory therapy, any department where practitioners gave direct care to patients, they came under my administrative oversight.*
Interviewer: *You hold the title of "Living Legend" in the American Academy of Nurses. Can you tell us about what that means and why you received this distinguished title?*
Manthey: *The American Academy of Nurses hands out the title of Living Legend to nurses who have made a significant contribution to the profession of nursing. It was a big honor; it was a huge honor. The fact that they were recognizing the impact*

of primary nursing on a nursing level, but that it really spearheaded a lot of growth and development, at the leadership level, throughout hospitals, and academia. It opened the door to look at a lot of old paradigms, and view nursing in new and different ways.

22.5.2 Nobody Suffers More than the Addicted Person

I had to quickly find some safe and good care for my two children who were 6 and 11, in New Haven, which I was still not quite familiar with, and find a treatment program. Everything came together and I had a good recovery program/process; nevertheless, about three or four weeks into the program, my employer came and told me that I was not going to come back to a job. I received 3 months' severance pay. I did not have savings, and now I also did not have a job, and I was scared to death that I was going to be "struck drunk" again because I didn't understand what was happening to me. I didn't understand how I had gotten to the point where I could not go a day without drinking.

Myth: *It's not normal to need substance use support long after they begin the recovery process.*
Truth: *Recovery is lifelong.*

The importance of this award as it relates to substance use disorder is that I spent almost 40 years in recovery by the time I received this honor. I had told everybody in my career world, my clients, my employees, about my alcoholism and my recovery. I knew I couldn't keep it a secret and stay sober. Early on in recovery I knew that relapse would likely occur if I did. I found that telling people about my experience often opened the door for a much more intimate conversation. I got to know my clients, either with their family or their nursing experience. My sobriety was not a secret, but I had never spoken about it publicly.

22.5.3 Advocacy is Essential

While in my recovery process, I was getting hints about the size of the problem within the nursing profession. Eventually, I became aware of the scope of the problem of substance use disorder within nursing. I have become very passionate about doing everything I can to help generate a new paradigm through which we can begin to understand that this is not a moral failure, it is a chronic disease.

The reason I'm talking about it now is that it shouldn't have been such a big deal, right? I had people coming up to me afterward who said, "Thank you so much for speaking about recovery," and, "I've been in AA for 18 years and I am the Dean of Nursing, and nobody knows that I am in recovery." The secrecy part of the disease, as we see it in the nursing profession, is a serious problem. There needs to be a major change in the paradigm of our understanding of this disease. The fact that it's still viewed as a moral failure is our problem to solve because it contributes to the conspiracy of silence, which results in secrecy, stigma, and shame.

22.5.4 Peer Support Programs Can Help

Interviewer: Please tell us about the Peer Support program in Minnesota and how it came about? How is it different from others?

Manthey: I was in my 35th or 36th year of recovery when I began to have an awareness to the depth of the problem of nurses in recovery versus being able to have the support and care that they needed, to resume their career once they were in recovery.

I really want you to understand that for 35–36 years I was deeply involved in my recovery. I went to five international recovery meetings that were held once every five years, I had a sponsor, I attended my home group regularly, and I also sponsored various individuals. On the other side, I was deeply involved with the growth of my professional career. I spoke frequently within the nursing community and at conferences, I worked with Creative Healthcare Management, and had written several articles. Both recovery and nursing are deep passions of mine that existed completely inside of my being but didn't connect at all.

The Texas peer support group is where I began to see what really happened within the profession. I was able to hear what the support group was doing and why they were doing it. After hearing their compelling stories, I took my place as the keynote speaker and said, for the first time among the nursing community, "My name is Marie, and I am an alcoholic." With over 35 years of experience, it was the first time I had said those words in that kind of setting. I see myself as a different kind of a being after going through recovery. I'm so grateful for it, but the two did not intertwine until that day in Texas. It was a total transformation; a wall came down that had created a barrier between those two worlds.

An individual who had started a similar group for physicians, dentists, pharmacists, and other licensed health professionals that didn't include nurses said, "I'm telling you, you need to get this going in nursing, you're the one that needs to do it!" The group could not be started by the Board of Nursing, there had to be trust between the nurse and those within the group. The first thing we did was to try and understand what was going on within the nursing community. I invited all those who were currently in recovery and who were also nurses, to an informative meeting at my house, and my living room ended up packed. We performed a check-in with everyone to see how their recovery was going. Halfway through the room, I was crying. My heart was broken hearing from individuals who had never said these things to a group of nurses, their own peers, before. Individuals who, for years, were applying for jobs, and were in complete recovery with a fully restored license. Because these individuals would admit that they were in recovery, they remained jobless. The stigma was real, and I could see it. The experiences individuals were *having with the board, the monitoring program, while nobody was trying to be mean to them, they still were awkward experiences that felt uncaring and difficult.*

Interviewer: *What barriers did you have to overcome to establish the Peer Support program?*

Manthey: *There was no question in my mind after that group, and I was completely charged up. I ended up getting a good committee of nurses together and we spent about a year studying lots of different ways of approaching the development of this group for licensed nurses. We reached out to recovery groups that existed here in the recovery community of Minnesota. Eventually, we ended up with the non-profit organization that we have now called The Nursing Peer Support Network. The name of the organization was chosen very carefully; it is about nursing, the health professionals. Most importantly, it is about peer support, which is a very special definition of a form of healing. A lot of things are called "peer support" that really aren't peer support. For this organization, the definition of peer support needs to be understood. We were not an association or a corporation, we were a network, a place where people could connect; and that was how we ended up doing our bylaws, developing our articles of incorporation, and creating the committees that we felt were needed to activate this kind of work.*

On average Minnesota currently has 13,000 nurses who are either struggling with addiction or in recovery. Over the years, the total number of individuals that we have touched ranges from 5000 to 8000 nurses. There's an online meeting that our program established on a platform that specializes in addiction recovery groups. On Tuesday nights, from 7 to 8 PM, the Minnesota peer support network has over 100 nurses coming online since the pandemic, and it has flourished! There are lives in America that we are touching and assisting with recovery.

22.5.5 Paradigms Need to Shift in the University, Professional, and Policy Spheres

Interviewer: *Marie, in your experience, what do faculty and academicians need to do to help shift the paradigm from moral failure to chronic disease?*

Manthey: *There needs to be a comprehensive curriculum incorporated into all prelicensure programs. This would include essential information that needs to be universally recognized and frequently discussed on the high-risk level for nurses and the devastating consequences of practice impairment. There is well-developed curriculum developed by a major university and available for everyone to use. Education is the key, and the level of ignorance among students and faculty is unacceptable. Open forums, frequent incorporation of SUD in nursing need to be incorporated in all content areas. Stop the conspiracy of silence. Lives will be saved.*

Interviewer: *Marie, from your experience, please share with us what clinicians need to do personally to shift the paradigm from moral failure to chronic disease?*

Manthey: *Educate oneself and one's team. Nurses are the worst and if we do not change our mindset the paradigm will not change. It has to be a conscious effort on* *our part. Nobody else can do it for us. This means treating the addict on the street with the same compassion as the person with terminal cancer. It is hard, but both are diseases.*

Interviewer: *Marie, from your experience, please share with us what healthcare leaders and leaders in professional organizations need to do to shift the paradigm from moral failure to chronic disease?*

Manthey: *A culture can be changed by having good leadership. Demonstrating a different thought process, having leadership treating and showing empathy toward our peers instead of "getting rid of a problem," this is how the paradigm can change. Instead of hiding a "problem," leadership can be open and honest about addiction and other issues nurses struggle with. It is very powerful to have someone in a leadership role come out and admit this, especially when one is told they will never make it if they ever are human and make a mistake.*

Interviewer: *What is the business model?*

Manthey: *The business model is a non-profit 501c3 with a Board of Directors, Articles of Incorporation, bylaws, and committees.*

As our program began to develop, it became clear that being free-standing was an important principle of our function. We decided we were not going to have an organizational relationship with either the Board of Nursing or with the Alternative Discipline monitoring program. Since the Minnesota Nurses Association is now officially a union, not a professional organization, the independence of NPSN was important. I strongly emphasize however, that in creating a space for this work we have maintained positive and supportive relationships with the BON, HPSP, and the MNA. We meet with each of them regularly and provide information to them as requested. MNA has been one of our strongest financial supporters and is supportive in other ways as well. Our program is not dependent on any one of the recovery institutions or agencies that exist within the state of Minnesota. We have our own organizing principles, our own structures, policies, and operating committee.

Those who participate feel safer because we are independent. Participants don't have to fear that what is said in a peer support meeting could be used against them. Our program consists of one part-time employee and the executive director; the rest of the work is completed by nurse volunteers. We currently have eight meetings, twice a month, statewide. During those meetings, there are usually two conveners who set the tone of the meeting, attend to management items that occur during the meeting, and close the meeting. Our program makes sure that everybody understands that conveners are not there to advise, counsel, or even to suggest. They're there to create an environment that makes it safe to talk and to provide the opportunity for nurses to help nurses. That is key! It is not about attending a group to have one's problems answered by a lead person. It's about the participants interacting with each other and sharing their addiction and recovery experiences. That is what produces healing and relieves stigma and shame. That is the primary purpose of our peer support network.

Attendees remain anonymous, and we do not collect personal information. We don't send email chains out, but if groups would like to, we encourage them to set up their own network and create their own WhatsApp group. Maintaining confidentiality makes it difficult for us to show outcome data, such as participation and attendance. For example, we could say ten new nurses participated in the Tuesday afternoon group session, but how would we know who were first-time attendees? We wouldn't. Not everything can be measured and sometimes, the experience of helping the individual outweighs the statistical measurement. There are other ways to measure success.

Interviewer: *Who can benefit from the program?*

Manthey: *First of all, anyone with a license, which includes Licensed Practical Nurses (LPNs), Registered Nurses (RNs), Advanced Nurse Practitioners (ANPs), and Certified Registered Nurse Anesthetist (CRNAs). The Program includes anyone who has been licensed, which includes those that might have lost or are attempting to reapply for their license. They are all welcome to attend the meeting. Certified Nursing Assistants (CNAs), although we've been asked to, are not included. We have thought about it, maybe someday we'll have a group of CNAs who are doing peer support for each other, but for now, it has been decided to stick with the individual.*

Interviewer: *What advice would you have for others who would like to start a similar program in their state?*

Manthey: *This question has been coming up a lot lately. These are the steps we took; I believe they have a generic quality that can be helpful to a peer support start-up in any state. Each state has different policies and practices already in place; therefore, each implementation process needs to be customized to each state's practices.*

First, we invited key individuals to join a formative task force. We looked for individuals who understand the nature and impact of SUD in nursing, and who are able to help create and support a new organization.

Steps that the task force needs to take include evaluating readiness, becoming informed about the problem in your state, and collecting data from other states to learn about different types of organizations.

The second step is to determine the key stakeholders and begin early communication. Information gathering is the major activity at this time, and support can come from a variety of individuals and institutions. As the task force members gather data, outreach to recovering nurses will be critical.

The third step is deciding the function and structure of the entity. Basic to this decision is the issue of whether to be independent or become a part of an already existing organization, such as the Board of Nursing, the state nurses' association, or an alternative to discipline program if one exists. This decision will drive many of the next major decisions, which is securing the funding source.

While these steps are in process, the internal structure, policies, service design, committees, and volunteer orientation can be planned.

This whole process in Minnesota took about a year, during which time we had invaluable support and guidance from a recovering person who helped other health professional groups (MDs, pharmacists, etc.) set up peer support groups of their own. This experience she shared was immensely helpful... she was our Guardian Guide.

One of NPSN's goals is to create a model that can be adapted so that other states can start a strong peer support program that can be adapted for all states and circumstances.

22.6 Conclusion

As a matter or workplace wellness, the issue of how to support healthcare professionals with substance use disorder is still a problem yet to be solved. It is imperative that healthcare leaders use a therapeutic approach toward encouraging acute treatment and recovery while maintaining licensure and employment. Advocating for independent statewide peer support programs is offered as one strategy for humanistic support of healthcare professionals with substance addictions.

Glossary

Alcoholism A chronic disease characterized by uncontrolled drinking and preoccupation with alcohol.

Chronic disease Conditions that last 1 year or more and require ongoing medical attention or limit activities of daily living.

Moral failure An act or thought that is carried out when one knows that one should not carry it out.

Substance use disorder The uncontrolled use of one or more substances despite harmful consequences which places the individual at risk of immediate harm.

Discussion Questions

1. How do universities approach the issue of substance abuse and the risk factors with students?
2. How can the negative thought process about addiction be changed within the profession/culture?
3. How can this issue become mainstream when most individuals are too afraid to mention their issue of addiction?

Discussion Leader Guide

1. *Should students be tested for risks? If they are high risk, do they enter into anonymous treatment? What would be the pos/neg effect? What education would work?*
   There will probably be many against this idea because of the stigma against those with high risk factors. Many might argue they will not get a job in a certain high stress area if they are positive for certain high risks. So what could the university's or hospitals do to make it safe? This could start an individual on a path that could assist them with handling those high stress areas. This also address the stigmas that are out there that many may think are not.
2. *Needs to start from within, but how? Start with the boards, there needs to be a way to take back the punitive culture against those who have a disease.*
   Many may feel that the punishment should fit the crime because it has yet to affect them. It is important to be clear and concise about the issues (depression, PTSD, anxiety), how it is not being addressed in a healthy way. How do the students and healthcare professionals feel that they are treated within their facility or unit? Is there empathy for mental health issues?
3. *The secrets need to stop. People need to be ok to speak about their struggles and not have it be held against them in order to have mainstream discuss it. Can this happen? Only time will tell.*
   Is there a way for healthcare professionals and students to feel supported if they have a substance abuse disorder? Do they feel that they can go to their professors and or leadership and receive help instead of being handed a pink slip (terminated)? What are some issues that the individuals see? What could be some steps to take in a positive direction to fix the negative punitive perspective and change to a disease/treatment-oriented approach?
4. *About the disparities specific to nursing: How can we change the system so that we are treated equitably to other healthcare professionals? How do we change the unintentional negative consequences of our social contract? How can we be accepted as humans prone to the same fallacies as other humans?*
   How can we change this image? Can we change the image and still be trusted individuals? Will there be grace given from the public if a mistake is made? How can the culture being changed?

Video for Discussion - Instructional Video: The online version contains supplementary material available at https://doi.org/10.1007/978-3-031-16983-0_22

References

1. Adams JM, Volkow ND. Ethical imperatives to overcome stigma against people with substance. AMA J Ethics. 2020;22(1):702–8.
2. Diane Kunyk P. Nurses, addictions and stigma. Faculty of Nursing, University of Alberta; 2015. https://www.ualberta.ca/nursing/nursing-news/2015/december/nurses-addictions-and-stigma.html.
3. National Academies of Sciences, Engineering, and Medicine, Health and Medicine Division, Board on Global Health; Global Forum on Innovation in Health Professional Education. In:

Forstag EH, Cuff PA, editors. A design thinking, systems approach to well-being within education and practice: proceedings of a workshop. Washington, DC: National Academies Press; 2018. Appendix B, The Importance of Well-Being in the Health Care Workforce. https://www.ncbi.nlm.nih.gov/books/NBK540859/.
4. Enforcement Data—Index. Sacramento: California Department of Consumer Affairs. https://www.dca.ca.gov/publications/2021_annrpt.pdf.
5. Fowler M. Guide to nursing's social policy statement: understanding the profession from social contract to social covenant. Silver Spring: American Nurses Association; 2015.

Differentiating Burnout from Depression 23

Sidney Zisook, Ami P. Doshi, Byron D. Fergerson, and Desiree N. Shapiro

Abbreviations

MDD Major depressive disorder
MDE Major depressive episode

Learning Objectives
1. Learn key characteristics, consequences, and management of burnout
2. Learn key characteristics, consequences, and management of major depressive disorder
3. Apply knowledge to differentiate burnout from major depressive disorder and recognize depression when both are present

---

Supplementary Information The online version contains supplementary material available at https://doi.org/10.1007/978-3-031-16983-0_23.

S. Zisook (✉)
Department of Psychiatry, UC San Diego, La Jolla, CA, USA
e-mail: zisook@health.ucsd.edu

A. P. Doshi
UC San Diego and Rady Children's Hospital—San Diego, San Diego, CA, USA
e-mail: adoshi@rchsd.org

B. D. Fergerson
Department of Anesthesiology, UC San Diego, La Jolla, CA, USA
e-mail: bfergerson@ucsd.edu

D. N. Shapiro
Department of Psychiatry, UC San Diego, La Jolla, CA, USA
e-mail: dlshapiro@health.ucsd.edu

23.1 Presentation of the Science

Health care workforce distress is increasingly recognized as a professional and public health crisis. High rates of suffering including burnout, substance abuse, secondary trauma or second victim phenomena, depression, and suicide are all receiving national attention and calls for action [1–3]. In turn, burnout and depression have serious consequences related to medical errors, absenteeism, presenteeism, turnover, patient satisfaction, and compassion [4–6]. To help address this health care crisis, enhancing provider wellness and mental health has become a national priority [5, 6].

This chapter will discuss two of the most prevalent mental health conditions in health care workers: burnout and major depressive disorder (MDD). After discussing key features, risks, and consequences of these conditions, we will describe ways to differentiate burnout from MDD, why the distinction is so critical, and how institutions and individual health care workers can apply this knowledge to foster resilience and enhance provider wellness and mental health.

23.1.1 Burnout

Case 1

Bill is a second-year resident in a demanding general surgery residency program. Bill had lived a charmed life, always in good health with an upbeat attitude, and enjoying a series of hard-earned successes. He had been a star athlete and straight "A" student in his hometown university, earning AOA and Gold Humanism honors in the same University's medical school. He was delighted to match with his first choice for a surgical residency on the other side of the country and maintained his customary record of superb achievement as a first-year resident. His second year was complicated by the COVID-19 pandemic. After weeks of working overtime covering the ER and ICU, he began feeling drained and depleted, unusually cynical and alienated, and totally ineffectual. No matter what he did, patients were getting sicker, several died on his watch, and more kept coming. Although his work-life was difficult, he managed to power-on, relying on the self-confidence he had developed throughout his education. He found himself resenting patients for not taking better care of themselves. He began wondering if being a doctor was worth it. To make matters worse, he learned that his father had contracted COVID-19. His father was hospitalized, placed on a ventilator, and was fighting for his life. He badly wanted to be there for his family but work responsibilities and travel restrictions made it impossible, which only increased his frustration. Despite all this, Bill found himself temporarily feeling better after being able to bike or jog. He felt considerably better once he finally had three days off, but dreaded coming back to work.

First described by Freudenberger [7], burnout is a psychological condition involving a prolonged response to enduring work stress. Manifestations described by Freudenberger included feeling hopeless, fatigued, bored, resentful, disenchanted, discouraged, confused, irritable, frustrated, and having a negative attitude. Freudenberger noted that burnout often occurred in contexts requiring large amounts of personal involvement and empathy, primarily among "the dedicated and the committed." Later, Maslach et al. [8] characterized burnout by three domains: emotional exhaustion (EE), depersonalization (DP), and a diminished sense of personal accomplishment (PA). In 2019, The World Health Organization (WHO) declared burnout as an "occupational phenomenon" in the *International Classification of Diseases, 11th Revision* (ICD-11), stating that burnout is a syndrome resulting from "chronic workspace stress that has not been successfully managed." [9] The WHO declaration recognized burnout as a serious health issue.

The prevalence of burnout is alarmingly high in all levels of medical training and practice, including among medical students [10], physician residents [11], and practicing physicians [12]. A survey of approximately 12,000 physicians conducted in 2020 demonstrated a burnout rate of 46%, with 47% of respondents noting that burnout has a strong or severe impact on their life and 79% noting their feelings of burnout preceded the COVID-19 pandemic [13]. Nurses may have a similarly high prevalence of burnout [14, 15].

For both doctors and nurses, the consequences of burnout are personal (poor physical and mental health, compassion fatigue), professional (poor quality of care, reduced patient satisfaction, poor compliance), and financial (more turnover, errors, resource utilization) [1, 12, 14]. A physician study, describing the relationship between turnover and burnout, found physicians to be 1.5 times more likely to turnover when they had high burnout [16]. Similarly, a 2018 National Survey of Registered Nurses found that among nurses who reported leaving their current employment (9.5% of sample), 31.5% reported leaving because of burnout [17]. Overall, about half of all physicians and nurses are dissatisfied with what they do, contemplate cutting back or leaving the field entirely, and do not recommend a medical career to their children.

When future health care professionals enter the profession, it is often with a sense of great purpose and fulfillment. Over the course of their training and practice, they rapidly begin to view their profession as a source of overwhelming distress. The logical question is "Why?" Several internal and external factors contribute to the problem of burnout. Key drivers of burnout include workload and job demands, control and flexibility, efficiency and resources, organizational culture and values, and social support and a sense of community at work [18]. Long work hours, heavy workloads, onerous health care system changes, lack of autonomy, and increased time spent on computers instead of with patients push health care workers toward burnout. Added to these workplace factors are a stoic culture of self-sufficiency and real and/or perceived barriers to help-seeking. Mental health issues thus often go unaddressed and potentially spiral into more severe, entrenched mental health problems [19–22].

In the case illustration above, Bill appears to be suffering from burnout. Some degree of perfectionism is a predispositional factor to developing burnout [23]. Being a star athlete with straight A's, honors, and "super-achievement" throughout his education suggests Bill has this characteristic. He is clearly overloaded with work responsibilities and exhibits little control over his time, both of which push individuals toward burnout. He is emotionally and physically "drained and depleted," consistent with the overwhelming exhaustion victims of burnout tend to suffer. This exhaustion leaves him feeling purposeless and "ineffectual," which he guards against by depersonalizing his patients through resentment thus "alienating" himself from his work. Despite all this, he powers-on, maintaining a small sense of self-esteem and self-worth. In addition, he remains interested and functional in other aspects of his life like recreation. The cause of all these problems is clear: the burden and stress of his residency. And the anecdote, taking time away from work, makes him feel better even though he maintains a sense of dread about returning.

23.1.2 Major Depressive Disorder

Case 2
Debra is a second-year resident in a family medicine residency program. Debra has always struggled with low confidence, social and performance anxiety, and feelings of insecurity, but, despite her self-doubts, has always performed well in school. Other than a few months of intermittent counseling as a teenager, she never received therapy or psychotropic medications. However, she recalls extended periods of low mood and thoughts of giving up in both college and medical school. Despite those periods, she plowed forward and never missed a day of school. Even her family and closest friends did not know how terrible and alone she felt. She was delighted to match with her first choice for a family medicine residency on the other side of the country and did well as a first-year resident despite lingering feelings of being out of her league, on the verge of being "found out" on many rotations, and persistent worries about just about everything. Her second year was complicated by the COVID-19 invasion. After weeks of working overtime covering the ER and ICU, she began feeling drained and depleted, unusually cynical and alienated and absolutely ineffectual. She felt overwhelmed by the workload, had trouble concentrating on her patient's needs, and the quality of her care and compassion had markedly diminished. No matter what she did, her patients were getting sicker, several passed away, and more kept coming. She found it difficult to get out of bed in the morning. She found herself resenting patients for not taking better care of themselves and began wondering if she was cut out to be a doctor. Her mood became considerably worse and she began having thoughts that she was a burden on her training program and her family. She often wished she could fall asleep and never wake back up to the pain she felt each morning. She felt she did not deserve to live but had no active suicidal plans or intent. Debra has lost the energy or will to stay connected with friends, make it to her daily yoga class, or experience any joy or relaxation during time off. When she finally had three consecutive days off duty, she found herself buried in her bed all day, each day, and felt even more hopeless.

Major depressive disorder (MDD) is a serious medical condition characterized by low mood (dysphoria) and/or inability to anticipate or experience pleasure (anhedonia) and a combination of other somatic (low energy, changes in sleep and appetite), psychomotor (slowing or activation), cognitive (low motivation, poor concentration, indecisiveness, guilt, feelings of worthlessness, suicidal thoughts), and behavioral (suicide attempts, suicide) disturbances. To qualify for the diagnosis of MDD, the mood symptoms must be present much of the time, most days, for at least two weeks and be associated with clinically meaningful distress or impairment in social, occupational, or other important areas of functioning [24]. More illustrative of what clinical depression is than a dry list of DSM symptoms are personal narratives of those with "lived experience." Three examples of such narratives come from well-known individuals who have struggled with depression:

> The pain is unrelenting, and what makes the condition intolerable is the foreknowledge that no remedy will come—not in a day, an hour, a month or a minute. It is hopelessness even more than pain that crushes the soul. So the decision making of daily life involves not, as in normal affairs, shifting from one annoying situation to another less annoying—or from discomfort to relative comfort, or from boredom to activity—but moving from pain to pain. One does not abandon, even briefly, one's bed of nails, but is attached to it wherever one goes.—William Styron [25]

> I am now the most miserable man living. If what I feel were equally distributed to the entire human race, there would not be one cheerful face left on earth.—Abraham Lincoln [26]

> It is a level of psychic pain wholly incompatible with human life as we know it. It is a sense of radical and thoroughgoing evil not just as a feature but as the essence of conscious existence. It is a sense of poisoning that pervades the self at the self's most elementary levels. It is a nausea of the cells and soul.—David Foster Wallace [27]

MDD is a highly prevalent, comorbid, disabling, and sometimes fatal disorder. In a national survey of 36,309 US adults, the 12-month and lifetime prevalence of major depressive disorder were 10.4% and 20.6%, respectively, with most being moderate (6–7 symptoms) or severe (8–9 symptoms) and associated with comorbidity and impairment [28]. The degree of workplace impairment is comparable to or greater than what has been reported in studies of chronic medical illness such as asthma, heart disease, and chronic obstructive pulmonary disease. The combination of its high prevalence and associated disability is why MDD now ranks as the leading cause of ill health and disability worldwide (https://www.who.int/news/item/30-03-2017%2D%2Ddepression-let-s-talk-says-who-as-depression-tops-list-of-causes-of-ill-health). In addition to work impairment, MDD is associated with a range of other negative consequences, such as a significantly increased risk of myocardial infarction, stroke, or developing diabetes. The co-occurrence of MDD with general medical conditions is associated with increased morbidity and mortality compared to the associated medical condition alone. Co-occurring MDD also is associated with greater health care utilization, lower adherence to prescribed regimens, and greater annual costs. The most serious consequence of MDD, especially untreated or insufficiently treated, is suicide. Suicide is the tenth leading cause of death in the United States. In 2019 alone, there was an estimated 1.38 million attempts and 47,511 individuals died by suicide. Other than a history of suicide attempts, MDD is greatest contributor to suicide risk [29]. Thus, every untreated MDD is a potentially preventable suicide.

Some studies have found higher rates of clinically meaningful depressive symptoms in medical students and physicians than in the general population [30], but there are not compelling data regarding comparative rates of MDD. A systematic review and meta-analysis of 195 studies involving 129,123 medical students in 47 countries found that 27% (range, 9–56%) of students screened positive for depression or depressive symptoms and that 11% (range, 7–24%) reported suicidal ideation during medical school. Only 16% of students who screened positive for depression reportedly sought treatment [31]. A systematic review and meta-analysis focusing on resident physicians showed a prevalence of depression or depressive symptoms in 29% (range, 21–43%, depending on the instrument used), and that depression was positively associated with increased time in training but not with medical specialty or country of training [32]. In an ambitious series of surveys of working physicians in the United States, the proportion of physicians screening positive for depression showed a modest but steady increase between 2011 and 2017 (2011, **38%** [2753 of 7213]; 2014, **40%** [2715 of 6818]; 2017, **42%** [2022 of 4854]; $p < 0.001$) [12]. Nurses and other health care providers also have impressive rates of depression and depressive symptoms which often evade mental health attention [32]. One large study of 1790 practicing nurses from 19 healthcare systems across the United States indicated that depression affected a third of the sample and was the leading cause of medical errors [33]. Despite their medical knowledge, resources, and generally good insurance coverage, health care workers do not appear more likely than the general population to seek mental health care for themselves [34], thus leaving them vulnerable to all the suffering and other ravages of untreated depression, including suicide.

Given her persistently low mood, low energy, sleep changes, feelings of worthlessness, poor concentration, lack of pleasure or anhedonia, isolation, and passive suicidal ideation, Debra is experiencing features of both burnout and MDD. Digging into her past, pervasive and longstanding self-doubt and insecurity paired with anxiety existed. She perseverated and suffered internally; but externally, she portrayed a picture of success, always working hard, present in the classroom, and eventually matching into her dream residency program. However, the cost of her achievements was substantial, including social isolation during what likely were multiple depressive episodes, described as lengthy periods of low mood and fantasizing about giving up or quitting. Debra had many missed opportunities to receive mental health support and create a proactive plan for her well-being. Transitioning to her role as a medical intern, she carried with her a significant vulnerability and history of mental illness. Had there not been barriers such as stigma, access, self-awareness, or limited support, she may have been able to seek treatment and manage, but not decrease entirely, the extensive workplace stress before her. Despite making it to residency, she was convinced she was an impostor, a fraud, and someone who was let in by mistake. Debra's narrative captures the pain and hopelessness that impaired all aspects of her life. The amotivation, apathy, and self-critical pessimistic ruminations overtook her ability to care for patients or herself. When she did get a break, she retreated to her home and spent days in bed, unable to bounce back like Bill. During the most intense depressive episode described, she was unable to seek or receive support from others and was passively suicidal, desperately wanting to relieve her perceived burden on others by not waking up in the morning.

23.1.3 Differentiating Burnout from MDD

Despite its prevalence, there is no concrete scientific definition nor classification system for burnout. In fact, there is an ongoing debate whether it represents a separate entity at all or is part of the MDD continuum [35–37]. One systematic review of 182 studies involving 109,628 physicians from 45 countries, found 142 unique definitions of "burnout" were used, resulting in overall burnout prevalence ranging from 0 to 81% [38]. MDD, as well, represents a broad and diverse constellation of symptoms and syndromes, with 227 possible ways to meet the DSM-5 definition of MDD [39]. Burnout and depression share several features in common, such as unhappiness, low energy, poor sleep, and a defeatist attitude, leading some investigators to speculate they are part of the same heterogeneous disorder [40]. Moreover, even biological parameters associated with stress disorders, such as heart rate variability and brain-derived neurotrophic factor, are similarly altered in both conditions [41]. Other investigators do not think the two conditions should be lumped together [42, 43] and emphasize the dangers inherent in conflating the two conditions [44]. The majority of people who have experienced both burnout and depression do not consider the conditions to be part of the same disorder [45]. Thus, differentiating burnout from MDD can be challenging.

There are several key aspects of burnout that are either more prominent than in MDD or completely distinct from it. It appears that most of the differences revolve around burnout as an externalizing emotional state as opposed to the internalizing state associated with MDD. People who suffer from burnout generally feel there is a distinct, external cause. For health care workers, that cause tends to be the dysfunctional system within which they work. With a distinct cause comes a clear treatment (in the case of health care workers, fixing the system or leaving their jobs) and thus leaving more room for optimism. Descriptions of burnout tend to be more associated with helplessness than hopelessness. This helplessness, derived from a sense that external circumstances are out of their control, often leave burnout sufferers anxious and angry. These symptoms are more "active" than the "heaviness" often associated with MDD. In addition, with a clear source, other aspects of one's life are less affected. Burnout sufferers are less likely to have disturbances in social, recreational, or other functional areas. Even at work, burnout sufferers are more functional, opting to "power-on." This functionality leaves the victim of burnout with more self-esteem and self-worth than those with MDD. Burnout sufferers, however, are not at their optimal functional level, enduring overwhelming exhaustion, and concentration and memory dysfunction [43, 46]. In fact, exhaustion is the cardinal feature of burnout. The cardinal features of MDD are persistent and pervasive unhappiness and lack of any ability to anticipate or experience pleasure. Similarly, other than specifically related to work, self-esteem is preserved in burnout, while feelings of worthlessness often predominate one's self-view in MDD. In contrast to the experiences of those with MDD, individuals with burnout often retain the capacity to laugh, to appreciate the comfort and support of relatives and neighbors, to be consoled, and to recognize that what they are going through will lessen in time.

To make matters more complicated, both burnout and MDD may coexist in the same person at the same time. Burnout may be an early manifestation or forerunner of MDD. MDD, in turn, affects one's capacity to cope with life stresses. Thus, an individual with MDD encountering prolonged job stress, especially in a field as demanding as health care, may be prone to all the symptoms and features of burnout. In addition, it is highly possible to miss the diagnosis of MDD in someone with all the manifestations of burnout. Individuals who are depressed frequently search for reasons why and may themselves mistakenly identify events occurring in proximity to the onset of the mood change, such as work stressors, as causes of the mood alteration [47]. When both symptoms of burnout and MDD coexist, it is easy to misattribute the suffering to burnout, ignoring the serious, but all-too-often stigmatized mental health condition, MDD. Furthermore, being in a depressed state may itself precipitate "dependent" or adverse life events, such as dropping out of school, leaving a job or a relationship, or exposing oneself to risky situations. In effect, depression often "recruits" misadventure, making judgments regarding cause and effect hazardous. Clinicians may join their patients' misidentification of MDD as something much more benign and "acceptable." Pies has coined the term, "*fallacy of misplaced empathy*," which refers to a well-intentioned clinician's paradoxically missing of the diagnosis of MDD, because he or she can "understand" that "anybody" undergoing a serious life stressor—whether becoming disabled, impoverished, terminally ill, humiliated, bereaved, or burned out at work—might be distraught and upset [48]. But it simply does not follow logically that, just because one's reaction to an event is "understandable," it cannot be pathological and, in many cases, severely debilitating. Such misplaced empathy may interfere with accurate diagnosis and much-needed treatment. The dilemma lies in knowing where to draw the line along the health–illness continuum.

23.1.4 Why It Matters?

The importance of differentiating burnout from depression may not be primarily an either/or proposition—is this burnout *or* MDD—but one of identifying when an individual who presents with features and symptoms of burnout may *also* have MDD. Failure to do so risks the potential of missing the detection and opportunity to provide effective treatment for individuals suffering a serious, if not life-threatening, mental disorder.

23.2 Application to Health Care Workers with Burnout and/or MDD

For "uncomplicated burnout" (i.e., without coexisting MDD), there are both institutional and individual interventions to enhance resilience and prevent or manage burnout. Resilience is protective against burnout, yet nearly 1/3 of physicians who have the highest possible resilience score still experience burnout, suggesting that it is a necessary but insufficient component of reducing burnout. Both individual and organizational strategies have been demonstrated to reduce burnout. However, organizational strategies are more effective, especially when directed at teamwork, communication, and autonomy. Individual-level strategies may thus be a part of the approach to address burnout, but ideally would be coupled with system-level interventions to maximize impact. Among individual strategies, cultivating a gratitude practice has been demonstrated to have myriad benefits including improving mood and resilience, decreasing burnout, and improving some dimensions of physical health. Practicing self-compassion, which involves mindfulness, self-kindness, and connectedness, has shown benefit in combating burnout and may be especially helpful in a situation such as Bill's when faced with a sense of inefficacy. Spending at least 20% of effort in the professional area they find most meaningful, protects physicians against burnout. This represents an opportunity as Bill may identify an area of work that is especially meaningful to him that could be integrated into his position with the support of his leadership. In addition, having his organization optimize workflow and streamline other processes may allow him to have time to participate in what he finds most meaningful. Workflow optimization efforts adopted at many institutions address burnout through their focus on improving efficiency by leveraging teamwork and flexibility to ensure that all health care team members are working at the top of their license. Local leadership and the wellbeing of local leaders directly and significantly impact physician burnout, accounting for nearly half of the difference in burnout scores among physicians. Wellness-centered leadership, which starts with the foundation of caring about people always, plays a pivotal role, and applied to Bill's situation may have mitigated his burnout had leadership given physicians a voice in determining travel restrictions, creating a coverage system to support physicians in their family needs, and allowing physician input and flexibility in defining work responsibilities under the circumstances. Lastly, Bill's sense of isolation is exacerbating his burnout and is worsened by the COVID-19 pandemic. Institutional efforts to address the isolation are warranted and could include provision of time or funds for structured physician small group meetings to build community and development of peer support programs to promote connection.

Returning to the case of Debra, she is facing a combination of both burnout and MDD. As described above, Debra clearly meets criteria for MDD with significant impairment in her personal and professional life. Working long hours with enormous work demands during the pandemic had led to her feeling drained, depleted, and cynical. Her capacity to practice with compassion and understanding is limited and an unfamiliar resentment toward her patients has emerged. These classic signs of burnout are distinct from MDD; however, her history of depression and recent depressive episode may have increased her likelihood to suffer from burnout. To best support Debra, both conditions must be acknowledged and addressed. Although beyond the purview of this chapter, providing effective treatment for Debra could involve confronting stigma about mental illness and treatment, eliminating roadblocks to care such as antiquated medical licensing procedure issues related to privacy and confidentiality, and attending to the national shortage of psychiatrists and other licensed mental health providers [2, 44]. But once those hurdles are addressed, effective, evidence-based psychotherapies and pharmacotherapies for MDD are available.

23.3   Opportunities for Future Research

Dyrbe et al. [1] outlined three broad areas regarding burnout that would benefit from further research. The same three recommendations are also true for depression: first, more research to identify individual, work-unit, health care organization/employer, and health care systems that contribute to risk for burnout and/or depression; second, longitudinal, controlled studies with reliable and valid measures of health care outcomes to advance our understanding of the professional consequences of burnout and treated versus untreated MDD; and, third, methodologically robust intervention studies to improve the work-lives, wellbeing, and mental health of health care professionals. For burnout, valuable investigation would look into ways this phenomenon can be productively discussed, assessed for in non-judgmental ways, and addressed with a menu of individualized options. For depression, more work is needed to better understand which of the many currently available evidence-based treatments are best for whom and under what circumstances; to make mental health care more accepted, available, and accessible; and to develop new treatments that are safe and effective for those individuals who cannot tolerate or do not have adequate outcomes with currently available treatment strategies, and that work more quickly with longer-lasting effects. Research should also explore any different manifestations or impact among health professionals from a wide array of cultures, backgrounds, genders, or other group identifications. The more information we gather about these conditions, the more information we can share with and offer our colleagues to collectively combat continued suffering.

Glossary

Burnout A syndrome conceptualized as resulting from chronic workplace stress that has not been successfully managed. It is characterized by three dimensions: (1) feelings of energy depletion or exhaustion; (2) increased mental distance from one's job, or feelings of negativism or cynicism related to one's job; and (3) reduced professional efficacy.

Major depressive disorder A mental disorder characterized by low mood (dysphoria) and/or inability to anticipate or experience pleasure (anhedonia) and a combination of other somatic (low energy, changes in sleep and appetite), psychomotor (slowing or activation), cognitive (low motivation, poor concentration, indecisiveness, guilt, feelings of worthlessness, suicidal thoughts), and behavioral (suicide attempts, suicide) disturbances.

Discussion Questions/Guide

- How do you diagnose depression in a health care worker who complains of work stress and has all the symptoms/features of burnout?
- What steps can the individual health care worker take to prevent or manage burnout and enhance their resilience, well-being, and emotional health?
- Why is it important to differentiate burnout from depression?
- What steps can the individual health care worker take to prevent or manage major depression and enhance their mental health?
- What steps can the health care institution take to enhance the work force's resilience, well-being, and emotional and mental health?

Discussion Questions

1. How would you differentiate burnout from depression?
2. What keeps health care workers who are depressed from receiving mental health care?
3. What organizational and institutional changes would you recommend to enhance well-being and reduce burnout among health care workers?
4. What interventions aimed at individual health care workers might enhance their well-being and reduce burnout?

Discussion Leader Guide

Video for Discussion - Instructional Video: The online version contains supplementary material available at https://doi.org/10.1007/978-3-031-16983-0_23

References

1. Dyrbye LN, Shanafelt TD, Sinsky CA, Cipriano PF, Bhatt J, Ommaya A, West CP, Meyers D. Burnout among health care professionals: a call to explore and address this underrecognized threat to safe, high-quality care (NAM Perspectives, Discussion Paper). Washington, DC: National Academy of Medicine; 2017. https://doi.org/10.31478/201707b.
2. Moutier CY, Myers MF, Feist JB, Feist JC, Zisook S. Preventing clinician suicide: a call to action during the COVID-19 pandemic and beyond. Acad Med. 2021;96(5):624–8. https://doi.org/10.1097/ACM.0000000000003972.

3. Davidson J, Mendis J, Stuck AR, DeMichele G, Zisook S. Nurse suicide: breaking the silence (NAM Perspectives, Discussion Paper). Washington, DC: National Academy of Medicine; 2018. https://doi.org/10.31478/201801a.

4. Linzer M, Guzman-Corrales L, Poplau S. Preventing physician burnout: improve patient satisfaction, quality, outcomes and provider recruitment and retention. AMA STEPSforward; 2018. https://edhub.ama-assn.org/steps-forward/module/2702509. Accessed 12 Dec 2020

5. Association of American Medical Colleges. Analysis in brief: burnout among U.S. Medical School Faculty. Washington, DC: AAMC; 2019. https://www.aamc.org/em/aib/aamc-february-2019-analysis-in-brief.pdf.

6. National Academies of Sciences, Engineering, and Medicine. Taking action against clinician burnout: a systems approach to professional well-being. Washington, DC: The National Academies Press; 2019.

7. Freudenberger HJ. The staff burn-out syndrome in alternative institutions. Psychothe Theory Res Pract. 1975;12(1):73.

8. Maslach C, Jackson SE, Leiter MP. Maslach burnout inventory. Scarecrow Education; 1997.

9. World Health Organization. Burn-out an "occupational phenomenon": international classification of diseases. Geneva: World Health Organization; 2019. https://www.who.int/news/item/28-05-2019-burn-out-an-occupational-phenomenon-international-classification-of-diseases. Accessed on 18 Sept 2021

10. Dyrbye LN, Thomas MR, Harper W, Massie FS Jr, Power DV, Eacker A, Szydlo DW, Novotny PJ, Sloan JA, Shanafelt TD. The learning environment and medical student burnout: a multicentre study. Med Educ. 2009;43(3):274–82.

11. Zhou AY, Panagioti M, Esmail A, Agius R, Van Tongeren M, Bower P. Factors associated with burnout and stress in trainee physicians: a systematic review and meta-analysis. JAMA Netw Open. 2020;3(8):e2013761.

12. Shanafelt TD, West CP, Sinsky C, Trockel M, Tutty M, Satele DV, Carlasare LE, Dyrbye LN. Changes in burnout and satisfaction with work-life integration in physicians and the general US working population between 2011 and 2017. Mayo Clinic Proc. 2019;94(9):1681–94.

13. Medscape. Physician, burnout and suicide report. 2021. https://www.medscape.com/sites/public/lifestyle/2021

14. Dyrbye LN, Shanafelt TD, Johnson PO, West CP. A cross-sectional study exploring the relationship between burnout, absenteeism, and job performance among American nurses. BMC Nurs. 2019;18(1):57.

15. Woo T, Ho R, Tang A, Tam W. Global prevalence of burnout symptoms among nurses: a systematic review and meta-analysis. J Psychiatr Res. 2020;123:9–20.

16. Willard-Grace R, Knox M, Huang B, Hammer H, Kivlahan C, Grumbach K. Burnout and health care workforce turnover. Ann Fam Med. 2019;17(1):36–41.

17. Shah MK, Gandrakota N, Cimiotti JP, Ghose N, Moore M, Ali MK. Prevalence of and factors associated with nurse burnout in the US. JAMA Netw Open. 2021;4(2):e2036469.

18. Shanafelt TD, Noseworthy J. Executive leadership and physician well-being: nine organizational strategies to promote engagement and reduce burnout. Mayo Clin Proc. 2017;92(1):129–46.

19. Moutier C. Physician mental health: an evidence-based approach to change. J Med Regul. 2018;104(2):7–13.

20. Davidson JE, Proudfoot J, Lee K, Terterian G, Zisook S. A longitudinal analysis of nurse suicide in the United States (2005–2016) with recommendations for action. Worldviews Evid Based Nurs. 2020;17(1):6–15.

21. Gold KJ, Schwenk TL. Physician suicide—a personal and community tragedy. JAMA Psychiat. 2020;77(6):559–60.

22. Yeh G, Davidson JE, Kim K, Zisook S. Physician death by suicide in the United States: 2012-2016. J Psychiatr Res. 2021;134:158–65.

23. Spagnoli P, Buono C, Kovalchuk LS, Cordasco G, Esposito A. Perfectionism and burnout during the COVID-19 crisis: a two-wave cross-lagged study. Front Psychol. 2021;11:4087.

24. American Psychiatric Association, American Psychiatric Association. Diagnostic and statistical manual of mental disorders: DSM-5. American Psychiatric Association; 2013.

25. Styron W. Darkness visible: a memoir of madness. Open Road Media; 2010.

26. Abraham Lincoln to John Stuart, January 23, 1841, House Divided: The Civil War Research Engine at Dickinson College. https://hd.housedivided.dickinson.edu/node/40485.
27. Wallace DF. Infinite jest. Hachette UK; 2011.
28. Hasin DS, Sarvet AL, Meyers JL, Saha TD, Ruan WJ, Stohl M, Grant BF. Epidemiology of adult DSM-5 major depressive disorder and its specifiers in the United States. JAMA Psychiat. 2018;75(4):336–46.
29. Cavanagh JT, Carson AJ, Sharpe M, Lawrie SM. Psychological autopsy studies of suicide: a systematic review. Psychol Med. 2003;33(3):395–405.
30. Joules N, Williams DM, Thompson AW. Depression in resident physicians: a systematic review. Open J Depress. 2014;3:89–100.
31. Rotenstein LS, Ramos MA, Torre M, Segal JB, Peluso MJ, Guille C, Sen S, Mata DA. Prevalence of depression, depressive symptoms, and suicidal ideation among medical students: a systematic review and meta-analysis. JAMA. 2016;316(21):2214–36.
32. Mata DA, Ramos MA, Bansal N, Khan R, Guille C, Di Angelantonio E, Sen S. Prevalence of depression and depressive symptoms among resident physicians: a systematic review and meta-analysis. JAMA. 2015;314(22):2373–83.
33. Melnyk BM, Orsolini L, Tan A, Arslanian-Engoren C, Melkus GDE, Dunbar-Jacob J, Rice VH, Millan A, Dunbar SB, Braun LT, Wilbur J. A national study links nurses' physical and mental health to medical errors and perceived worksite wellness. J Occup Environ Med. 2018;60(2):126–31.
34. Melnyk BM. Burnout, depression and suicide in nurses/clinicians and learners: an urgent call for action to enhance professional well-being and healthcare safety. Worldviews Evid Based Nurs. 2020;17(1):2–5.
35. Mehta SS, Edwards ML. Suffering in silence: mental health stigma and physicians' licensing fears. Am J Psychiatry Residents' J. 2018;13:2–4.
36. Bianchi R, Verkuilen J, Schonfeld IS, Hakanen JJ, Jansson-Fröjmark M, Manzano-García G, Laurent E, Meier LL. Is burnout a depressive condition? A 14-sample meta-analytic and bifactor analytic study. Clin Psychol Sci. 2021;9(4) https://doi.org/10.1177/2167702620979597.
37. Bianchi R. Do burnout and depressive symptoms form a single syndrome? Confirmatory factor analysis and exploratory structural equation modeling bifactor analysis. J Psychosom Res. 2020;131:109954.
38. Rotenstein LS, Torre M, Ramos MA, Rosales RC, Guille C, Sen S, Mata DA. Prevalence of burnout among physicians: a systematic review. JAMA. 2018;320(11):1131–50.
39. Zimmerman M, Ellison W, Young D, Chelminski I, Dalrymple K. How many different ways do patients meet the diagnostic criteria for major depressive disorder? Compr Psychiatry. 2015;56:29–34.
40. Schonfeld IS, Bianchi R. Burnout and depression: two entities or one? J Clin Psychol. 2016;72(1):22–37.
41. Orosz A, Federspiel A, Haisch S, Seeher C, Dierks T, Cattapan K. A biological perspective on differences and similarities between burnout and depression. Neurosci Biobehav Rev. 2017;73:112–22.
42. Parker G, Tavella G. Distinguishing burnout from clinical depression: a theoretical differentiation template. J Affect Disord. 2021;281:168–73.
43. Summers RF. The elephant in the room: what burnout is and what it is not. Am J Psychiatry. 2020;177(10):898–9.
44. Oquendo MA, Bernstein CA, Mayer LE. A key differential diagnosis for physicians—major depression or burnout? JAMA Psychiat. 2019;76(11):1111–2.
45. Tavella G, Hadzi-Pavlovic D, Parker G. Burnout: re-examining its key constructs. Psychiatry Res. 2020;287:112917.
46. Schaufeli WB, Bakker AB, Hoogduin K, Schaap C, Kladler A. On the clinical validity of the Maslach Burnout Inventory and the Burnout Measure. Psychol Health. 2001;16(5):565–82.
47. Shuchter SR, Downs N, Zisook S. Biologically informed psychotherapy for depression. Guilford Press; 1996.
48. Pies R. From context to phenomenology in grief versus major depression. Psychiatr Ann. 2013;43(6):286–90.

Risk Detection and Suicide Prevention in the Workplace

Christine Yu Moutier and Maggie G. Mortali

Abbreviations

ACEP	American College of Emergency Physicians
AFSP	American Foundation for Suicide Prevention
AMA	American Medical Association
APA	American Psychiatric Association
FSMB	Federation of State Medical Boards
ISP	Interactive Screening Program
WHO	World Health Organization

Learning Objectives

Upon completion of this chapter, readers will be able to:

1. Describe the prevalence, risk and protective factors of suicide
2. Identify individual and organizational strategies to reduce suicide risk
3. Convey opportunities for future research

Supplementary Information The online version contains supplementary material available at https://doi.org/10.1007/978-3-031-16983-0_24.

C. Y. Moutier (✉) · M. G. Mortali
American Foundation for Suicide Prevention, New York, NY, USA
e-mail: cmoutier@afsp.org; mmortali@afsp.org

© The Author(s), under exclusive license to Springer Nature Switzerland AG 2023
J. E. Davidson, M. Richardson (eds.), *Workplace Wellness: From Resiliency to Suicide Prevention and Grief Management*, https://doi.org/10.1007/978-3-031-16983-0_24

24.1   Presentation of the Science

Suicide is a global health problem. According to the World Health Organization (WHO), over 700,000 people die by suicide every year worldwide [1]. According to the Centers for Disease Control and Prevention (CDC), suicide is currently the tenth leading cause of death in the United States; however, among people of working age (16–64 years), suicide is the fourth leading cause of death [2]. While these numbers change every year, the CDC reports that in 2019, the most recent year for which complete data are available, 47,511 Americans died by suicide, with over 37,000 of those who died by suicide being people of working age [2]. Many of those who die by suicide are employed at the time of death [3].

Suicide rates are known to vary widely across occupational groups; however, data are limited. A 2020 CDC report provides suicide rates by industry and occupational group among working-age decedents [4]. Using data from the 32 states participating in the 2016 National Violent Death Reporting System (NVDRS), suicide rates were significantly higher in six major occupational groups, including: construction and extraction (males: 49.4 per 100,000; females: 25.5 per 100,000); installation, maintenance, and repair (males: 36.9 per 100,000); arts, design, entertainment, sports, and media (males: 32.0 per 100,000); transportation and material moving (males: 30.4 per 100,000; females: 12.5 per 100,000); protective service (females: 14.0 per 100,000); and health care support (females: 10.6 per 100,000) [4]. Data collection and surveillance of suicide to determine suicide rates among specific health disciplines are limited; however, there are clear signals that suicide rates among nurses and physicians (especially female physicians), and veterinarians are elevated when compared with age-matched general population cohorts [5–7].

People who die by suicide represent a fraction of those who consider or attempt suicide. While there is no complete count of suicide attempt data in the United States, since 2008, the National Survey on Drug Use and Health (NSDUH) respondents aged 18 or older have been asked if at any time during the past 12 months they had thought seriously about trying to kill themselves (serious thoughts of suicide). Adults who reported serious thoughts of suicide in the past 12 months were asked whether they made a plan to kill themselves (suicide plan) or tried to kill themselves (suicide attempt) in that period [8]. Among adults aged 18 or older in 2019, 4.8% (or 12.0 million people) thought seriously about trying to kill themselves in the past year, 1.4% (or 3.5 million people) made a suicide plan, 0.6% (or 1.4 million people) made a nonfatal suicide attempt, and 0.1% (or 217,000 people) attempted suicide without a suicide plan [8].

There is no single cause for suicide, but rather there are multiple, intersecting factors that come together to create risk. The multifactorial nature of suicide risk includes biological factors, psychological factors, and social and environmental factors (see Fig. 24.1). However, it is important to note, many risk and protective factors do not fall exclusively into one category. For example, a strong family history of suicide likely indicates genetic, family environment, and psychological risk factors all playing a role in the outcome of multiple suicides within one family.

Fig. 24.1 Interacting risk
and protective factors [9]

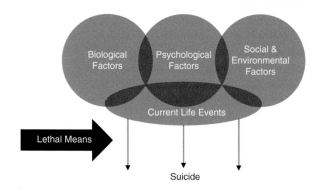

24.1.1 Biological Factors

The first of the three general categories of suicide risk factors are biological in nature—factors that are related to the biological makeup of a person, which can include everything from genes to brain functions like stress response. The most significant risk factors for suicide are chronic mental health conditions which likely arise from a combination of biological, psychological, and environmental factors [10, 11]. When left untreated, mental disorders carry a significant risk of disability and death [12]. Research has shown that 85–95% of people who die by suicide have a diagnosable mental health condition at the time of their death [13].

According to the 2019 National Survey on Drug Use and Health (NSDUH), approximately 51.5 million adults aged 18 or older (20.6% of all US adults) reported experiencing a mental health condition within the past 12 months [8]. Of the 51.5 million adults aged 18 or older who experienced a mental health condition, 23.8 million (61.9%) reported being currently employed (full-time: 23.8 million; part-time: 8.1 million) [8]. In that same year, 13.1 million adults aged 18 or older experienced a serious mental health condition [8]. This number represented 5.2% of all US adults [8].

Despite the prevalence of mental health conditions and suicide risk among adults, approximately two-thirds of people with symptoms of clinical criteria for mental and substance use disorders do not receive treatment [14]. There are a number of reasons people in various occupational groups do not seek treatment. Pervasive social stigma and lack of awareness of resources and their effectiveness are among the most common from keeping employees from seeking care [12]. Professionals with mental health conditions often face work-related discrimination or fear such discrimination—fears such as limits on independence, increase in supervision, jeopardized job-security, or restriction on their career advancement. This often results in individuals taking great lengths to ensure that co-workers and managers do not find out about their mental health conditions, which includes avoiding employee assistance programs and effective treatment options.

Mental health conditions are not the only health factors that are associated with suicide risk. In addition to research in neurophysiology and genetics/epigenetics, early research is finding associations between suicidal behavior and numerous "physical health" areas, including inflammatory, immunological, and gut–brain biome systems. Many chronic conditions such as chronic pain, heart disease, chronic pulmonary disease, traumatic brain injury, and HIV/AIDS are associated with increased suicide risk [15]. These health conditions are not necessarily known to elevate suicide risk in isolation, but rather more likely contribute to suicide risk in combination with other suicide risk factors.

Data shows that physical and mental health of students entering health professions are similar to age-matched controls; however, there is a body of research demonstrating higher rates of various distress, certainly including higher rates of burnout among health professionals across many disciplines, sleep deprivation among clinicians and trainees, and also higher rates of clinical depression, anxiety, PTSD, and other health conditions among health professionals. While one might assume that health professionals would be more likely to seek treatment for mental health and physical health conditions, data show that some health professionals, such as physicians, are actually less likely to seek professional mental health care than the general population. Therefore, reducing barriers to mental health care is one of the clearly established targets for suicide prevention among health professionals.

24.1.2 Psychological Factors

Particular psychological risk factors are also known to increase suicide risk. Traits such as perfectionism, sense of identity as a caregiver to others, or more rigid cognitive style, for example, are shown to contribute to higher risk for suicide. Note that these traits such as diminished ability to tolerate conflict are not a sign of potential suicide risk when considered in isolation. Instead, these risk factors come into play when they intersect with other risk factors and stressors, such as a current major depressive episode or a personal or professional setback or loss.

For some individuals, the psychological impact of transitions in relationship status, occupation, or financial status can diminish one's resilience reserve, which can lead to greater negative impact of other risk factors on mental health and coping, which in turn can lead to a sense of hopelessness and worthlessness that can increase suicide risk. Similarly, individuals experiencing shame and humiliation related to a current stressor—for example, legal or work-related—can have a sense of failure, rejection, and disconnection from their support network.

Among health professionals, there may be psychological traits that contribute to self-selection into the helping and healing professions. Some of these traits may be beneficial during patient care and for academic achievement or career advancement but may actually work against optimizing one's own mental health. Traits such as perfectionism, exaggerated sense of responsibility, eagerness to please others, or difficulty in taking time to process conflict or traumatic events, are examples of psychological traits that have been documented by Glenn Gabbard and Michael Myers related to physicians and other health professionals' reluctance toward self-care [16].

24.1.3 Social and Environmental Factors

Social and environmental factors (including early life trauma, neglect/abuse, or experiences of racial discrimination, and current experiences such as bullying, relationship, and financial or cultural factors) also contribute as risk factors for suicide. Social and environmental factors can also be job-related, such as isolated or demanding occupations, stressful work environments, and work–home imbalance. Any prolonged stress, including harassment, workplace bullying, legal problems, and unemployment, can also serve as social/environmental risk factors. One of the most significant environmental risk factors is access to a method for killing oneself, which is referred to as access to lethal means. Every type of lethal means that has been studied has found similar results: When access to lethal means becomes lessened in almost any way, suicide risk decreases. This is true for methods including the detoxification of the domestic gas supply in the United Kingdom, bans on toxic pesticides in Sri Lanka, and decreases in household firearm ownership in the United States, in which all were followed by significant reductions in method-specific suicides as well as overall suicide rates in these countries [17].

The combination of biological, psychological, social, and environmental risk factors contributes to an individual's risk for suicide. Current life stressors may intersect with a person's underlying risk factors. For example, a person who loses their job (social/environmental) and job-centered identity and self-worth (psychological) may also be experiencing a mental health condition (biological plus) and tend to have inflexible cognition. Therefore, this person may see no way out of the situation. These factors can come together to lead to hopelessness, and a lack of problem solving or hope for the future. This, combined with prolonged occupational stress, paired with access to lethal means, creates a high-risk situation for suicide. Strategic programs and policies can be designed by workplace leaders with their own industry or setting-specific unique features in mind. Proactive approaches that decrease stigma and enhance help-seeking can lead to a mentally healthier workforce.

The environment of both training and practice in health professions has been implicated as a key component in the "set up" for unattended mental health outcomes including suicide risk. Environmental factors related to these outcomes include shaming culture, rationalizing significant distress as "part of the job," perpetuating stigma related to distress or help-seeking, and leadership that is complicit to toxic or harassing behaviors in the workplace or training environment [18]. All of these factors, many of which have been discussed as part of the "hidden curriculum," create an environment that is not conducive to help-seeking, perpetuate outdated, harmful views toward mental health, and which are actively being addressed with new standards by leading organizations such as the AMA, American Psychiatric Association, American Psychological Association, American Nursing Association, and the National Academy of Sciences workgroup on Clinician Wellbeing [19]. Efforts that accentuate protective factors such as sense of community, support, interpersonal connections, and accessing effective mental health care are all evidence-based strategies to decrease suicide risk.

24.1.4 Identifying Suicide Risk and Facilitating Support

A long history of discriminatory practices related to health professionals' mental health have led to overwhelming avoidance of help-seeking based on fear of negative repercussions and avoidance of treatment, even in the face of life-threatening health conditions [18]. Therefore, it is necessary to shift the balance toward methods that encourage safe ways for individuals to recognize signs of distress and to have multiple avenues for dialog, support, and seeking treatment. While screening may seem like an obvious step, great care must be taken to utilize screening methods that prioritize a sense of safety so that mental health distress and suicide risk are not driven underground. Further, safe screening is needed so that the field does not inadvertently take a step backward with regard to the progress going on at the national and local levels related to health professional mental health and suicide prevention.

One program that has evidence for identifying risk and enhancing connection to support is the American Foundation for Suicide Prevention's Interactive Screening Program. Implemented within in a variety of health care settings, the Interactive Screening Program provides a unique method for health professionals and trainees to participate in an anonymous online screening. Using an individualized and interactive approach, a designated program counselor (assigned by the health care setting) reviews participant questionnaires and posts a confidential response on the secure program website, which participants can retrieve using their self-assigned user ID and password. Via the program website, participants have the option of exchanging online dialogue messages with the counselor and are encouraged to set up an appointment or referral to meet with a counselor in person. Among the many approaches to address health professional and trainee well-being and suicide prevention, the Interactive Screening Program seeks to reduce individuals' barriers to help-seeking by connecting them to a counselor who can "meet" individuals where they are, process their concerns or assumptions about the implications of getting help, and engage them into mental health services. While this program is not a clinical intervention, it has been demonstrated to have high rates of engagement and enhancing motivation and readiness for high-risk individuals to engage in mental health services. In one study of the program, among 6115 health professionals who voluntarily took the screening questionnaire, 30% engaged in dialogue with the program coordinator, 17% endorsed current suicidal ideation, plans, or behaviors, and 85% of them were not in treatment [20]. Many health institutions are reporting success with the Interactive Screening Program in reaching those who would otherwise be suffering in silence to engage in dialogue and/or treatment.

Please see Sect. 24.2 for practical suggestions to create a culture of safety/support that can contribute to suicide prevention.

24.2   Application of Principles into Wellness Practice

24.2.1 Pre-Licensure Application in the Academic Environment

- Review and update policies of the academic institution to optimally reduce trainees' real and perceived barriers to help-seeking, support, and mental health treatment.
- Maximize access for students/trainees to mentorship, support, and mental health care without punitive consequences, e.g., build in debriefs following critical incidents, encourage therapy, and to optimize resilience, allow for access to treatment within and outside of the home institution when feasible.
- Be transparent about institutional policies and procedures; communicate clearly about how trainee challenges are handled.
- Prioritize and promote a growth mindset: e.g., *"Every professional and trainee struggles at times. It is a sign of strength to address challenges. It is commendable not to wait until the point of crisis to get help."*
- Continuously provide information about how trainees and staff can access support, guidance, and mental health treatment. Resources can be listed on the back of ID cards, on program websites, etc.
- Introduce self-care early in the curriculum as a practice linked to professionalism that can be cultivated throughout one's career.
- Model mental health literacy by disclosing human struggles when appropriate, and by mentioning that we as leaders regularly lean on others for support or treatment. Provide opportunities for storytelling to set new norms with hopeful narratives for addressing struggles.
- Enhance peer support by teaching trainees how to reach out and respond to distressed peers, cultivate active listening skills, and utilize available resources for support.

24.2.2 Clinical Application Post-Licensure

- Cultivate daily habits of self-care by being curious and learning about the internal and external factors in your life that lead to improved resilience or deterioration in mental health. Practice the activities that lead to positive outcomes.
- Realize that mental health is a dynamic part of human health for each of us, which means we can have some influence over our own mental health outcomes, e.g., staying on effective treatment for depression or anxiety is an obvious way to positively impact mental health.
- Do not fall prey to assuming that accomplished peers have it together and do not ever struggle; check in on your strong friends.

344

- Look out for your colleagues; realize that subtle changes in behavior can be the "tip of the iceberg" indicating more significant struggles beneath the surface.
- Learn how to have caring conversations with peers that invite deeper disclosure.
- When dialoguing with a distressed colleague, remember with distress comes negative cognitive distortions, so it is important to state the obvious: that you respect them, think well of them for getting help, are willing to help them connect with treatment, and will continue to be there for them. If you have struggled previously, you may have special empathy that can be marshalled to help them understand they are not alone.

24.2.3 Leadership Application (Structural and Organizational Considerations)

- Develop initiatives for staff and trainees that safely address barriers to addressing suicide risk and mental health concerns, e.g., the Interactive Screening Program of the American Foundation for Suicide Prevention, now implemented by academic institutions, health systems, and even state professional associations [20].
- Follow the recommendations of the FSMB, AMA, APA, ACEP, and others to refrain from asking questions in licensing and privileging processes about health professionals' mental health [21–24]. This practice of asking intrusive questions about diagnoses and treatment history has been shown to be an ineffective way to detect impairment and protect public safety; it is also at odds with the American with Disabilities Act in many instances [25]. Moreover, intrusive questioning drives treatable health issues underground and prevents scores of health professionals from accessing effective treatment that *can*, in fact, protect both patient safety and the health and careers of the providers themselves [18]. Policy changes at a national level to stop asking these questions during licensing and privileging is a critical step in dismantling a toxic infrastructure that has perpetuated fear of getting help for too long. In 2021, the American Medical Association released a brief endorsing the elimination of mental health questions from licensing and reaccreditation procedures (https://www.ama-assn.org/print/pdf/node/77416).
- Institutions can develop a suicide response (postvention) plan prior to a suicide occurring. If the institution already has a protocol for death of a trainee/employee, take steps to ensure it specifically addresses suicide. There are some unique aspects of suicide loss that require consideration to facilitate healthy grieving and mitigate potential for suicide contagion. Having a plan in place will facilitate a coordinated response by a team of individuals who can support each other. Toolkits with this specialized guidance are freely available for download to guide leaders for postvention response after suicide [26].

24.3 Opportunities for Future Research

While the literature is clear about overall levels of distress including burnout, depressive symptoms, anxiety, and suicidal thoughts being generally higher among several health disciplines than the general population, data is lacking in the following areas:

- Suicide rates among most health disciplines are mostly unknown due to lack of research and surveillance efforts. Suicide surveillance is improving in the United States for the general population, but occupational data is imprecise. Developing systematic suicide surveillance mechanisms for various occupational and trainee populations would fill a gap in the science and surveillance related to suicide risk. For example, to date, there is no systematic surveillance of US medical student suicides.
- While many suicide risk factors are well demonstrated among health professionals, research should focus on protective factors and prevention efforts.
- Suicide preventive programmatic efforts (policies, programs, and education) warrant greater attention to evidence-informed development as well as evaluation of outcomes.
- Given the increased risk of suicide especially among nurses and women physicians, more information about specific risks and interventions for these populations is warranted.
- Intersectionality such as racial, gender, and sexual minority identities among health care professionals warrants further research in terms of suicide risk and prevention.

Glossary

AFSP The American Foundation for Suicide Prevention (AFSP) is the leading voluntary health organization that gives those affected by suicide a nationwide community empowered by research, education, and advocacy to take action against this leading cause of death.

ISP The Interactive Screening Program (ISP) is an online program utilized by mental health services at institutions of higher education, including medical and professional degree schools, hospitals and health systems, law enforcement agencies, and organizations and workplaces through their Employee Assistance Programs (EAPs).

Discussion Questions

1. Suicide is clearly not the result of just one thing in any instance. What did you learn about risk factors for suicide in this chapter?
2. How do these suicide risk factors potentially impact people in health professions?
3. Distressing experiences such as depression, anxiety, and suicidal thoughts are more prevalent among some groups of health professionals who have been studied, than in the general population. Does this resonate with your experience?
4. Are there protective factors for suicide risk as well?
5. What are some of the barriers—institutional or individual—for health professionals to open up and proactively address mental health concerns?
6. Are there examples of programs or groups you are aware of that are contributing to improvements in culture around mental health and suicide prevention?

Discussion Leader Guide

Prepare to lead a discussion on the topic of health worker/trainee suicide prevention:

Know that in any group, there are individuals who have been personally touched by suicide. Suicide loss, lived experience of a suicidal struggle or attempt, and/or having a loved one who struggled are common experiences. Acknowledge these experiences as a potential part of the group's collective experience.

You can start by saying something like:

"We know that science is growing, providing more knowledge related to suicide risk and prevention. Suicide, while complex, is a health issue. We need to be able to discuss mental health and suicide prevention in our own profession to make improvements. Each of us in this occupation are human beings with our own family histories, early experiences, health, and environmental impacts.

We can each exert an influence on the environment around us and help create a culture of safety and support within the spaces where we work and live. And we need to learn the facts to do that best. Suicide is not a one-cause effect phenomenon as there are many risk factors that influence suicide. There are many opportunities to make a difference to reduce suicide risk. We also know that many people (55% in AFSP's most recent Harris poll) are personally touched by suicide. Many of us may have experienced the loss of a family member, friend, patient, or colleague to suicide. We may also know people who have struggled—past or present—with suicidal thoughts or attempts. And we ourselves may have experienced mental health struggles. And so, to make progress in this important health issue, let us engage in a discussion to learn more about the issue. Please be aware that others in the group may have had experiences that make this topic sensitive, and we want to ensure that the discussion is a supportive environment where everyone has a chance to contribute."

- Use language that is up-to-date related to suicide.
- Avoid the phrase "commit suicide" since it connotes a morally reprehensible act rather than a complex health outcome. Instead, use the term "died by suicide" or other plain language phrases.
- Avoid calling suicide attempts "successful" or "failed." The term "suicide attempt" is clear on its own to express that the person did not die by suicide.
- Avoid other pejorative language such as "manipulative attempt" or "gesture."
- Be specific about the term "survivor." To indicate someone who was bereaved by suicide, the terms "suicide loss survivor" or "suicide bereaved" are recommended. To indicate someone who has survived an attempt, use the term "suicide attempt survivor" or a person with "lived experience of suicide" (which usually indicates a history of suicide attempt but can also include experience of loss).
- Learn more at afsp.org/hcp.
  - On this web page you can review FAQs on physician, nurse, and veterinarian mental health and suicide prevention to prepare for questions and discussion.
  - Consider showing the 4-min short film *Make the Difference: Preventing Medical Trainee Suicide* as part of an educational session.
  - Become familiar with suicide postvention; consider utilizing some of the messaging templates and tips from "AFSP's After Suicide" toolkits in your presentation/discussion.

Video for Discussion - Instructional Video: The online version contains supplementary material available at https://doi.org/10.1007/978-3-031-16983-0_24

References

1. World Health Organization. Suicide. Geneva: WHO; 2020. https://www.who.int/health-topics/suicide. Accessed 1 Nov 2021
2. Centers for Disease Control and Prevention. Injury prevention & control. Atlanta: CDC; 2016. https://www.cdc.gov/injury/wisqars/fatal.html. Accessed 1 Nov 2021
3. Yip PS, Caine ED. Employment status and suicide: the complex relationships between changing unemployment rates and death rates. J Epidemiol Community Health. 2011;65(8):4.
4. Centers for Disease Control and Prevention. Suicide rates by industry and occupation. National violent death reporting system, 32 states, 2016. Atlanta: CDC; 2020. https://wwwcdcgov/mmwr/volumes/69/wr/pdfs/mm6903a1-Hpdf. Accessed 1 Nov 2021
5. Davidson JE, Proudfoot J, Lee K, Zisook S. Nurse suicide in the United States: analysis of the Center for Disease Control 2014 National Violent Death Reporting System dataset. Arch Psychiatr Nurs. 2019;33(5):16–21. https://doi.org/10.1016/j.apnu.2019.04.006.
6. Duarte D, El-Hagrassy MM, Couto TCE, Gurgel W, Fregni F, Correa H. Male and female physician suicidality: a systematic review and meta-analysis. JAMA Psychiat. 2020;77(6):587–97. https://doi.org/10.1001/jamapsychiatry.2020.0011.
7. Witte TK, Spitzer EG, Edwards N, Fowler KA, Nett RJ. Suicides and deaths of undetermined intent among veterinary professionals from 2003 through 2014. J Am Vet Med Assoc. 2019;255(5):595–608. https://doi.org/10.2460/javma.255.5.595.
8. Center for Behavioral Health Statistics and Quality. Results from the 2019 National Survey on Drug Use and Health: detailed tables. Rockville: SAMHSA; 2020. https://www.samhsa.gov/data/ Accessed 1 Nov 2021

9. Moutier CY, Pisani AR, Stahl SM, editors. Suicide prevention, Stahl's handbooks. Cambridge: Cambridge University Press; 2021.
10. Kessler RC, Borges G, Walters EE. Prevalence of and risk factors for lifetime suicide attempts in the National Comorbidity Survey. Arch Gen Psychiatry. 1999;56(7):10.
11. Nock MK, Borges G, Bromet EJ, Alonso J, Angermeyer M, Beautrais A, Bruffaerts R, Chiu WT, de Girolamo G, Gluzman S, de Graaf R, Gureje O, Haro JM, Huang Y, Karam E, Kessler RC, Lepine JP, Levinson D, Medina-Mora ME, Ono Y, Posada-Villa J, Williams D. Cross-national prevalence and risk factors for suicidal ideation, plans and attempts. Br J Psychiatry. 2008;192(2):98–105. https://doi.org/10.1192/bjp.bp.107.040113.
12. World Health Organization. Preventing suicide: a resource at work. Geneva: WHO; 2006.
13. Cavanagh JT, Carson AJ, Sharpe M, Lawrie SM. Psychological autopsy studies of suicide: a systematic review. Psychol Med. 2003;33(3):395–405. https://doi.org/10.1017/s0033291702006943. Erratum in: Psychol Med 2003;33(5):947
14. Wang PS, Simon GE, Avorn J, Azocar F, Ludman EJ, McCulloch J, Petukhova MZ, Kessler RC. Telephone screening, outreach, and care management for depressed workers and impact on clinical and work productivity outcomes: a randomized controlled trial. JAMA. 2007;298(12):1401–11. https://doi.org/10.1001/jama.298.12.1401.
15. Ahmedani BK, Peterson EL, Hu Y, Rossom RC, Lynch F, Lu CY, Waitzfelder BE, Owen-Smith AA, Hubley S, Prabhakar D, Williams LK, Zeld N, Mutter E, Beck A, Tolsma D, Simon GE. Major physical health conditions and risk of suicide. Am J Prev Med. 2017;53(3):308–15. https://doi.org/10.1016/j.amepre.2017.04.001.
16. Myers MF, Gabbard GO. The physician as patient: a clinical handbook for mental health professionals. Arlington: American Psychiatric Publishing; 2008.
17. Gunnell D, Miller M. Strategies to prevent suicide. BMJ. 2010;341:2.
18. Moutier C. Physician mental health: an evidence-based approach to change. J Med Regul. 2018;104(2):7.
19. Moutier CY, Myers MF, Feist JB, Feist JC, Zisook S. Preventing clinician suicide: a call to action during the COVID-19 pandemic and beyond. Acad Med. 2021;96(5):624–8. https://doi.org/10.1097/ACM.0000000000003972.
20. Mortali M, Moutier C. Facilitating help-seeking behavior among medical trainees and physicians using the interactive screening program. J Med Regul. 2018;104(2):27–36.
21. Federation of State Medical Boards. Policy on physician wellness and burnout. Euless: FSMB; 2018. https://www.fsmb.org/siteassets/advocacy/policies/policy-on-wellness-and-burnout.pdf. Accessed 1 Jan 2021
22. American Medical Association. Policy on access to confidential health services for medical students and physicians H-295.858. Chicago: AMA; 2019. https://policysearch.ama-assn.org/policyfinder/detail/physician%20suicide?uri=%2FAMADoc%2FHOD-295.858.xml. Accessed 2 Jan 2021
23. American Psychiatric Association (2015) APA official action: position statement on inquiries about diagnosis and treatment of mental disorders in connection with professional credentialing and licensing. https://www.psychiatry.org/File%20Library/About-APA/Organization-Documents-Policies/Policies/Position-2015-Inquiries-about-Diagnosis-and-Treatment-of-Mental-Disorders-in-Connection-with-Professional-Credentialing-and-Licensing.pdf. Accessed 7 Jan 2021
24. American College of Emergency Physicians (2020) Mental health and emergency medical experts encourage support for clinicians health during pandemic. https://www.emergency-physicians.org/press-releases/2020/6-2-20-mental-health-and-emergency-medical-experts-encourage-support-forclinicians-health-during-pandemic Accessed Jan 2, 2021
25. Jones JTR, North CS, Vogel-Scibilia S, Myers MF, Owen RR. Medical licensure questions about mental illness and compliance with the americans with disabilities act. J Am Acad Psychiatry Law. 2018;46(4):458–71. https://doi.org/10.29158/JAAPL.003789-18.
26. Dyrbye L, Konopasek L, Moutier C, for the American Foundation for Suicide Prevention. After a suicide: a toolkit for physician residency/fellowship programs. https://www.datocms-assets.com/12810/1578318836-after-a-suicide-a-toolkit-for-physician-residency-fellowship-program.pdf. Accessed Oct 11, 2021

Identifying and Intervening with a Suicidal Colleague

25

Sharon Tucker

Learning Objectives
1. Review the evidence for suicide risk assessment to identify an individual in suicidal crisis.
2. Discuss key elements of providing mental health first aid for a clinician or peer in distress, including self-care for the helper.
3. Cultivate confidence in crisis intervention strategies demonstrated to assist a person in crisis.

25.1 Presentation of the Science

25.1.1 Introduction

The reality of burnout, increased perceived and actual stress levels, anxiety, depression, and substance abuse among healthcare clinicians demand vigilance to the possibility of suicidality and/or suicide ideations among overwhelmed healthcare staff. The actual prediction of who will go on to attempt suicide or end their life by suicide is challenging given the dynamic nature of suicidal thoughts and research method limitations [1]. The ideal method of assessment would be to conduct a prospective study monitoring all individuals screened for suicide ideation and follow

---

Supplementary Information The online version contains supplementary material available at https://doi.org/10.1007/978-3-031-16983-0_25.

S. Tucker (✉)
College of Nursing, The Ohio State University, Columbus, OH, USA
e-mail: tucker.701@osu.edu

them long-term. This would require a multisite, longitudinal, multistate, or national study given that the base rate of suicide is low (thankfully). Even then, given the dynamic nature of suicidal thoughts and individual risk factors, constant assessment and vigilance is needed for someone in mental health distress. *As a non-mental health clinician helping a colleague in mental health distress, your role is to provide empathic listening, keep them safe, and get them connected with professional mental healthcare as soon as possible.*

In this chapter, readers will find a review of latest research findings concerning suicide risk assessment, prevention, and intervention. This includes review of evidence-based suicide prevention training programs that can guide non-mental health experts and healthcare leaders in identification of someone in distress and strategies for approaching and helping them.

This chapter concludes with discussion of strategies for self-care of the helper in managing suicidal crises.

25.1.2 Suicide Assessment, Prevention, and Intervention State of the Science

As discussed in earlier chapters in this book, suicide rates in the United States (US) have continued to climb since the turn of the century, while they have been declining in most other countries [2]. This is alarming given the major research and prevention programs that have been implemented. Predicting suicide is highly challenging given the complexity for any individual person as well as the reality that suicide prevention is hard to study. Instruments and approaches to suicide assessment are important for aiding a clinician who might be in a suicidal crisis. Understanding the state of the science in these areas can offer non-mental health experts insights about suicide risk assessment and prevention.

Instruments for the assessment of suicide risk have been examined, yet studies are of low quality making it difficult to draw conclusions to determine sufficient diagnostic accuracy [3]. Nelson et al. (2017) conducted a systematic review of suicide risk assessment and prevention among veterans [4]. They evaluated 19 studies that used 19 different approaches and found fair or better diagnostic accuracy for most methods, but most had high rates of false positives and many of the studies included methodological limitations making applicability of findings weak. Nonetheless, the commonly used in clinical practice 9-item Patient Health Questionnaire (PHQ-9) that includes a suicide ideation question was associated with 75% increased risk of suicide in a sample of nearly 400,000 VA patients [5].

Given the challenges in rigorously studying suicide assessment and prevention, recent research has applied sophisticated models using population-level data and machine learning to evaluate whether identification of risk factors can be improved for suicide prevention. For example, Belsher et al. (2019) conducted a systematic review evaluating the diagnostic accuracy of suicide prevention models in predicting suicide attempts and suicide [6]. Reviewing 17 papers that met inclusion criteria with high quality, they concluded that the accuracy of predicting an event is near zero. Whiting and Fazel evaluated three systematic reviews that examined suicide risk assessment current tools and models derived from machine learning approaches, one of which was the Beshler et al. review [7]. Whiting and Fazel argued that while there are indeed limitations to predictive models, it is important to consider use of machine learning with clinician assessment. That is, perhaps machine learning tools can guide risk stratification and aid clinical decision-making that can improve efficiency and consistency in real world settings that have a finite pool of mental health resources. Such approaches can also anchor assessments with evidence and improve clinician confidence and time to focus on interventions where most needed.

Doupnik et al. (2020) completed a systematic review and meta-analysis to examine the association of brief acute care suicide prevention interventions with patient subsequent suicide attempts, linkages to follow-up care and depression symptoms at follow-up [8]. These interventions included brief encounters such as telephone calls, post-cards, and letters; care coordination; safety planning interventions; and other brief therapies. Safety planning interventions included: (1) identifying personalized warning signs; (2) determining coping strategies to counter suicidal thoughts; (3) identifying support persons and places that can help distract from thoughts and provide support; (4) listing mental health resources including crisis locations; and (5) counseling on environmental safety including eliminating lethal means. Fourteen studies were included in the review, representing 4270 patients. Findings indicated that brief suicide prevention interventions were associated with reduced subsequent suicide attempts and increased linkages to follow-up care, but not associated with reduced depression symptoms at follow-up. These findings indicated that a single in-person encounter focused on safety planning may be effective in reducing future suicide attempts and getting individuals into mental healthcare for more comprehensive assessment and treatment.

Researchers are beginning to expand the standard suicide risk assessments of "are you suicidal or thinking of killing yourself" and "what is your plan" and bringing contemporary and changing recommendations for suicide risk assessment. There are multiple reasons for this including that we do not seem to be reversing the suicide rates in the US with the current approaches and with other evidence about the dynamic nature of suicidality, the complexity of suicidal cognitions [8, 9], and what individuals reveal and to whom about suicidal thoughts [10]. Craig Bryan, PhD, a psychologist in the Department of Psychiatry and Behavioral Health at The Ohio State University, is a leader in this work, which grew from his experiences with military and veteran populations. Bryan outlines limitations with traditional suicide risk assessment approaches, instead pointing out three major factors that invite a different approach to suicide risk assessment. Consider these three factors when approaching and intervening with a clinician in acute mental distress.

1. First, be informed that suicide risk is dynamic and changes constantly.
2. Second, suicide risk can be sudden and also discontinuous. Data indicate that over 50% of suicide decedents deny suicide ideation or do not share suicidal thoughts in the time leading up to their deaths. Thus, the belief that there are always warning signs may be misguided in preventing suicide and can leave survivors with much guilt.

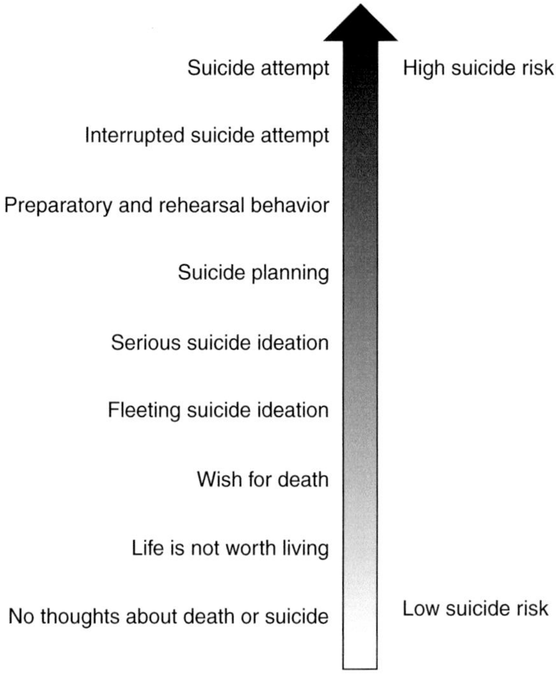

Fig. 25.1 Low-to-high
suicide risk behaviors

Suicide attempt — High suicide risk

Interrupted suicide attempt

Preparatory and rehearsal behavior

Suicide planning

Serious suicide ideation

Fleeting suicide ideation

Wish for death

Life is not worth living

No thoughts about death or suicide — Low suicide risk

3. Third, suicidal thinking is heterogeneous, and there is not one-way that individuals in crisis think. Suicide cognitions that relate to suicide ideations indeed vary from person to person and may be a better predictor of a future suicide attempt. Thoughts such as "It is unbearable when I get this upset" or "I don't deserve to live another moment" are examples of concerning thoughts that need to be explored in clinicians who appear in distress. An individual may deny they are having suicidal thoughts but may be having these cognitions that may progress to suicidal thoughts and behavior.

Bryan also presents that there are distinct differences between someone at high vs low risk of suicide (see Fig. 25.1). Thus, thinking of suicidal behaviors on a continuum of low to high risk of suicide may be more effective than the dichotomous "suicidal" or "not suicidal." This type of perspective can guide work with clinicians in distress through a thoughtful discussion of their thoughts and behaviors, past and present.

Bryan and Rudd [9] present a framework for suicide risk assessment that helps generate a profile that can guide understanding level of risk for suicide and immediate steps forward. This framework includes thinking about factors that can cumulatively increase the stress one is facing coupled with their internal capabilities and external resources that can increase or decrease the amount of distress that could lead to suicidal behavior. Factors include:

1. Baseline risk factors such as prior attempts
2. Activating events such as relationship or financial problems

3. Symptoms such as guilt or depression
4. Suicide-specific beliefs such as hopelessness or thinking of oneself as a burden
5. Impulse control and dysregulation such as non-suicidal self-harm or alcohol use
6. Protective factors such as reasons for living and hope

These factors can be assessed when assisting a clinician in distress. For example, take a clinician with a history of depression and past suicide attempt who has made a medical error that led to patient harm. She is on unpaid leave while the case is being investigated and she is feeling great guilt, fear, and anxiety which add to her depression. She is worried about her job and license and is drinking to numb her anxiety and depression. She is divorced, living alone and has limited hope for the future. She stops into the manager's office to be interviewed again. This presents an opportunity for an assessment given the multiple stress factors that would raise concerns and a need to intervene with this nurse to prevent a suicide attempt.

It is now known that both physicians and nurses have more job-related problems known prior to death by suicide than others. These job-related problems are often tied to job loss or the threat of losing a job or license due to mental health issues that are uncontrolled, uncontrolled pain leading to job loss, or substance use and investigations [11, 12].

25.1.3 Recommendations for Crisis Intervention with Clinicians in Suicidal Distress

Major Points for Intervening in a Potential Suicidal Crisis
1. Understand that suicidal thoughts are dynamic and occur in persons feeling very alone and isolated in a moment. They may also feel very ambivalent, and their thoughts and emotions could change in a moment.
   (a) Repeated assessment is important in an acute crisis period; including after the person appears stabilized until next steps are initiated.
2. Note patterns of suicide cognitions, suicide-related thoughts and if they are increasing.
3. Be informed that people who are suicidal may have a very narrow lens in the moment where they are not perceiving that living is better than dying. They may be in incredibly significant mental and emotional pain and cannot see a way out of it.

25.1.4 Actions for Intervening in a Potential Suicidal Crisis [10, 13]

Step 1: Build a Therapeutic Alliance With a Person in Crisis
1. Use active listening.
2. Ask the person in distress about their situation, showing empathy and compassion, and an authentic desire to understand their experience (see Fig. 25.2 for example questions to ask).

- Tell me about your thoughts of suicide. How long have these been going on? Have you acted on these right now?
- What has recently happened that brings you to suicidal thoughts?
- What feelings are you having right now?
- How do you feel physically in your body?
- How are you managing your suicide thoughts? How about in the past?
- Have you ever acted on these thoughts and tried to kill yourself?
- Do you have any plans to kill yourself? Tell me about those.
- Do you have access to firearms, medicines that could kill you?
- Who is most important to you and supports you? Do they know about your suicidal thoughts?
- What are some reasons to be hopeful and to stay alive? What makes your life worth living?
- What things would you like to change in your life?
- What has helped you in the past when you have struggled?
- How can I best help?

Fig. 25.2 Possible questions to assess a peer/staff person for suicidality

3. Ask them about their thoughts, what they are experiencing and feeling, and what the hardest thing is for them right now.
4. Ask direct questions about suicidal thoughts.
   (a) Given what you are experiencing right now, I wonder if you have had any thoughts of killing yourself?
   (b) Or, that you would be better off dead?
   (c) Sometimes with the stress and the hopelessness people experience, they may see the only solution is suicide. What about you?
5. Assure them you are not leaving as you care and are deeply concerned about their safety.
6. Convey hope—there are options even though they cannot see them right now; ask them to give life a chance and share that the fact that they are still alive shows they are not sure, and that life may still have a chance.
   (a) I can see things have been very challenging for you lately.
   (b) It seems that you have really been struggling.
   (c) It has to be frustrating to be going through your experience.
7. Be willing to be present no matter what the individual says unless there is a threat to your safety; then seek emergency assistance.
8. Plan to solicit additional resources to help such as managers, directors, security, and emergency room help.
9. Be aware of your attitudes about suicide and how they may impact your ability to help.
10. Know that your beliefs may differ from those of the person in crisis and the goal is not to change beliefs but to honor them as you are able while protecting the safety of the person in crisis.

Step 2: Identify Risk Factors to Guide Step 3

As a non-mental health clinician, *you are not responsible for determining level of risk* but knowing what is going on with the person in the moment through talking with them and being an active listener can give some direction about what the safest next step is.

1. Baseline risk factors such as prior attempts
2. Activating events such as relationship, job, or financial problems
3. Symptoms such as guilt or depression
4. Suicide-specific beliefs such as hopelessness or thinking of oneself as a burden
5. Impulse control and dysregulation such as non-suicidal self-harm or alcohol use
6. Protective factors such as reasons for living and hope
7. Withdrawal from friends/family
8. *Access to lethal means…, e.g., substances or firearms (major concern)*
9. Poor reasoning/judgment
10. Recent dramatic change in mood
11. Other illnesses and treatment adherence
12. Ethnicity, gender, race or cultural risk group (any group that may feel marginalized, minoritized, or stigmatized with resulting social isolation could have increased risk)
13. Family history
14. Trauma experience
15. Hallucinations
16. Recent admission/ED visit
17. Disability or impairment
18. Information from family/friends lending concern
19. Circle of support
20. Housing situation

Step 3: Decide on a Plan Forward

1. Call family/friend to be with person
2. Have person call suicide hotline with you present, for additional assessment and expertise in hotline assessment
3. Take the person to the emergency room if you are at a hospital or call 911
4. Call security if any threats to harm self or others

Know that some people die by suicide no matter what others do to try and the degree of help received. This can be very traumatizing for all involved. Seeking help for processing this trauma may be essential to the individuals who tried to help and the coworkers of the person who has died. Group process debriefing is advocated and a sign of caring in leadership when organized [14].

These videos can help you to learn the skills of identifying a colleague at risk and holding a discussion that will lead to accessing mental health treatment (Video 25.1).

25.1.4.1 Self-Care for the Helper/Intervener

It is essential to pause after helping a staff member of clinician through a suicidal crisis, regardless of the outcome [15, 16]. Working with someone in a mental distress crisis is highly emotionally charged and can initiate a major stress response that needs debriefing and de-escalation for the helper. A number of recommended strategies can help take care of the helper.

1. Focus on what you as a helper did, not what you did not. While natural to think about what happened and what you might have done differently, such thoughts can create stress and anxiety. Whatever you were able to offer the person in crisis is positive and meant to support the person.
2. Give yourself space to feel emotions. A gamut of emotions during and after the incident are likely. You may also feel physically exhausted given the stress response and chemicals released. Whatever you feel is natural and acceptable and can just be accepted without judgment. Follow up with a professional is indicated when distress does not go away.
3. Set boundaries for yourself, whether you have to say no to opportunities/invitations or reduce some of your current demands, so that you can meet your needs for well-being.
4. Share your emotions, thoughts, and experience with others you trust and feel safe with. Again, you might well have a lot of mixed feelings and thoughts and whatever is present can be processed with others. Sometimes just saying the words aloud can help immensely.
5. Remember that you are not responsible for the outcome; this is shared by many. Do not take on this burden. Use others to debrief and share your experience.
6. Make time for yourself. Do something that helps you feel relaxed, nurtured, and cared for and/or that you enjoy. This will differ from person to person. Examples include: taking a walk in nature, listening to music, journal, taking a hot bath, treat self to a massage or other relaxing therapy, drinking some tea, exercise, meditate, or allow yourself to nap. Remember that having fun and laughing are normal human experiences that reduce stress and bring peace and joy.
7. Consider your lifestyle and what behaviors can help support your health and well-being: quality nutrition, adequate exercise and sleep, clarity about purpose, doing leisure activities, spending time with friends and family, moderating use of alcohol and other drugs, nurturing spirit/soul/faith, and engaging in your community.
8. Know that seeking professional counseling to help process the incident and your experience is normal. Secondary trauma following crisis intervention can be overwhelming and require professional help to process.

25.2 Application of Principles into Wellness Practice

25.2.1 Pre-Licensure Application in the Academic Environment

Students at the undergraduate and graduate level consistently report suicidal thoughts and behaviors. Faculty and staff who work with healthcare students can bring important assessment and communication skills to prevent suicide and help identify treatment and support for underlying mental health conditions. While the stressors may be different between students and clinicians, as well as the available resources, the assessments and crisis intervention will be the same. The vulnerability of the student may also implicate the types of actions an intervener might take. For example, a student who is in danger of self-harm may need to have their parents contacted, depending on federal, state and school laws and policies, regardless of whether the student consents to this or not. The important concepts will be to collaborate with the student, demonstrate empathy and active listening, and avoid judgmental statements. Promoting overall safety, functioning, recovery, and sense of well-being are key elements to suicide assessment and intervention. Faculty need to be aware of institution-specific resources for crisis intervention and counseling and add these contacts to their phones for ease of referral. Holding group forums to emotionally process difficult situations exposed to during clinical rotations will support the whole cohort of students. Milestones such as the first death, the first death of a patient similar to oneself, the first exposure to violence from a patient or family all warrant acknowledgment with support from academic colleagues.

25.2.2 Clinical Application Post-licensure

Over the past 10 years, a growing body of evidence and awareness has emerged regarding the mental health of licensed clinicians. Stress, long hours, competing demands, and burnout have become recognized as major consequences for clinicians with suicide as one emerging crisis. Depression, anxiety, and substance abuse are growing problems in clinicians requiring a call to action at the national level. The National Academy of Medicine released a report in 2019 titled *Taking action against clinician burnout: A systems approach to professional well-being.* This report puts forward that clinician burnout is a strong signal that the nation's healthcare system is failing to achieve its aims for system-wide improvement and advocates for positive, healthy work and learning environments to support the professional well-being recognized as essential to the therapeutic alliance among clinicians, patients, and families in delivering high quality healthcare. Promoting well-being of clinicians includes suicide assessment, prevention, and intervention when relevant. Take the time to participate in risk screening if offered by your organization. Request and attend emotional process debriefings following significant events in the workplace. Participate in workplace wellness activities to bolster resilience. Take action when you see a colleague in distress using the steps outlined above.

25.2.3 Leadership Application (Structural and Organizational Considerations)

A model for suicide prevention in the US has been proposed by the National Alliance for Suicide Prevention [17]. This model is called the Zero Suicide (ZS) Model and offers an integrated, system-wide strategy for suicide prevention. The model includes four clinical care components: Identify, Engage, Treat, and Transition; and three administrative components: Lead, Train, and Improve. The model offers a framework for clinical care: Assess, Intervene, and Monitor for Suicide Prevention (AIM-SP). Within the three elements of AIM are 10 steps. These steps recommend active assessment of ideations and behaviors; identification of risk factors: focus on safety; develop a collaborative safety plan; facilitate coping behaviors; implement specific suicide-specific targets in treatment; increase monitoring; involve social support; and enlist clinician support. Organizations are being called to offer integrated programs such as this to enhance employee and patient well-being and safety.

Two additional programs for training in mental health crisis intervention that would prepare individuals in healthcare settings are *Mental Health First Aid* and *Gatekeeper Programs.* Each of these are briefly reviewed.

25.2.3.1 Mental Health First Aid

Several strategies can help healthcare organizations and individuals be prepared to help a clinician or healthcare staff member who is in psychological distress and at risk for suicide. *Mental Health First Aid (MHFA)* is a course that teaches how to identify, understand, and respond to signs and symptoms of mental illnesses including substance use disorders. Individuals who attend training learn knowledge, skills, and approaches to help persons in distress or approaching a crisis [18]. The program originated in Australia in 2000 created by Betty Kitchener, an educator and mental health consumer, and Anthony Jorm, a mental health literacy researcher. It was adopted by the US in 2008, one of the 24 countries delivering MHFA across the globe. In 2021, the MHFA program changed its name to Mental Health First Aid from the National Council for Mental Wellbeing. The key approach of MHFA is the use of the ALGEE mnemonic:

A = Approach, assess for risk of suicide or harm
L = Listen nonjudgmentally
G = Give reassurance and information
E = Encourage appropriate professional help
E = Encourage self-help and other support strategies

Becoming trained and certified in MHFA provides a foundation for identifying, responding to and helping a clinician in distress.

25.2.3.2   Gatekeeper Training for Suicide Prevention

The gatekeeper programs emerge from the idea that certain individuals in a community can be influential to community health and well-being because they have face-to-face contact with a large number of community members as part of their usual routine. Gatekeepers may be trained as people who identify individuals at risk for suicide. These roles can be found in the military and several civilian sectors. For example, many schools have someone deemed a gatekeeper for identifying youth at risk. Military programs have provided some evidence of effects of gatekeeper programs on suicidal ideation, suicide attempts, and death by suicide [19]. The RAND corporation conducted an extensive review of gatekeeper training programs for suicide prevention [20]. They concluded the following:

1. Evidence exists for the effectiveness of these programs for improving knowledge, beliefs/attitudes, self-efficacy, and reluctance to intervene.
2. The transfer of these attributes to actual intervention behavior is, however, unstudied.
3. Individual and contextual factors may influence gatekeeper behavior.
4. More research is needed on the success of gatekeeper programs for suicide.

Leaders have the responsibility to set up the structure and resources for risk screening, referral, and non-punitive treatment of those who need mental health resources. Knowing that job-loss, threat of unemployment, and threat or actual loss of license are risk factors for physician and nurse suicide, it is important that leaders identify and refer those at risk during involuntary job transitions. New systems/processes may need to be put into place to routinely add suicide risk screening to the process of job termination. Preserving employment while on leave (vs. termination) during treatment for mental health issues may reduce the risk of suicide.

25.3   Opportunities for Future Research

Multiple research opportunities exist in the space of crisis intervention for suicide prevention. As presented in this chapter, there are changing models for how suicide assessment and risk can be approached. These models build on past research and need continued testing to demonstrate reduction in national suicide rates. Specific programs such as MHFA and Gatekeeper need additional research, particularly in how the programs affect suicide ideation, suicide attempts, and deaths by suicide. Research is needed to identify best practices for suicide prevention in the healthcare environment targeted toward suicide reduction among healthcare workers. The impact of teaching non-mental healthcare workers how to detect a colleague at risk warrants quantification.

Glossary

Lethality Degree of likelihood of harm in a method or plan of suicide a person has created; violent (e.g., firearms) and nonviolent methods (e.g., ingestion, suffocation) are included.

Safety plan A prioritized written list of coping strategies and sources of support to be used by individuals before or during a suicidal crisis.

Suicidality Risk of suicide, usually includes suicide ideation or intent, especially when accompanied by well-elaborated plan; also includes actual suicide attempts.

Suicide ideation Thoughts or ideas about suicide, includes a range of contemplations, wishes, and preoccupations with death and suicide.

Discussion Questions

1. What are the key principles for non-mental health professionals when helping a clinician in mental distress?
2. How has suicide risk assessment advanced?
3. What are the key steps to helping a peer in mental health distress?
4. Why is self-care of the helper important and what does this mean?

Discussion Leader Guide

1. What are the key principles of helping a clinician in mental distress for non-mental health professionals?
   (a) Being a good listener and talking with a person to understand their cognitions, emotional state, behaviors, and physical experiences is a first step.
   (b) Always assessing the safety of the person in distress and yourself is critical.
   (c) Demonstrating empathy, caring, nonjudgment, hope, and truly wanting to help are essential.
   (d) Seeking professional help will be the ultimate goal.
   (e) Self-awareness about your own thoughts and attitudes is important to being an effective helper.
2. How has suicide risk assessment advanced?
   (a) Persons in mental distress were once viewed as either suicidal or not. Rather, the nature of suicide can be viewed on a continuum that recognizes suicide risk is dynamic, can change in a moment, and suicidal thinking is heterogeneous. Knowing cognitions in general related to suicidal thinking is important.
   (b) Previous attempts increase risk profile.

(c) Activating events are often triggers such as relationship problem, financial stress, real or perceived loss, job loss, negative memories, or strong and distressing physical sensations. Clinicians and healthcare staff experiencing these events with other stressors might have suicidal thoughts and plans. You can be an important person to intervene and help the person get professional help.

3. What are the key steps to helping a peer in mental health distress?
   (a) Develop therapeutic relationship with person in distress; active listening and learning about what is going on cognitively, emotionally, behaviorally, and physically.
   (b) Assess a number of risk factors to help decide the best plan forward for getting professional help.
   (c) If in doubt, call 911 or take to emergency services.
   (d) Do not leave a distressed person alone, get someone present if you need to leave.
   (e) Work with others at the organization to find appropriate help.
   (f) Seek self-care following a crisis.

4. Why is self-care of the helper important and what does this mean?
   (a) Working with someone in a mental distress crisis is highly emotionally charged and can initiate a major stress response that needs debriefing and de-escalation for the helper.
   (b) Self-care along several dimensions includes acknowledging things you did right, giving self-space to debrief, talking with others onsite, focusing on reducing stress response, performing health behaviors, and seeking professional help as needed.

Video for Discussion - Instructional Video: The online version contains supplementary material available at https://doi.org/10.1007/978-3-031-16983-0_25

References

1. Sublette ME. Grappling with suicide risk. Mayo Clin Proc. 2018;93(6):682–3.
2. Weir K. Worrying trends in U.S. suicide rates. APA Monitor Psychol. 2019;50(3):24. https://www.apa.org/monitor/2019/03/trends-suicide.
3. Runeson B, Odeberg J, Pettersson A, Edbom T, Jildevik Adamsson I, Waern M. Instruments for the assessment of suicide risk: A systematic review evaluating the certainty of the evidence. PLoS One. 2017;12(7):e0180292. https://doi.org/10.1371/journal.pone.0180292.
4. Nelson HD, Denneson LM, Low AR, Bauer BW, O'Neil M, Kansagara D, Teo AR. Suicide risk assessment and prevention: a systematic review focusing on veterans. Psychiatr Serv. 2017;68(10):1003–15. https://aquila.usm.edu/fac_pubs/17635.
5. Louzon SA, Bossarte R, McCarthy JF, Katz IR. Does suicidal ideation as measured by the PHQ-9 predict suicide among VA patients? Psychiatr Serv. 2016;67(5):517–22. https://doi.org/10.1176/appi.ps.201500149.
6. Belsher BE, Smolenski DJ, Pruitt LD, Bush NE, Beech EH, Workman DE, Morgan RL, Evatt DP, Tucker J, Skopp NA. Prediction models for suicide attempts and deaths: a system-

atic review and simulation. JAMA Psychiat. 2019;76(6):642–51. https://doi.org/10.1001/jamapsychiatry.2019.0174.

7. Whiting D, Fazel S. How accurate are suicide risk prediction models? Asking the right questions for clinical practice. Evid Based Ment Health. 2019;22:125–8. https://doi.org/10.1136/ebmental-2019-300102.

8. Doupnik SK, Rudd B, Schmutte T, Worsley D, Bowden CF, McCarthy E, Eggan E, Bridge JA, Marcus SC. Association of suicide prevention interventions with subsequent suicide attempts, linkage to follow-up care, and depression symptoms for acute care settings: a systematic review and meta-analysis. JAMA Psychiat. 2020;77(10):1021–30. https://doi.org/10.1001/jamapsychiatry.2020.1586.

9. Bryan CJ, Rudd MD. Advances in the assessment of suicide risk. J Clin Psychol. 2006;62(2):185–200.

10. Hom MA, Stanley IH, Podlogar MC, Joiner TE Jr. "Are you having thoughts of suicide?" Examining experiences with disclosing and denying suicidal ideation. J Clin Psychol. 2017;73(10):1382–92. https://doi.org/10.1002/jclp.22440.

11. Gordon YY, Davidson JE, Kim K, Zisook S. Physician death by suicide in the United States: 2012–2016. J Psychiatr Res. 2021;1(134):158–65.

12. Davidson JE, Ye G, Parra MC, Choflet A, Lee K, Barnes A, Harkavy-Friedman J, Zisook S. Job-related problems prior to nurse suicide, 2003-2017: A mixed methods analysis using natural language processing and thematic analysis. J Nurs Regul. 2021;12(1):28–39.

13. Sadek J. A clinician's guide to suicide risk assessment and management. Springer; 2019.

14. Howard MS, Buck M, Carpenter H, McMillan K. Nativating the loss and grief of a nurse suicide. Am Nurse J. 2021;16(3):14–6.

15. Beyond Blue. Self-care for the supporter. 11 Oct 2021. https://www.beyondblue.org.au/the-facts/suicide-prevention/worried-about-someone-suicidal/self-care-for-the-supporter.

16. SANE Australia. Self-care after someone discloses suicidal thoughts. The SANE Blog. 6 Feb 2017 https://www.sane.org/information-stories/the-sane-blog/suicide-prevention/self-care-after-someone-discloses-suicidal-thoughts.

17. Brodsky BS, Spruch-Feiner A, Stanley B. The zero suicide model: applying evidence-based suicide prevention practices to clinical care. Front Psych. 2018;9:33. https://doi.org/10.3389/fpsyt.2018.00033.

18. Morgan AJ, Ross A, Reavley NJ. Systematic review and meta-analysis of mental health first aid training: effects on knowledge, stigma, and helping behaviour. PLoS One. 2018;13(5):e0197102. https://doi.org/10.1371/journal.pone.0197102.

19. Isaac M, Elias B, Katz LY, Belik SL, Deane FP, Enns MW, Sareen J, Swampy Cree Suicide Prevention Team. Gatekeeper training as a preventative intervention for suicide: a systematic review. Can J Psychiatry. 2009;54(4):260–8. https://doi.org/10.1177/070674370905400407.

20. Burnette C, Ramchand R, Ayer L. Gatekeeper training for suicide prevention: A theoretical model and review of the empirical literature. RAND National Defense Research Institute; 2015.

Grief and Grieving Part 1: Grieving Our Patients, Rituals that Heal

Allison Kestenbaum and Kristopher Halsey

Learning Objectives
1. Understand and apply advice for grieving losses in clinical care, including patient deaths.
2. Identify and address cumulative grief through personal and communal rituals in the workplace.
3. Recognize and engage with colleagues who may need treatment to deal with prolonged grief.

26.1 Presentation of the Science

This chapter will focus on rituals as a critical resource for addressing personal, professional and communal grief and loss for medical providers [1]. Grief is "the anguish experienced after significant loss, usually the death of a beloved person." It may include physiological, emotional, spiritual reactions or take other forms [2–9]. Medical trainees and clinicians must address the emotional interplay between the losses that they witness at the bedside and those in their own personal life [10, 11]. Grief can be felt in response to a death, or the loss of a role, opportunity, dream,

Supplementary Information The online version contains supplementary material available at https://doi.org/10.1007/978-3-031-16983-0_26.

A. Kestenbaum (✉)
University of California, San Diego Health Spiritual Care Services, San Diego, CA, USA
e-mail: akestenbaum@health.ucsd.edu

K. Halsey
Halsey Life Coaching Solutions, Philadelphia, PA, USA

hope, etc. [12]. Some people experience cumulative grief, which is when many losses are experienced in a short period of time [13]. Losses that were assumed to be resolved long ago may be reawakened by a devastating clinical situation or the loss of a colleague [14]. Recognizing that grief can show itself in myriad ways can help clinicians and faculty to be compassionate and attentive to ourselves and others we work with [15]. Knowing the signs of grief in trainees, colleagues, or team members can help to identify those who may be struggling and need specialized help. Other people may experience spiritual distress, feeling as if they are being punished. They may feel guilty or suddenly feel disconnected from a sense of purpose in their life or work [16–18].

> Grief is not a disorder, a disease or sign of weakness. It is an emotional, physical and spiritual necessity, the price you pay for love. The only cure for grief is to grieve. [19]

Institutional administrators, credentialed clinicians, and trainees can normalize the holistic impact of grief by suspending judgment and offering support. One way to do this is to teach all team members that individuals may experience disruptions in functioning for some time after loss, but only a minority of people experience chronic, long-term grief reactions. As we will outline below, rituals help with grief. There are also types of grief, including complicated or hidden, disenfranchised, and ambiguous loss, which may pose challenges to rituals, but adaptations can be made [6, 20]. For example, those experiencing disenfranchised grief, which is a grief that may not fall into what is considered acceptable in a specific culture, may find that communal and public rituals may not be possible [21]. Ritual in ambiguous loss may need to be modified because some aspect of the loss is unclear [22].

Although the word ritual may be perceived as having a religious connotation, rituals are simply "a symbolic activity that is performed before, during, or after a meaningful event in order to achieve some desired outcome—from alleviating grief to winning a competition to making it rain." [23] Administrators and those making a case to their leaders to recognize grief institutionally, should take notice that this definition is offered by Harvard Business School professors advocating for the role of rituals in helping team members to regain a sense of control through ritual in the face of change or loss. Ritual is an empowering, embodied action that allows humans to process and work through experiences and concepts that may be hard to understand intellectually [24].

> Ritual ... has been one of the most practical and efficient ways to stimulate the safe healing required by both the individual and the community. Ritual...is a tool to maintain the delicate balance between body and soul. [25]

Rituals are a way to address the experience of feeling that a person's world has shattered or has fundamentally changed due to a loss or stressful event [26]. Rituals can be effective when they include:

1. Concrete steps for recovery
2. Reduce feelings of anxiety, depression, and helplessness

3. Encourage support from community, as the individual defines it
4. Encourages acceptance and compassion for oneself
5. Elements of spiritual resources [27]

All cultures have rituals. To that end, we recommend combining rituals related to loss with the regular activities and tasks your clinical caregiving environment already has in place. By building these into the culture, it supports resilience while considering inevitable losses of clinical care, without adding significant time burden for already busy team members.

For example, rituals for healing grief can be performed individually or in groups; in person or online; and anywhere—from a hospital breakroom to a beach. If available at your institution, healthcare chaplains who are extensively trained in facilitating and customizing ritual can help you. However, staff and trainees of all disciplines should feel empowered to lead rituals. Rituals may occur several times a day (e.g., a moment of mindfulness while washing hands), daily (e.g., an inspiring quote at team huddle), weekly, monthly, annually (e.g., setting aside time for a holiday celebration). Grief rituals in healthcare settings are most effective when they rely on universal themes that people of all backgrounds can relate to. Examples include love, peace, forgiveness, hope, light/darkness, community, remembering, and dedication. Although individuals may benefit from personal rituals that draw from their cultural or spiritual background, teams in healthcare are served best by rituals with universal themes that avoid cultural appropriation [28]. If you plan to lead a longer ritual or service, such gatherings are most effective when the arc of experience is taken into consideration. This means that participants benefit from an easing into the ritual as they transition from "work mode." They are given an opportunity to engage with their depth of feeling and then are prepared to gradually go back into the non-ritual space (see Fig. 26.1).

Often, grief rituals in clinical and teaching environments take a hybrid approach in that the ritual itself is an educational opportunity about loss and grieving. For example, when facilitating a grief support ritual for a medical division that had recently experienced the sudden and shocking death of lead faculty, the chaplain took the opportunity to educate the dozens of physicians and faculty assembled

Fig. 26.1 The arc of ritual

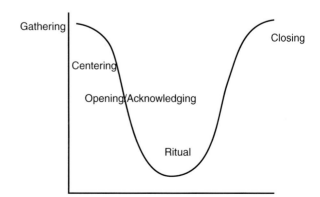

about the basics of grief and complicated bereavement. Faculty reflected on how setting aside time to grieve this loss would allow them to also grieve the cumulative losses of the prior year, which coincided with the COVID-19 pandemic. With the hybrid approach to grief rituals in clinical settings, we can also teach and role model for clinicians and trainees how to commit to and maintain their own personal, ongoing grief rituals.

In addition, some clinicians find that dealing with illness and loss every day leads to compounded emotional reactions to personal loss. Others may be surprised to learn that information they know about grief and how to address it will be temporarily forgotten in the initial shock of a new personal loss. In these situations, it can be helpful to have colleagues and friends who can provide reminders about resources for coping. Even disciplines that are accustomed to mental health and psycho/spiritual treatment cannot rely on treating themselves. Having insight into your limitations and boundaries and seeking professional grief support with openness and relaxed convictions can be useful. Another consideration is the impact of daily loss witnessed by clinicians on their families. Clinicians may need to provide "instructions" to loved ones about how to provide support, especially if the clinician is often leaned upon in their own family system for support. Clinicians are, of course, also entitled to being vulnerable and may need to name this and ask for compassion in their family. Some clinicians establish simple rituals for themselves that help them transition from the stressful clinical environment back to their home after their shifts. An example is to briefly pause as they exit the hospital and mentally offer healing wishes for everyone in building.

Because grief can feel amorphous, many people rely on metaphors, symbols, music, etc., to make sense of what they are feeling [29]. When trainees, clinicians, faculty, and administration engage in a personal ritual or facilitating for others, they may benefit from drawing upon one of these metaphors to help colleagues access their full array of coping strategies:

Waves—Some people describe grief as coming in waves; you feel stable and then suddenly the grief comes in a big wave, as if you were standing on the shore, and knocks you off your feet. The nature of grief ebbs and flows, just like the sea.

The ball & the box—When we first experience a loss, it feels like a huge ball that is constantly hitting up against the edges of the box, causing us to feel pain. But over time, the ball gets smaller, or some believe the box (i.e., our hearts) grows bigger so that we are not constantly reminded of the pain of the loss. The pain remains but we notice it less frequently [30].

Spiral—There is no particular end point to grief. Many people find that over time, they have a sense of feeling better and that their grief feels less raw and more incorporated into their identity and memory. However, a stressful event or difficult time may occur and cause them to feel that they have regressed or gone right back to where they started when they first experienced the prior loss. In reality, grief is more like a spiral. There is a sensation of moving backward but in fact, there has just been a temporary dip and after which moving "up" in the spiral of healing will be possible.

Favorite shirt—You wore your favorite shirt every day until you realized that there is a hole. You take the shirt to the tailor and ask them to fix the hole. They explain that they cannot fix the hole, but that they can smooth out the tattered edges and make the shirt into a different shape. Like grief, the hole cannot be filled but the sharp painful edges of the grief can be reshaped and smoothed out over time.

26.2 Application of Principles into Wellness Practice

All the recommendations to follow for addressing grief through regular practice and rituals can be helpful across all stages of training and clinical practice.

26.2.1 Pre-Licensure Application in the Academic Environment

In general, learners in health sciences may be younger, and death and loss in the training environment may be some of the first that they have personally experienced. Learners will be helped by a culture that normalizes grief as well as basic empathy from instructors, preceptors, and mentors about the newness of the proximity to loss. One way to address this is to "ritualize" discussion about loss by including it as a standing agenda item in mentoring or group process sessions. Here is an example of how a mentor may respond to a learner's reflections about loss:

Learner: "I haven't ever had a loved one die and I feel so unprepared to communicate with family members of a dying patient. I have no experience to draw on."
Mentor: "It is natural to feel helpless when witnessing loss. Even I still feel helpless at times when caring for grieving family members. I have seen that you are a very caring person, and you know what it is like to lose something you care about."

One of the most effective ways to teach grief rituals to learners is for faculty and trainers to prioritize these by setting an example. While faculty and trainers have their own outlets and rituals to process grief, expressing grief in the clinical environment can be healing for all. There is a Buddhist story about Master Shaku Soen, who was seen crying with a bereaved family when witnessing a tragic loss in a nearby village. An onlooker noticed "and remarked, rather shaken on seeing the famous master crying with them: "I would have thought that you at least were beyond such things [crying]." "But it is this which puts me beyond it, replied the master with a sob." Although crying is not a requirement for teaching about grief rituals in the clinical environment, do not stifle tears when they occur. Crying can be a natural reaction to loss. The act of shedding tears embodies vulnerability and may support the grieving process to take its natural course. Learners also benefit from learning how to empathize with others in the laboratory of their training so that they can then apply this skill to future clinical work.

Learners, like all of us, come to experiences with traumatic or unresolved losses from their life experience. For those who have experienced significant losses, new grief can also remind them of rituals and coping strategies that have been helpful in the past. Learners may take comfort from knowing they have healed from loss in the past and can do so again. We recommend that knowledge about how and where to refer peers and colleagues be built into the training program.

Some people come to see their regular sessions with a therapist, mental health counselor, etc., to be a ritual that helps them find support, rejuvenation, and release. We recommend framing counseling support as a regular ritual that helps with clinician resilience. As some trainees may be new to receiving mental health support, this is an opportunity for them to prioritize finding a helper that is right for them. Just as with any ritual, trainees can be taught that factors like cadence, match, tone, accessibility, and method and finding the right fit for them can help them to develop a meaningful and healing therapeutic ritual practice.

Another way to ritualize personal exploration and reflection about loss, mortality, and death is by building in reflective writing or discussion activities into the curriculum. These can include prompt questions like: What is your greatest fear concerning loss? For yourself? In caring for others? What does a good helping relationship related to loss look like? Some academic and training programs do this through assignments that require students to complete their own advance directive or life review. In one exercise, participants are asked to:

1. Write down 5 people you love the most
2. Write down 5 things you most enjoy doing
3. Write down 5 places that give you the most comfort

The instructor then removes the paper and destroys it in some way in front of the learner. The group engages in discussion. What did you feel when your paper was taken from you? When it was destroyed? How might this experience inform your empathy toward those in your clinical care?

26.2.2 Clinical Application Post-Licensure

Education and practice about grief rituals in post in post-licensure settings is primarily about facilitating sustainability and building these rituals into normal clinical practice. Many busy clinicians and leaders fear that pausing to honor grief through ritual will open a floodgate and interrupt workflow. While it is important for people to grieve and adopt rituals that feel authentic in settings that feel safe to them, not addressing and processing grief at all makes clinicians more susceptible to burnout, compassion fatigue, and exhaustion. While there are many systemic factors that are not in the direct control of clinicians, determining how, when, and with whom they process their grief is something that is very much within clinicians' control.

...Grant me the serenity to accept the things I cannot change, courage to change the things I can, and the wisdom to know the difference, living one day at a time; enjoying one moment at a time; taking this world as it is and not as I would have it... —Reinhold Niebuhr

We recognize that time is a precious commodity and most post-licensure clinicians are managing the many demands of professional and personal life. We recommend that clinicians seek out opportunities that allow them to address grief while meeting other needs. They may avail themselves of offerings in the workplace, such as mindfulness, yoga, or other reflective practices that support healthy grieving. Continuing education activities that address clinical practices related to grief or those that focus explicitly on self-care and restoration can be helpful. One example of this is Schwartz Rounds which are hosted at many medical centers around the country. Holding oneself accountable to taking sick and vacation time that is allotted is another important ritual practice that clinicians can engage in. If clinicians feel reluctant about taking time off, they can be encouraged to write down the obstacles and how to overcome them. Some obstacles may include:

- Personal expectations that may not match that of the institution
- Departmental culture
- Perceptions about staff restraints, being short-staffed
- Financial restraints on "traveling"; undervaluing "staycations"
- Saving up sick time for retirement

26.2.3 Leadership Application (Structural and Organizational Considerations)

Learners and licensed clinicians are more likely to prioritize rituals for grief if institutional leadership models this in meaningful ways. When leaders normalize grief support and rituals, it becomes more commonplace for stakeholders at all levels. Some ways that departmental and institutional leadership can model this include:

1. Collaborate with HR for wellness activities and designate paid time off for activities and continuing education that support healthy grieving.
2. Incorporate brief rituals and acknowledgment about loss as a standing agenda item into high profile gatherings such as town halls, monthly department meetings, stake/shareholder/board meetings.
3. Host system-wide days of remembering, co-facilitated by spiritual care staff.
4. Work to destigmatize grief with leaders and managers. Provide concrete, appropriate examples of what authentic grief expressions look like from leadership, so staff can learn from this.
5. For leaders who have influence over continuing education requirements, advocate for activities that offer the required educational rigor along with teaching about practices that support clinician's healing and resilience regarding grief and loss.

6. Implement a Nurse Coaching Process to Support Bereaved Staff, like the ELNEC (End-of-Life Nursing Education Consortium) which entails learning how to reach out, support each other, as well as set and implement goals related to healthy grieving [31].
7. Announce deaths of colleagues so that their legacy can be celebrated, and staff can begin to process grief.

Managers of a unit or leaders of a hospital service can prioritize rituals for healing by approving setting aside time to grieve and remember, as well as attending and actively participating. An example of this is an outpatient clinic at an academic teaching hospital that developed a ritual of sharing information about patient deaths once a month, for 30 min. Each patient was remembered for about 2–5 min by team members discussing what they will remember or miss about the patient, while placing a stone into a large vase. All members of the team participated, regardless of "rank" and were gently reminded that it was not a medical discussion, but rather a reflection on the loss. Once each year, the team brought all the stones to a nearby beach. The chaplain led a ritual and reflection where all in attendance returned the stones to the ocean, thus having time away from the clinical setting for reflection and for an embodied practice of letting go. Other examples for these kinds of "letting go" rituals include butterfly release, regular memorial services, writing names on seashells and realizing into water, writing down losses on rice paper and dissolving in water. Other teams appreciate rituals that start with an empty vessel, with everyone bringing some object of beauty such as flowers and an empty vase or a memory board in a communal place for staff, with everyone coming together to build a meaningful memorial. Whatever is chosen, advocacy and support from leadership to set aside time on a regular basis will be critical to the ritual's longevity and success.

26.3   Opportunities for Future Research

While some research has been conducted about the impact of personal rituals on healthcare workers, most of this has been in the context of hospice of end-of-life care [24]. Further exploration on questions about professional satisfaction and resilience related to rituals in all corners of healthcare education and clinical practice could be a promising next step for research. In addition, research that explores the impact of institutional and team/group rituals is also lacking. As described in this chapter, there are many rituals that can be built into the normal flow and functioning of training programs, as well as clinical and institutional operations. A further empirical basis for these practices could help to bring legitimacy to strategies that positively impact quality of life and wellness measures for clinicians and help them to heal.

Glossary

Burnout Reduction in energy related to work that may present as exhaustion, frustration, lack of meaning in work.

Compassion fatigue The physical, psychological, emotional, and spiritual impact of helping others.

Empathy The ability to understand and share the feelings of another.

Grief The physical, psychological, spiritual, and emotional pain experienced most often after the death of a loved one but can be for any kind of loss. Terms have been established to recognize grief experiences including compounded, complicated, hidden, ambiguous, and disenfranchised.

Rituals Actions that are performed to mark a significant event or to bring meaning to an experience.

Self-care The act of engaging in activities or behaviors that help one achieve or maintain good physical or mental health, especially to mitigate the effects of stress or trauma.

Spirituality The aspect of humanity that refers to how individuals seek and express meaning, and how they experience connectedness to the moment, self, others, nature, and to the sacred.

Discussion Questions

1. What are ways that you have collaborated on grief rituals? How can chaplains/spiritual care counselors help?
2. How are interprofessional grief rituals, across the training and clinical practice spectrum helpful?
3. What is the appropriate cadence for rituals in the areas where you teach, work, or lead at your healthcare institution? Daily, weekly, monthly, annually, other?
4. What are additional strategies that take into the unique culture of your institution that can be instituted in your healthcare organization that will support and encourage the importance of grief rituals?
5. Practicing grief rituals can be a form of restorative self-care. Knowing this, what are some self-care tips you have practiced that have become rituals for you or your team?

Discussion Leader Guide

Video for Discussion - Instructional Video: The online version contains supplementary material available at https://doi.org/10.1007/978-3-031-16983-0_26

References

1. Wojtkowiak J, Lind J, Smid GE. Ritual in therapy for prolonged grief: a scoping review of ritual elements in evidence-informed grief interventions. Front Psych. 2020;11:623835.
2. American Psychological Association. APA dictionary of psychology. 2020. https://dictionary. apa.org/grief. Accessed 29 Sept 2021.
3. O'Connor M-F. Grief: a brief history of research on how body, mind, and brain adapt. Psychosom Med. 2019;81(8):731–8.
4. Burke L, Neimeyer R. The inventory of complicated spiritual grief: assessing spiritual crisis following loss. Religions (Basel). 2016;7(6):67.
5. Burke LA, Neimeyer RA, Young AJ, Bonin EP, Davis NL. Complicated spiritual grief II: a deductive inquiry following the loss of a loved one. Death Stud. 2014;38(1–5):268–81.
6. Zisook S, Shear K. Grief and bereavement: what psychiatrists need to know. World Psychiatry. 2009;8(2):67–74.
7. Bonanno GA, Wortman CB, Lehman DR, Tweed RG, Haring M, Sonnega J, et al. Resilience to loss and chronic grief: a prospective study from preloss to 18-months postloss. J Pers Soc Psychol. 2002;83(5):1150–64.
8. Park CLH, J. Religion and spirituality in adjusting to bereavement: grief as burden, grief as gift. In: Neimeyer R, Harris D, Winokuer H, Thornton G, editors. Grief and bereavement in contemporary society. New York: Routledge; 2011. p. 353–63.
9. Puchalski CM, Vitillo R, Hull SK, Reller N. Improving the spiritual dimension of whole person care: reaching national and international consensus. J Palliat Med. 2014;17(6):642–56. https://doi.org/10.1089/jpm.2014.9427.
10. Saunders JM, Valente SM. Nurses' grief. Cancer Nurs. 1994;17(4):318–25.
11. Sikstrom L, Saikaly R, Ferguson G, Mosher PJ, Bonato S, Soklaridis S. Being there: a scoping review of grief support training in medical education. PLoS One. 2019;14(11):e0224325.
12. Doehring C. The practice of pastoral care: a postmodern approach. Louisville: Westminster/ John Knox Press; 2015.
13. Marino PA. The effects of cumulative grief in the nurse. J Intraven Nurs. 1998;21(2):101–4.
14. Spencer L. How do nurses deal with their own grief when a patient dies on an intensive care unit, and what help can be given to enable them to overcome their grief effectively? J Adv Nurs. 1994;19(6):1141–50.
15. Boston PH, Mount BM. The caregiver's perspective on existential and spiritual distress in palliative care. J Pain Symptom Manage. 2006;32(1):13–26.
16. Becker G, Xander CJ, Blum HE, Lutterbach J, Momm F, Gysels M, et al. Do religious or spiritual beliefs influence bereavement? A systematic review. Palliat Med. 2007;21(3):207–17.
17. Greenspan M. Healing through the dark emotions. Boston: Shambhala; 2004.
18. Burke LA, Neimeyer RA. Inventory of Complicated Spiritual Grief (ICSG). In: Neimeyer RA, editor. Techniques of grief therapy: assessment and intervention. Routledge; 2016. p. 76–80.
19. Grollman EA. Living when a loved one has died. London: Souvenir Press; 1996.
20. Iglewicz A, Shear MK, Reynolds CF 3rd, Simon N, Lebowitz B, Zisook S. Complicated grief therapy for clinicians: an evidence-based protocol for mental health practice. Depress Anxiety. 2020;37(1):90–8.
21. Doka KJ. In: Stroebe MS, Hansson RO, Schut H, Stroebe W, editors. Disenfranchised grief in historical and cultural perspective. American Psychological Association; 2008. p. 223–40.
22. Boss P. Ambiguous loss: learning to live with unresolved grief. London: Harvard University Press; 2009.
23. Norton MI, Gino F. Rituals alleviate grieving for loved ones, lovers, and lotteries. J Exp Psychol Gen. 2014;143(1):266–72.
24. Montross-Thomas LP, Scheiber C, Meier EA, Irwin SA. Personally meaningful rituals: a way to increase compassion and decrease burnout among hospice staff and volunteers. J Palliat Med. 2016;19(10):1043–50.

25. Patrice M. The healing wisdom of Africa: finding life purpose through nature, ritual and community. London: Thorsons; 1999.
26. Parkes CM, Prigerson HG. Bereavement: studies of grief in adult life. 4th ed. New York: Routledge; 2013.
27. Achterberg J, PhD D, RN, Kolkmeier, RN. Rituals of healing: using imagery for health and wellness. New York: Bantam Books; 1994.
28. Unitarian Universalist Association. Considerations for cultural borrowing. 1996–2021. https://www.uua.org/multiculturalism/introduction/misappropriation/23371.shtml. Accessed 29 Sept 2021.
29. Nadeau JW. Metaphorically speaking: the use of metaphors in grief therapy. Illn Crisis Loss. 2006;14(3):201–21.
30. HospisCare. Why grief is like a ball in a box. 2020. https://www.hospiscare.co.uk/how-we-help/advice-support/talking-about-death-and-dying/why-grief-is-like-a-ball-in-a-box/. Accessed 29 Sep 2021.
31. AACN ELNEC support for nurses during COVID-19American Association of Colleges of Nursing. [cited 2021 Sep 29]. http://AACNNURSING.ORG/ELNEC/COVID-19.

Losing a Patient or Colleague to Suicide

27

Sidney Zisook, Joan M. Anzia, Alana Iglewicz, and Deepak Prabhakar

Learning Objectives
1. Learn common reactions to losing a patient to suicide
2. Appreciate ways reactions suicide loss differ from other losses and causes of death
3. Apply individual, organizational, and institutional strategies to help clinicians cope with death of a patient from suicide

27.1 Presentation of the Science

Every clinical specialty has its own high risk patient challenges that threaten to undermine the clinician's well-being, professional identity, and sense of competence. In mental healthcare, it is patient suicide, an all-too frequently encountered

Supplementary Information The online version contains supplementary material available at https://doi.org/10.1007/978-3-031-16983-0_27.

S. Zisook (✉)
Department of Psychiatry, UC San Diego, La Jolla, CA, USA
e-mail: szisook@health.ucsd.edu

J. M. Anzia
Department of Psychiatry and Behavioral Sciences, Feinberg School of Medicine, Northwestern University, River Forest, IL, USA
e-mail: janzia@nm.org

A. Iglewicz
Veterans Affairs San Diego Healthcare System, La Jolla, CA, USA

D. Prabhakar
Sheppard Pratt, Baltimore, MD, USA
e-mail: dprabhakar@sheppardpratt.org

consequence of severe mental illness that may leave the clinician bereft, perplexed, guilt-ridden, and uncertain of their suitability for the profession. This chapter describes common responses to the death by suicide of a patient, evidence-based approaches to enhancing education about this all-too-often avoided aspect of clinical care, and the provision of support and treatment to those who lose a patient to suicide.

Suicide is among the leading causes of death worldwide, with more deaths due to suicide than to malaria, HIV/AIDS, breast cancer, or war and homicide. More than one in every 100 deaths (1.3% in the 20 years between 2000 and 2019) was due to suicide. According to the Centers for Disease Control and Prevention (CDC) WISQARS Leading Causes of Death Reports, in 2019 suicide was the tenth leading cause of death overall in the United States, claiming the lives of over 47,500 people. Suicide was the second leading cause of death among individuals between the ages of 10 and 34, and the fourth leading cause of death among those ages 35–44 [1].

The underlying vulnerability of suicidal behavior is the subject of intense research scrutiny, and includes biological, social, and psychological underpinnings [2, 3]. Among the best studied and replicated risks for suicide is mental illness. Over 90% of those who die by suicide have a diagnosable mental health condition at the time of their death. While depression and bipolar disorder are the most common disorders among people who attempt suicide, those who attempt suicide may also suffer from substance abuse disorders or other psychiatric disorders such as schizophrenia and may feel that suicide is the only way to end an unbearable pain they may be feeling as the result of their mental illness, trauma, or a significant loss, rejection, or disappointment [3]. Additionally, a history of suicide attempts is the best predictor for future attempts [4]. Common themes among people who attempt suicide are feelings of hopelessness, despair, and isolation from family and friends. Despite loved ones' and professionals' best efforts to support them in their suffering, those who attempt suicide often are unable to think clearly and rationally through their pain.

In 2019, 4.8% (~12.0 million people) of adults ages 18 or higher thought seriously about trying to kill themselves, 1.4% (~3.5 million people) made a suicide plan, 0.6% (~1.4 million people) made a nonfatal suicide attempt, and 0.1% (~217,000 people) attempted suicide without a suicide plan. Almost half of adults with any mental illness receive some kind treatment, even more so in adults with "serious" mental illness (i.e., diagnosis of a mental illness which results in serious functional impairment that substantially interferes with or limits one or more major life activities). In 2019, among the 13.1 million adults with serious mental illness, 8.6 million (65.5%) received mental health treatment [5]. Thus, it is no surprise that mental healthcare professionals, providing that care, are vulnerable to losing patients to suicide. Indeed, some have called losing a patient to suicide an occupational hazard for psychiatrists [6].

First and foremost, clinicians are human beings. The customary human response to the death of someone we hold close is grief. Thus, when a clinician loses a patient to suicide, they are not immune to the burdens associated with losing an important person in their lives. In general, bereavement from suicide is similar to bereavement experiences with other traumatic losses. But suicide loss survivors, including clinicians losing patients to suicide, often also face unique challenges that differ from those who have been bereaved by other types of death. In addition to the inevitable grief, sadness, and disbelief typical of all grief, overwhelming guilt, confusion, rejection, shame, blame, anger, and the perceived need to conceal the cause of the death also are often prominent [7–10]. These painful experiences may be further complicated by the effects of stigma [11, 12] and trauma [13].

Several common themes that characterize suicide bereavement differ qualitatively from other forms of bereavement and may lead to delays in survivors' healing [13, 14]. These themes also apply to healthcare providers losing patients to suicide. These include the role of stigma, the need to understand, guilt, feelings of responsibility, rejection, perceived abandonment, anger, and, in some cases, trauma and are exemplified in the following case:

Case

Mr. H., a patient who suffered from severe, recurrent Major Depressive Episodes, died by suicide by overdose two months ago. Dr. Smith is the psychiatrist who was providing mental healthcare to Mr. H. over the past three years, initially during Dr. Smith's last year of residency training when she saw Mr. H. for weekly therapy sessions, then in the outpatient clinic where Dr. Smith has been employed since she graduated from residency and where Dr. Smith saw Mr. H. on a monthly basis for pharmacotherapy and supportive psychotherapy sessions.

Dr. Smith has been struggling with Mr. H.'s death. When she first learned the news, she was utterly shocked. For, Mr. H. had been doing clinically better. At their last appointment, Mr. H. seemed brightened and lighter. He recently got engaged to his girlfriend of five years. He had started a new job that sounded meaningful and promising. There had been times in the past few years when Mr. H.'s depressive episodes were severe, and Dr. Smith worried about Mr. H.'s suicide risk. Importantly, this was not that time. Quite the contrary, rather than worrying about Mr. H., Dr. Smith was impressed and pleased with how Mr. H. had been doing.

Since learning of Mr. H.'s death by suicide, Dr. Smith cannot help but ruminate about how she missed "the signs" and "didn't see this coming." She is consumed by the "if only's" and "should have's," focusing on how Mr. H.'s use of dark humor at their last appointment was not salient to her at that time, but should have been and that if only she picked up on it, she could have intervened and prevented this tragic death. Dr. Smith blames herself for missing "cues" and is embarrassed to discuss Mr. H.'s death with colleagues, fearing that they will think less of her clinical skills and will regret hiring her into their practice.

The image of Mr. H.'s fiancée finding him unresponsive on the bathroom floor at their house haunts Dr. Smith. This image, combined with her ruminative self-blaming thoughts, interferes with her ability to restfully sleep. Dr. Smith has also started to worry about being sued over Mr. H.'s death. For the past two years, she had been working a weekly shift in the emergency department for additional income. This work often entails assessing patients' suicide risk and determining if they should be admitted to the psychiatric hospital. Since Mr. H.'s death, Dr. Smith feels incapable of doing her job. She is overthinking each clinical decision and is highly contemplating quitting this part of her job, feeling ineffective at making the needed clinical decisions and unworthy of this weighted responsibility.

Dr. Smith's anger at herself was initially intertwined with anger toward the clinical practice in which she worked and was eventually directed toward Mr. H. She became frustrated that the clinic in which she worked did not allow her to see her patients on a weekly basis for therapy, but rather limited her visits to a total of 20 minutes spaced at a maximum frequency of every four weeks. She pondered if only she could have continued weekly therapy with Mr. H., maybe he would not have died. With time, she started to acknowledge her anger toward Mr. H. himself. She felt rejected by him and kept asking why her care for him was not enough. Did he not care that she would be haunted by the fact that he died of an overdose using the medications she prescribed to him? The moment she would experience anger toward Mr. H., guilt would immediately wash over her. She questioned how she could feel anger toward a man who suffered profoundly, a question which led to further self-recriminations.

27.1.1 The Need to Understand, Guilt, and Responsibility

Most suicide loss survivors are plagued by the need to make sense of the death and to understand why the suicide completers made the decision to end their life. Over half of completed suicides occur in individuals not considered high risk, leaving family members and clinicians to ruminate endlessly about clues they may have missed. Even when a clearly "at risk" individual dies by suicide, clinicians still may haunt themselves with asking "why," "why now," and "why under my watch." Related to this is a clinician's tendency to overestimate their own level of responsibility as well as guilt for not having been able to do more to prevent such an outcome. Clinician survivors may see a patient an hour a week, or often less frequently, and often are unaware of the many factors occurring between sessions that may have contributed to the suicide, and in retrospect see things they may have not been aware of before the event. Clinicians who have lost a patient to suicide will often replay events up to the last moments of their patients' lives, digging for clues and warnings that they blame themselves for not noticing or taking seriously enough. They might recall past disagreements, interventions gone array, plans not fulfilled, calls not returned, words not said, and ruminate on how if only they had done or said something differently, maybe the outcome would have been different. While guilt is not a grief response specific to death by suicide, it is not uncommon for a clinician to view the suicide as an event that could and should have been prevented. Therefore, it is easy for clinicians to get caught up in self-blame [8, 14].

Understanding that most suicide completers were battling serious and life-threatening psychiatric illnesses for which even our most experienced and dedicated clinicians, using the best and most evidence-based interventions sometimes are just not always enough when a patient reaches a suicide crisis helps some clinician survivors make sense of the death and can decrease self-blame.

27.1.2 Rejection, Perceived Abandonment, and Anger

Clinicians may feel rejected or abandoned by their deceased patient because they see the deceased as choosing to give up and leave their "caring and compassionate" clinician behind. They are often left feeling bewildered, wondering why their relationship with the person was not enough to keep them from taking their lives. One clinician felt reassured when an "at risk" patient promised to never act upon their suicidal thoughts without reaching out to them first. When that patient took her own life, the clinician not only felt abandoned but also deceived. She felt angry about this perceived deception, and that her patient put her through the pain of dealing with her patient's family after the suicide. Anger is a common emotion among many survivors of suicide. It can be experienced as anger at the person who died, at themselves, at the patient's family members or acquaintances, at other providers, at God, or at the world in general. Often survivors feel angry at themselves for feeling angry, as they also recognize that the deceased was suffering greatly when deciding to die.

27.1.3 Stigma

Unlike other modes of death, suicide is stigmatized, despite recent valiant strides to destigmatize mental illness and suicide. Many bereaved clinicians report that it can be difficult to talk to others about their loss because, either because of their own self-blame, fear or shame, or because others often feel uncomfortable talking about suicide. This can leave the bereaved clinician feeling alone and isolated [11].

27.1.4 Trauma

> **Case (Continued)**
> In the above case of Mr. H., imagine if Mr. H.'s death by suicide occurred in the clinic's bathroom and John, a nurse involved in Mr. H.'s care, was the first to find his body. Further imagine that John had prior traumas in his life and how evocative and triggering the experience of finding Mr. H.'s body would be.

After a death by suicide, themes of violence, victimization, and volition (i.e., the choice of death over life, as in the case of suicide) are common and may be intermixed with other aspects of grief. Disbelief, despair, anxiety symptoms, preoccupation with the deceased and the circumstances of the death, withdrawal, hyper arousal, and dysphoria are more intense and more prolonged than they are under non-traumatic circumstances [10].

Resonating with these suicide-loss themes, Gutin et al. [15] interviewed several psychotherapists who had lost a patient to suicide and found the following responses and concerns:

- **Treatment-specific relationships**: clinicians reviewed and reconstructed some of their work with the patient, particularly their last session, and spoke about contact with the patient's family
- **Relationships with colleagues**: this proved to be one of the most complicated experiences and included contacts with the clinician's personal analyst or psychotherapist, supervisors, peers, trainees, and other institutional staff
- **Risk management concerns**: many had to do with potential for being sued
- **Grandiosity, shame, humiliation, guilt, judgment, and blame**: clinicians sought to understand their own ongoing internal response and their projected fear about how others would respond to them as "the person whose patient killed himself or herself"
- **Affective responses**: crying, sadness, anger, grief, and fear or anxiety about the consequences
- **Traumatic responses**: dissociation, traumatic intrusion, avoidance, somatic symptoms participants associated with the suicide, and dreams (nightmares) about the patient
- **Effect on work with other patients:** clinicians spoke about how they were changed for better and, at times, for worse in their work with other patients; some spoke of no longer accepting suicidal patients for treatment, or quickly moving into management and action rather than seeking to deepen the relationship and understand the suicidal patient; a few felt calmer in the face of suicidal crises with patients.
- **A sense of crisis**: trainees were uncertain about their work and choice of a specialty; others felt unsure that they wanted to continue work, feeling that psychotherapy exposed them and their patients to an unsettling vulnerability.

27.1.5 Other, Less Common Responses

As with other suicide loss survivors, clinicians who loss a patient to suicide may be vulnerable to worsening of pre-existing mood or anxiety disorders, or, less often, new onset Major Depressive Disorder, PTSD or Prolonged Grief Disorder [7–10]. Prolonged Grief Disorder is now recognized by both the ICD-11 and the DSM-5-TR as a clinical condition [16]. The DSM-5-TR diagnosis stipulates that if after a year there remain intense levels of distressing symptoms of acute grief, which significantly interfere with functioning and are out of keeping with that person's cultural and religious expectations, then a diagnosis of Prolonged Grief Disorder may be warranted. The gateway features are yearning, longing, and/or preoccupation with the loved one. Other associated symptoms include identity disruption (e.g., feeling as though part of oneself has died), marked sense of disbelief about the death, avoidance of reminders that the person is dead, intense emotional pain (e.g., anger, bitterness, sorrow) related to the death, difficulty with reintegration (e.g., problems engaging with friends, pursuing interests, planning for the future), emotional numbness, feeling that life is meaningless, and intense loneliness (i.e., feeling alone or detached from others) [16, 17]. More on Prolonged Grief Disorder can be found below in the section on management/support/treatment.

27.2 Education

When each of this chapter's authors were psychiatry trainees, nary a word about coping with patient suicide was spoken during our training. Looking back, it was a forbidden topic. As far back as the mid-1980s, the Association of Directors of Psychiatry Residency Training's core curriculum committee expressed concern about the need for, and lack of, training in suicide care, coping with patient suicide. That led to Lomax propose a comprehensive core curriculum on suicide care for psychiatry trainees [18] that integrated didactics, supervision, clinical experiences, and evaluation. The curriculum included attention to the residents' personal reactions to a patient's suicide attempts or completed suicide. For residents who treat a patient who dies by suicide, individual supervision will help the resident deal with the event. But since not all residents lose a patient to suicide, an important educational component of the curriculum must focus on postvention (the response to a person who has attempted or completed suicide). Lomax suggested small group meetings, organized as journal clubs, that include faculty members who have experienced patient suicides themselves. An important part of these sessions is self-revelation on the part of the faculty member or more senior residents about their own personal experiences and the mechanisms they used in coping with these, as well as the behaviors that made the process more difficult. Almost two decades later, in a survey of psychiatric residents, only a third of residents acknowledged receiving training on the impact of patient suicide [19]. It is no surprise then that a 2004 survey of psychiatrists who experienced patient suicide in training revealed that 71% felt helpless, 69% reported the patient suicide had a significant impact on them, 55% experienced recurrent feelings of horror, and 44% developed significant anxiety following the event [20]. Still, years later, a 2009 national survey of chief residents of psychiatry training programs across the United States found less than 20% felt prepared for the possibility of having to manage the aftermath of a patient suicide. As of today, there remains no requirement for residency training in patient suicide by the Psychiatry Common Program Requirements.

To help provide a "model curriculum" on suicide postvention that could be readily transported to all psychiatry training programs, Prabahaker et al. [21] described a single session, 90-min seminar which featured a recorded program called Collateral Damages. The program consists of (1) a video program that includes introductory comments; five brief vignettes from clinicians (two from senior faculty, two from junior faculty, and one from a trainee) on their patients who killed themselves and their immediate emotions, thoughts, and behaviors; a panel discussion of the five psychiatrists who have provided their narratives and two senior training directors that focuses on universal themes, processes, and procedures to follow after a patient suicide, principles of dealing with families, critical incident review, risk management, and the roles of counseling/supporting trainees and colleagues; and closing comments; (2) a PowerPoint presentation emphasizing suicide-related basic epidemiological facts, emotional reactions to patient suicide, and a brief overview of resources available to grieving individuals; (3) a patient-based case learning exercise covering Accreditation Council for Graduate Medical Education (ACGME) competencies as a means to stimulate discussion; and (4) pre- and post-questions [22]. Collateral Damages is available to residency training programs on the AADPRT website and educators by request from the AFSP.

Educators at UC San Francisco proposed a curriculum consisting of a biennial half-day workshop for all trainees plus an "as-needed curriculum" used after a completed suicide. The workshop is designed to teach trainees how to manage both the logistical and emotional aspects of patient suicide. It has three components: (1) a large group lecture, (2) small group discussions, each led by faculty members who have experienced a patient suicide, and (3) a reconvening of the large group with a guest speaker who had experienced the loss of a relative by suicide. The overall goal of the lecture is to help learners develop a basic understanding of issues that arise when a patient completes suicide. Topics covered include discoverability and confidentiality, risk management, and malpractice insurance, whether to contact the family, what to do with unpaid bills, and documentation. It also reviews relevant institutional policies of the university and hospital and provides guidelines to follow when in independent practice. Last, the lecture covers common emotional reactions of clinicians and their colleagues after a patient suicide [23].

In the aftermath of a series of patient suicides, the University of Colorado established a four-session seminar given early in the internship year which consists of a 4-h course that was developed to address both safety assessment and patient suicide. The course discusses safety assessments, provides a packet of resident resources, and the institution's response to patient suicide. This course also includes two written cases and a role-playing exercise, which are each followed by a group discussion. At the end of the course, a panel of psychiatrists with different levels of experience discusses their experiences with patient suicide [24].

At Ohio State, training begins early in the first year of training with a mandatory 11/2-h Brief Emotional Support Team training experience for all residents and faculty involved in resident supervision. The training uses evidence-based training and therapy customized to assist first responders and healthcare professionals to respond effectively in a crisis while also engaging in skills that build resilience to cope with chronic exposure to stress. It aims to strengthen the peer and supervisor support provided to residents who experienced patient suicide. Next, a communication tree was disseminated to all faculty, residents, and staff that outlined the necessary steps to follow if anyone (e.g., faculty, resident, staff, nursing) receives notification that a patient has completed suicide. It formalized the procedure for delivering the news to a resident to ensure a supervisor and/or training director is able to provide immediate support. A third component of the curriculum was a 1-h faculty panel composed of supervisors who had experienced a patient suicide during training. This allowed residents an opportunity to hear faculty share their personal experiences with patient loss and engage in an open dialogue if trainees had questions about the experience. Following this, two related published manuscripts were emailed to residents: (1) "Losing a patient to suicide: What we know" [25], (2) "Losing a patient to suicide: Navigating the aftermath" [26]. The final portion of the curriculum involved having the residents meet with an attorney from the hospital's Risk Management division and a faculty member who served as the department's Associate Chief Quality Officer. This interactive discussion session reviewed the root-cause analysis process conducted after a patient's suicide, as well as the medical-legal implications [27].

What each of the programs described above have in common is a recognition of the importance of breaking through the shroud of silence surrounding patient suicide, destigmatize and universalize the experience, provide support and community, and provide relevant information, resources, and processes to follow. The next steps may be ACGME guidelines for all psychiatry training programs, similar attention to this important aspect of training in other disciplines, mental health specialties, and attention to coping with patient suicide in continuing education courses.

27.3   Death By Suicide of a Colleague

Physicians and nurses are at higher risk for suicide than is the general population (references needed). This is especially the case for female physicians and even more so for female nurses. Resultantly, it is not uncommon for health professionals to have a colleague die by suicide at some point in their careers. The death of a patient by suicide can be layered, painful, and confusing, as delineated above. The death of a colleague by suicide can be even more so. The following expansion of the case of Mr. H. highlights common themes inherent in colleague deaths by suicide.

Case (Continued)
In the original case of Mr. H.'s death by suicide, imagine a scenario in which Mr. H. was a colleague, not a patient. During a busy day at work, John, a nurse colleague of Mr. H.'s, went to use the hospital staff bathroom. Immediately upon entering the bathroom, John found Mr. H.'s unresponsive body on the bathroom floor, a floor littered with scattered pills. A letter outlining the reasons Mr. H. chose to die by suicide was found at the side of his body. John tried to resuscitate Mr. H.'s body, to no avail.

For the weeks after Mr. H.'s death, John could not stop thinking about how he missed the signs of his colleague's despair. Images of finding Mr. H.'s body kept him up at night and invaded his dreams. He avoided using the staff bathroom in which the death occurred and when he needed to use the bathroom, he would disrupt his day by walking an extra five minutes to a different restroom in the hospital. John was confused about what he could and could not disclose to his colleagues. Confusion and shame led John to keep his thoughts and feelings to himself rather than process Mr. H.'s death with friends and colleagues at work.

Further imagine the layered complexities surrounding the handling of Mr. H.'s death if Mr. H.'s family did not want the cause of death shared. Similarly, envision how, bound by HIPAA, colleagues involved in resuscitation efforts cannot immediately discuss the circumstances of the death with those not involved in the medical care. Who would provide them with support? Would they have a place to process their colleagues' death? How should their supervisors handle the legalities and support needs?

27.4   Management/Support/Treatment

Considering that grief is a normal, adaptive response to loss, a clinician's grief after losing a patient to suicide does not warrant any formal intervention in most circumstances. However, in light of the above delineated stigma, anger, and guilt so often associated with suicide loss, reassurance, support, and information from colleagues, supervisors, and leaders is often not available or sufficient. Too often, these events are shrouded in silence, leaving the clinician to suffer alone. Thus, reaching out to a colleague who has lost a patient to suicide to provide that support may be beneficial, especially if it comes from another clinician who can share their own "lived" experience with a patient suicide. The universality of their experiences provides great reassurance that they are not alone in their feelings and that others have faced similar experiences and have come out not only intact but often stronger. Through such support, individuals may receive helpful suggestions for taking care of real-life obligations such as dealing with families, risk management, other members of the healthcare team, patients, and lawyers if necessary.

One example of a programmatic approach to supporting clinicians after a patient death by suicide is the UC San Diego Psychiatry Residency's SAVE (Suicide and AdVerse Events) program. Whenever a patient attempts or completes suicide the Program Director, Chief Resident and the resident's immediate service chief and supervisor are immediately contacted along with a cascade of support interventions, including caring conversations with an assigned "ombudsman," debriefs for the staff, and the offer of time off and mental health counseling for the involved resident. The SAVE program also provides support to the affected resident and others during Morbidity and Mortality conferences which formerly were sources of major stress, finger-pointing (often at the resident), shame and humiliation rather than of support and compassion. Many other training programs have similar mechanisms to provide support, but others have maintained the destructive code of silence.

For those whose responses are especially intense, persistent, pervasive, or disabling, formal treatment beyond simple support may be indicated. Focus treatment on the grief as well as any co-occurring conditions that may have been triggered or amplified by the loss. Include recommended combinations of education, psychotherapy, and pharmacotherapy with a focus on loss, depression, guilt, and trauma [14].

Assess for the presence of thoughts and behaviors that are indicative of Prolonged Grief Disorder [16, 28, 29] with the use of a clinical interview. Intense grief is not pathologic; however, grief that is inordinately intense, disabling, and prolonged beyond the individual's social, cultural, or religious norms triggers a more detailed assessment. Since providers are not only ashamed of losing a patient to suicide but also by their persistently intense grief, it is important for clinicians to ask direct questions in a sensitive and empathic way. The inquiry can be aided by screening questionnaires, such as the Brief Grief Questionnaire [30] or the Prolonged Grief-13-Revised Scale (PG-13-R) [31]. A tutorial on how to make a differential diagnosis can be found online (Resources for Clinicians | Center for Reseh on End-of-Life Care (cornell.edu)). When recognized and appropriately diagnosed, Prolonged Grief Disorder can be successfully treated. A short-term approach called complicated grief treatment [32] is the treatment that has been most extensively studied to date. A therapy tutorial, developed at the Center for Complicated Grief at the Columbia School of Social Work, can be found online (https://prolongedgrief. columbia.edu. If this therapy is not available, a reasonable approach is an intervention that provides information about adaptation to grief and includes strategies to reduce avoidance of reminders of the loss and strategies for behavioral activation [14, 33].

Postvention refers to activities which reduce risk and promote healing after a suicide death. Gutin [25] provided several examples of postvention protocols for clinicians [34–36], clinical staff [37], and agencies [38, 39]. These protocols have several recommendations in common. Emphasize information about suicide loss, including its likelihood and potential aftermath, in clinicians' general education and training. Incorporate suicide postvention policies and protocols into institutional policy and procedure manuals, and stress that legal, institutional, and administrative needs be balanced with the emotional needs of affected clinicians and staff, as well as those of the surviving family. Table 27.1 provides key components of such policies and protocols. Gutin stresses that having comprehensive and supportive postvention policies in place maximizes the potential for clinicians who lose a patient to suicide to emerge with personal and professional growth: becoming more knowledgeable about optimal interventions for patients who are at risk; increasing sensitivity to patients and suicide-loss survivors; learning from omissions and commissions; and reducing grandiosity and omnipotence along with a more realistic appraisal of one's humanness and limitations [25, 26].

Table 27.1 Postvention policies and protocols

Having a proactive, written policy, and procedure to follow before the crisis occurs	Postvention protocol available before the incident occurs Clearly delineate who is responsible for what
Education on universal feelings, thoughts, behaviors, and themes often encountered after a patient, colleague, or student suicide	Grief is a human response to loss Shame, doubt, guilt, blame often accentuated and disproportional after suicide Opportunity and potential for growth
Principles of dealing with families	Compassionate family contact reduces liability and facilitates healing for both parties Respect Health Insurance Portability and Accountability Act (HIPAA) laws When in doubt, do what's right
Supportive debriefs for those affected	Group and individual as requested or needed Focus on sharing emotional reactions rather than details, finding faults, or fixing problems
Critical incident review/morbidity mortality conference	Not immediately after the event Focus on identifying gaps in institution/department/agency procedures and training and improving pre- and postvention procedures Students and trainees should be accompanied by supportive mentors, supervisors, and leaders Within supportive environment
Consulting with legal representation and/or Risk Management	Clarify procedures for chart completion and review Clarify the specific information to be shared both within and outside of the institution, and how to address the needs of current patients, trainees, staff, faculty, and family
Roles of counseling/supporting trainees and colleagues	Time off usual duties offered for a brief period (hours to days as needed/requested Opportunity to debrief with a neutral supporter Peer support, especially from someone with "lived experience" ("A trouble shared is a trouble halved") Grief counseling and/or therapy as needed or requested

In addition to individual, staff and agency guidelines, toolkits for schools [40], medical schools [41], and residencies [42] available on the AFSP website (https://afsp.org) provide procedures, strategies, checklists, and pragmatic resources for programs and institutions after a suicide loss. The toolkits serve as practical handbooks to consult at the time a suicide death does occur. The details are beyond the scope of this chapter, but the toolkits include tips on: gathering information; communicating with the deceased's emergency contact; notifying the community; helping affected students/trainees, as well as faculty and staff, cope; dealing with the practical consequences on schedules and workflow; and coordinating and planning a memorial. They also include tips for talking about suicide, sample scripts to be used in face-to-face communication and sample email death notifications, a memorial service planning checklist, a sample media statement, and key messages for the media spokesperson.

27.5   Application of Principles into Wellness Practice

Clinicians treating patients with mental illnesses need to be prepared for patients who, despite their best efforts, end their lives to suicide. They need to recognize that mental disorders are serious business which can be fatal. Suicide is not a signal that the treating clinician was not good enough, skilled enough, or compassionate enough. Suicide risk is too complex and multi-dimensional to be reduced to an overly simplistic cause-and-effect model. We cannot predict if or when a patient may take their own life, and we cannot always prevent it. The best we can do is to know risk factors and warning signs and apply the most compassionate and evidenced-based treatments available to us. But that is not always enough. Suicide is health outcome in the same way that many complex health outcomes are. Just as a cardiologist does not take the meaning of prevention related to cardiac mortality to mean that they know who will die or when, nor to assume that no one with risk factors for heart disease who receives appropriate treatment and makes efforts with diet, exercise, and stress reduction will die of heart disease, or the oncologist does not feel they are to blame when a patient dies of the cancerous diseases they treat, the mental health practitioner is not to blame for a patient succumbing to their illness [43]. This message is an important one and deserves to part of the early education of mental health clinicians, repeated throughout training and in post-training continuing medical education and coupled with support and self-compassion when they have a patient who dies by suicide. The conspiracy of silence regarding suicide so long a part of our mental health culture is no longer acceptable. We owe it to ourselves, our colleagues, and our patients to keep the dialogue open.

27.6   Opportunities for Future Research

Innovative educational programs and supportive interventions aimed at helping mental health clinicians who lose patients to suicide are now being implemented, but few have been multi-centered, controlled, or evaluated for effectiveness, transportability, impact, or sustainability. Such studies will be a welcome addition to ensuring the wellness of our workforce as we move forward.

Glossary

Prolonged Grief Disorder: DSM-5-TR A persistent, pervasive and impairing grief response characterized by persistent longing or yearning and/or preoccupation with the deceased accompanied by at least 3 of 8 additional symptoms that include disbelief, intense emotional pain, feeling of identity confusion, avoidance of reminders of the loss, feelings of numbness, intense loneliness, meaninglessness or difficulty engaging in ongoing life. The grief response has persisted for an atypically long period of time following the loss (more than 6 months for the ICD-11 and more than one year for the DSM5-TR) and clearly exceeds expected social, cultural or religious norms for the individual's culture and context.

Suicide The act of intentionally causing one's own death.

Discussion Guide

- What are the expected responses and reaction of a mental health clinician to the death by suicide of a patient? Why might this differ from a cardiologist losing a patient to heart disease or an oncologist losing a patient to cancer?
- How can individual clinicians and institutions help clinicians cope with the loss of a patient to suicide?

Discussion Leader Guide

Video for Discussion - Instructional Video: The online version contains supplementary material available at https://doi.org/10.1007/978-3-031-16983-0_27

References

1. Hedegaard H, Curtin SC, Warner M. Suicide mortality in the United States, 1999-2019. NCHS Data Brief. 2021;398:1–8.
2. Turecki G, Brent DA. Suicide and suicidal behaviour. Lancet. 2016;387(10024):1227–39.
3. Bachmann S. Epidemiology of suicide and the psychiatric perspective. Int J Environ Res Public Health. 2018;15(7):1425.
4. Simon GE, Johnson E, Lawrence JM, Rossom RC, Ahmedani B, Lynch FL, Beck A, Waitzfelder B, Ziebell R, Penfold RB, Shortreed SM. Predicting suicide attempts and suicide deaths following outpatient visits using electronic health records. Am J Psychiatry. 2018;175(10):951–60.
5. Substance Abuse and Mental Health Services Administration. Key substance use and mental health indicators in the United States: results from the 2019 National Survey on Drug Use and Health (HHS Publication No. PEP20-07-01-001, NSDUH Series H-55). Rockville: Center for Behavioral Health Statistics and Quality, Substance Abuse and Mental Health Services Administration; 2020. https://www.samhsa.gov/data/
6. Chemtob CM, Bauer GB, Hamada RS, Pelowski SR, Muraoka MY. Patient suicide: occupational hazard for psychologists and psychiatrists. Prof Psychol Res Pract. 1989;20(5):294.
7. Iglewicz A, Tal I, Zisook S. Grief reactions in the suicide bereaved. In: Bui E, editor. Clinical handbook of bereavement and grief reactions. Cham: Humana; 2018. p. 139–60.
8. Shear MK, Zisook S. Suicide-related bereavement and grief. In: Koslow SH, Ruiz P, Nemeroff CB, editors. A concise guide to understanding suicide: epidemiology, pathophysiology, and prevention. Cambridge University Press; 2014. p. 66–73. https://doi.org/10.1017/CBO9781139519502.010.
9. Young IT, Iglewicz A, Glorioso D, Lanouette N, Seay K, Ilapakurti M, Zisook S. Suicide bereavement and complicated grief. Dialogues Clin Neurosci. 2012;14(2):177.
10. Tal I, Mauro C, Reynolds CF III, Shear MK, Simon N, Lebowitz B, Skritskaya N, Wang Y, Qiu X, Iglewicz A, Glorioso D. Complicated grief after suicide bereavement and other causes of death. Death Stud. 2017;41(5):267–75.

11. Sudak H, Maxim K, Carpenter M. Suicide and stigma: a review of the literature and personal reflections. Acad Psychiatry. 2008;32(2):136–42. https://doi.org/10.1176/appi.ap.32.2.136.
12. Evans A, Abrahamson K. The influence of stigma on suicide bereavement: a systematic review. J Psychosoc Nurs Ment Health Serv. 2020;58(4):21–7.
13. Jordan JR. Bereavement after Suicide. Psychiatr Ann. 2008;38(10):679–85.
14. Iglewicz A, Shear MK, Reynolds CF III, Simon N, Lebowitz B, Zisook S. Complicated grief therapy for clinicians: an evidence-based protocol for mental health practice. Depress Anxiety. 2020;37(1):90–8.
15. Gutin N, McGann VL, Jordan JR. The impact of suicide on professional caregivers. In: Jordan JR, McIntosh JL, editors. Grief after suicide: understanding the consequences and caring for the survivors. London: Routledge; 2011. p. 123–42.
16. Prigerson HG, Kakarala S, Gang J, Maciejewski PK. History and status of prolonged grief disorder as a psychiatric diagnosis. Annu Rev Clin Psychol. 2021;7(17):109–26.
17. Mauro C, Reynolds CF, Maercker A, Skritskaya N, Simon N, Zisook S, Lebowitz B, Cozza SJ, Shear MK. Prolonged grief disorder: clinical utility of ICD-11 diagnostic guidelines. Psychol Med. 2019;49(5):861–7.
18. Lomax JW. A proposed curriculum on suicide care for psychiatry residency. Suicide Life Threat Behav. 1986;16(1):56–64.
19. Pilkinton P, Etkin M. Encountering suicide: the experience of psychiatric residents. Acad Psychiatry. 2003;27(2):93–9.
20. Ruskin R, Sakinofsky I, Bagby RM, Dickens S, Sousa G. Impact of patient suicide on psychiatrists and psychiatric trainees. Acad Psychiatry. 2004;28(2):104–10.
21. Prabhakar D, Anzia JM, Balon R, Gabbard G, Gray E, Hatzis N, Lanouette NM, Lomax JW, Puri P, Zisook S. "Collateral damages": preparing residents for coping with patient suicide. Acad Psychiatry. 2013;37(6):429–30.
22. Prabhakar D, Balon R, Anzia JM, Gabbard GO, Lomax JW, Bandstra BS, Eisen J, Figueroa S, Theresa G, Ruble M, Seritan AL. Helping psychiatry residents cope with patient suicide. Acad Psychiatry. 2014;38(5):593–7.
23. Lerner U, Brooks K, McNiel DE, Cramer RJ, Haller E. Coping with a patient's suicide: a curriculum for psychiatry residency training programs. Acad Psychiatry. 2012;36(1):29–33.
24. Whitmore CA, Cook J, Salg L. Supporting residents in the wake of patient suicide. Am J Psychiatry Resid J. 2017;12(1):5–7.
25. Gutin NJ. Losing a patient to suicide: navigating the aftermath. Current Psychiatry. 2019;18(11):17–24.
26. Gutin NJ. Losing a patient to suicide: what we know: suicide loss can impact clinicians' professional identities, relationships with colleagues, and clinical work. Curr Psychiatry. 2019;18(10):15–25.
27. McCutcheon S, Hyman J. Increasing resident support following patient suicide: assessing resident perceptions of a longitudinal, multimodal patient suicide curriculum. Acad Psychiatry. 2021;45(3):288–91.
28. Shear MK. Complicated grief. N Engl J Med. 2015;372:153–60.
29. Zisook S, Reynolds CF III. Complicated grief. Focus. 2017 Oct;15(4):12s–3s.
30. Shear K, Essock S. Brief grief questionnaire. University of Pittsburgh; 2002.
31. Prigerson HG, Boelen PA, Xu J, Smith KV, Maciejewski PK. Validation of the new DSM-5-TR criteria for prolonged grief disorder and the PG-13-Revised (PG-13-R) scale. World Psychiatry. 2021;20(1):96–106.
32. Shear MK, Reynolds CF, Simon NM, et al. Optimizing treatment of complicated grief: a randomized clinical trial. JAMA Psychiat. 2016;73(7):685–94.
33. Zisook S, Shear MK, Reynolds CF, Simon NM, Mauro C, Skritskaya NA, Lebowitz B, Wang Y, Tal I, Glorioso D, Wetherell JL. Treatment of complicated grief in survivors of suicide loss: a HEAL report. J Clin Psychiatry. 2018;79(2):17m11592.
34. Grad OT. Therapists as survivors of suicide loss. In: Wasserman D, Wasserman C, editors. Oxford textbook of suicidology and suicide prevention. Oxford, UK: Oxford University Press; 2009. p. 609–15.

35. Quinett P. What to do if a patient dies by suicide: guidelines for professionals. www.clinician-survivor.org.
36. Sung JC. Sample individual practitioner practices for responding to client suicide. www.sprc.org/resources-programs/sample-individual-practitioner-practices-responding-client-suicide.
37. Grad OT. Guidelines to assist clinical staff after the suicide of a patient. www.cliniciansurvivor.org
38. Quinnett P. Postvention guidelines for agency suicides: QPR Institute administrative directory. Spokane, WA: QPR Institute; 1999.
39. Sung JC. Sample agency practices for responding to client suicide. www.sprc.org/resources-programs/sample-agency-practices-responding-client-suicide
40. American Foundation for Suicide Prevention and Suicide Prevention Resource Center. After a suicide: a toolkit for schools. 2nd ed. Waltham: Education Development Center; 2018.
41. Dyrbye L, Moutier C, Wolanskyj-Spinner A, Zisook S. After a suicide: a toolkit for medical schools. American Foundation for Suicide Prevention; 2018.
42. Dyrbye L, Konopasek L, Moutier C. After a suicide: a toolkit for physician residency/fellowship programs. American Foundation for Suicide Prevention (AFSP) and the Mayo Clinic; 2017.
43. Moutier CY. Innovative and timely approaches to suicide prevention in medical education. Acad Psychiatry. 2021;45(3):252–6.

Printed in the United States
by Baker & Taylor Publisher Services